Venous Thromboembolism in Critical Care

Guest Editor

KENNETH E. WOOD, DO

CRITICAL CARE CLINICS

www.criticalcare.theclinics.com

Consulting Editor
RICHARD W. CARLSON, MD, PhD

October 2011 • Volume 27 • Number 4

SAUNDERS an imprint of ELSEVIER, Inc.

W.B. SAUNDERS COMPANY
A Division of Elsevier Inc.

Elsevier Inc. • 1600 John F. Kennedy Blvd., • Suite 1800 • Philadelphia, Pennsylvania 19103-2899

http://www.theclinics.com

CRITICAL CARE CLINICS Volume 27, Number 4
October 2011 ISSN 0749-0704, ISBN-13: 978-1-4557-1093-5

Editor: Patrick Manley

Critical Care Clinics (ISSN: 0749-0704) is published quarterly by Elsevier Inc., 360 Park Avenue South, New York, NY 10010-1710. Months of issue are January, April, July, and October. Business and Editorial Offices: 1600 John F. Kennedy Blvd., Suite 1800, Philadelphia, PA 19103-2899. Customer Service Office: 6277 Sea Harbor Drive, Orlando, FL 32887-4800. Periodicals postage paid at New York, NY and additional mailing offices. Subscription prices are $193.00 per year for US individuals, $463.00 per year for US institution, $94.00 per year for US students and residents, $238.00 per year for Canadian individuals, $574.00 per year for Canadian institutions, $278.00 per year for international individuals, $574.00 per year for international institutions and $137.00 per year for Canadian and foreign students/ residents. To receive student/resident rate, orders must be accompanied by name of affiliated institution, date of term, and the signature of program/residency coordinator on institution letterhead. Orders will be billed at individual rate until proof of status is received. Foreign air speed delivery is included in all *Clinics* subscription prices. All prices are subject to change without notice. POSTMASTER: Send address changes to *Critical Care Clinics*, Elsevier Periodicals Customer Service, 11830 Westline Industrial Drive, St. Louis, MO 63146. **Customer Service: 1-800-654-2452 (US). From outside of the US, call 1-314-447-8871. Fax: 1-314-447-8029. E-mail: journalscustomerservice-usa@elsevier.com (for print support) or journalsonlinesupport-usa@elsevier.com (for online support).**

Reprints. For copies of 100 or more of articles in this publication, please contact the Commercial Reprints Department, Elsevier Inc., 360 Park Avenue South, New York, NY 10010-1710. Tel.: 212-633-3813; Fax: 212-462-1935; E-mail: reprints@elsevier.com.

Critical Care Clinics is also published in Spanish by Editorial Inter-Medica, Junin 917, 1er A, 1113, Buenos Aires, Argentina.

Critical Care Clinics is covered in *MEDLINE/PubMed (Index Medicus)*, *EMBASE/Excerpta Medica, Current Concepts/ Clinical Medicine, ISI/BIOMED*, and *Chemical Abstracts*.

Printed and bound by CPI Group (UK) Ltd, Croydon, CR0 4YY

Transferred to Digital Print 2011

Contributors

CONSULTING EDITOR

RICHARD W. CARLSON, MD, PhD
Chairman Emeritus, Department of Medicine, Maricopa Medical Center; Director, Medical Intensive Care Unit; Professor, University of Arizona College of Medicine; Professor, Department of Medicine, Mayo Graduate School of Medicine, Phoenix, Arizona

GUEST EDITOR

KENNETH E. WOOD, DO
Chief Medical Officer, Geisinger Medical Center, Danville; Clinical Professor of Medicine, Temple University School of Medicine, Philadelphia, Pennsylvania

AUTHORS

JULIA A.M. ANDERSON, MD
Consultant Hematologist, Department of Clinical and Laboratory Hematology, Royal Infirmary of Edinburgh, Scotland, United Kingdom; Associate Professor (P/T), Department of Medicine, McMaster University, Hamilton, Ontario, Canada

ROBERT BERCOVITCH, MD
Fellow, Division of Pulmonary and Critical Care Medicine, Department of Medicine, University of California, San Diego, San Diego, California

LINDSAY M. FAIRFAX, MD
Surgical Critical Care Fellow, Department of Surgery, Carolinas Medical Center, Charlotte, North Carolina

PETER FEDULLO, MD
Clinical Professor of Medicine, Division of Pulmonary and Critical Care Medicine, Department of Medicine, University of California, San Diego, San Diego, California

WILLIAM GEERTS, MD
Thromboembolism Service, Department of Medicine, Sunnybrook Health Sciences Centre; Faculty of Medicine and Centre for Patient Safety, University of Toronto, Toronto, Ontario, Canada

STAVROS KONSTANTINIDES, MD
Department of Cardiology, Democritus University of Thrace, University General Hospital, Alexandroupolis, Greece

MAREIKE LANKEIT, MD
Department of Cardiology and Pulmonology, Georg August University of Göttingen, Germany

MARISA MAGAÑA, MD
Assistant Clinical Professor, Division of Pulmonary and Critical Care Medicine, Department of Medicine, University of California, San Diego, San Diego, California

FADI MATTA, MD
Department of Research, St. Mary Mercy Hospital, Livonia; Department of Internal Medicine, College of Osteopathic Medicine, Michigan State University, East Lansing, Michigan

ANNE G. MCLEOD, MD, MSc
Thromboembolism Service, Department of Medicine, Sunnybrook Health Sciences Centre; Faculty of Medicine, University of Toronto, Toronto, Ontario, Canada

TIMOTHY A. MORRIS, MD, FACCP
Professor of Medicine, Division of Pulmonary and Critical Care Medicine, Department of Medicine, University of California, San Diego School of Medicine, San Diego, California

RONALD F. SING, DO, FACS, FCCM
Clinical Associate Professor of Surgery, University of North Carolina School of Medicine, Chapel Hill; Attending, Division of Trauma and Surgical Critical Care, Department of Surgery, Carolinas Medical Center, Charlotte, North Carolina

PAUL D. STEIN, MD
Department of Research, St. Mary Mercy Hospital, Livonia; Department of Internal Medicine, College of Osteopathic Medicine, Michigan State University, East Lansing, Michigan

VICTOR F. TAPSON, MD
Professor of Medicine, Division of Pulmonary and Critical Care Medicine; Director, Center for Pulmonary Vascular Disease, Duke University Medical Center, Durham, North Carolina

THEODORE E. WARKENTIN, MD, FRCP(C), FACP
Professor, Department of Pathology and Molecular Medicine, and Department of Medicine, McMaster University; Regional Director, Transfusion Medicine, Hamilton Regional Laboratory Medicine Program; Hematologist, Division of Clinical Hematology, Department of Medicine, Hamilton Health Sciences, Hamilton, Ontario, Canada

JEFFREY I. WEITZ, MD
Professor of Medicine, Biochemistry, and Biomedical Sciences, McMaster University; Executive Director, Thrombosis and Atherosclerosis Research Institute, Hamilton, Ontario, Canada

KENNETH E. WOOD, DO
Chief Medical Officer, Geisinger Medical Center, Danville; Clinical Professor of Medicine, Temple University School of Medicine, Philadelphia, Pennsylvania

Contents

Venous Thromboembolism Prophylaxis in Critically Ill Patients   765

Anne G. McLeod and William Geerts

Venous thromboembolism (VTE) is a frequent but often silent complication of critical illness that has a negative impact on patient outcomes.
The prevention of VTE is an essential component of patient care in the
intensive care unit (ICU) setting, and is the focus of this article. The use
of anticoagulant thromboprophylaxis significantly decreases the risk of
VTE in ICU patients and is discussed at length.

Vena Cava Interruption   781

Lindsay M. Fairfax and Ronald F. Sing

Anticoagulation has been proven to be effective in preventing and
treating deep vein thrombosis and pulmonary embolus. However, many
critically ill patients are unable to receive anticoagulation or suffer
recurrent venous thromboembolism despite adequate treatment. This
article examines the use of vena cava filters in the critically ill. Indications for, techniques, and complications of vena cava filter insertion are
reviewed. The importance of vena cava filters with the option to be
retrieved and bedside insertion in the intensive care unit is emphasized.

Heparin-Induced Thrombocytopenia in Critically Ill Patients   805

Theodore E. Warkentin

Critically ill patients commonly evince thrombocytopenia, either evident
on admission to the intensive care unit (ICU) or that develops during
their stay. Heparin-induced thrombocytopenia (HIT) explains thrombocytopenia in only approximately 1/100 critically ill patients; also, only 1
or 2 in 10 ICU patients with a positive PF4-dependent enzyme immunoassay has "true" HIT. Thus, there is major potential for overdiagnosis
of HIT in the ICU. A recent study showing that dalteparin is associated
with a reduced frequency of HIT indicates that critically ill patients too
can benefit from the HIT-reducing potential of this low molecular weight
heparin preparation.

challenging. Differentiating PE from other life-threatening cardiopulmonary disorders can be exceedingly difficult. This article will review a
structured pathophysiologic approach to the diagnostic, resuscitative
and management strategies related to PE in the ICU.

The proportion of hospitalized patients with pulmonary embolism (PE) is
increasing. Whether this represents more admissions with PE or more
diagnoses made in hospitalized patients is uncertain. The proportion of
hospitalized patients with deep venous thrombosis has decreased
precipitously as a result of home treatment. Asians and Native Americans have a lower incidence of PE than whites or African Americans.
The incidence of PE increases exponentially with age, but no age
group, including infants and children, is immune. Several medical
illnesses have now been shown to be associated with a higher risk for
venous thromboembolism. Epidemiologic data and new information on
risk factors provide insight into making an informed clinical assessment
and evaluation for antithrombotic prophylaxis.

Hypercoagulable states can be inherited or acquired. Inherited hypercoagulable states can be caused by a loss of function of natural
anticoagulant pathways or a gain of function in procoagulant pathways.
Acquired hypercoagulable risk factors include a prior history of thrombosis, obesity, pregnancy, cancer and its treatment, antiphospholipid
antibody syndrome, heparin-induced thrombocytopenia, and myeloproliferative disorders. Inherited hypercoagulable states combine
with acquired risk factors to establish the intrinsic risk of venous
thromboembolism for each individual. Venous thromboembolism occurs when the risk exceeds a critical threshold. Often a triggering factor,
such as surgery, pregnancy, or estrogen therapy, is required to increase the risk above this critical threshold.

Acute venous thromboembolism remains a frequent disease, with an
incidence ranging between 23 and 69 cases per 100,000 population per
year. Of these patients, approximately one-third present with clinical
symptoms of acute pulmonary embolism (PE) and two-thirds with deep
venous thrombosis (DVT). Recent registries and cohort studies suggest
that approximately 10% of all patients with acute PE die during the first
1 to 3 months after diagnosis. Overall, 1% of all patients admitted to

hospitals die of acute PE, and 10% of all hospital deaths are PE-related. These facts emphasize the need to better implement our knowledge on the pathophysiology of the disease, recognize the determinants of death or major adverse events in the early phase of acute PE, and most importantly, identify those patients who necessitate prompt medical, surgical, or interventional treatment to restore the patency of the pulmonary vasculature.

THE CLINICS ARE NOW AVAILABLE ONLINE!

Access your subscription at:
www.theclinics.com

Preface

Venous Thromboembolism in Critical Care

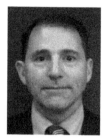

Kenneth E. Wood, DO
Guest Editor

Despite significant advances in the understanding of the pathophysiology of venous thromboembolism (VTE), multiple trials evaluating and comparing VTE diagnostic modalities, and a myriad of new anticoagulants, VTE in the intensive care unit (ICU) remains difficult to detect and challenging to treat. Unfortunately, many of the diagnostic and therapeutic advances in VTE that have been made in the outpatient arena may not be applicable to the complicated ICU patient with multiple comorbidities and organ system failures and the intensivist is left to devise diagnostic and therapeutic strategies tempered by limitations in transport to diagnostic modalities, bleeding risks, and uncertain outcome data. Against this background, this issue of the *Critical Care Clinics* seeks to address the issue of VTE in critical care medicine by reviewing the natural history of VTE, prophylactic measures, and diagnostic and therapeutic approaches, while addressing complications of and alternatives in treatment. The authors hope that this issue will assist in mitigating some of the uncertainty surrounding VTE in the ICU.

I would like to express my genuine appreciation to all of the contributing authors who took time from their many other activities and obligations to contribute to this issue and to Patrick Manley from Elsevier, whose ongoing vigilance assured the *Clinics* completion.

Kenneth E. Wood, DO
Geisinger Medical Center
100 North Academy Avenue
Danville, PA 17822, USA

E-mail address:
kewood@geisinger.edu

Crit Care Clin 27 (2011) xi
doi:10.1016/j.ccc.2011.10.001
0749-0704/11/$ – see front matter © 2011 Elsevier Inc. All rights reserved.

Venous Thromboembolism Prophylaxis in Critically Ill Patients

Anne G. McLeod, MD, MSc[a,b],*, William Geerts, MD[a,c]

KEYWORDS
- Venous thromboembolism • Thromboprophylaxis
- Prevention • Critical care

Venous thromboembolism (VTE) is a frequent but often silent complication of critical illness that has a negative impact on patient outcomes.[1] The prevention of VTE is an essential component of patient care in the intensive care unit (ICU) setting, and is the focus of this review.

Critically ill patients present a number of important challenges with respect to VTE and its prevention. First, ICU patients have greater heterogeneity in their risk of thrombosis than do other hospitalized patient groups. Second, a clinical suspicion of possible VTE is very common (often daily) in these patients because of tachycardia, desaturation, patient anxiety, limb swelling, and fever. Third, symptoms and signs commonly associated with deep vein thrombosis (DVT) or pulmonary embolism (PE) are not reliable indicators of VTE in critical care patients.[2,3] Fourth, ICU patients frequently have compromised cardiopulmonary function and, therefore, relatively small pulmonary emboli could have dire consequences. Autopsy studies have shown that PE is found in up to 25% of these patients and is sometimes the cause of their death.[3] Finally, although critically ill patients often have multiple risk factors for VTE, they are frequently also at increased risk for bleeding because of recent surgery, trauma, intracranial or gastrointestinal bleeding, thrombocytopenia, and renal insufficiency. Despite these challenges, studies in trauma, surgery and acutely ill medical patients, as well as recently published studies in critical care patients, allow clinicians to provide effective and safe thromboprophylaxis.

Dr McLeod and Dr Geerts have both received program and personal support from Bayer Healthcare, Boehringer-Ingelheim, Pfizer and Sanofi Aventis.

[a] Thromboembolism Service, Department of Medicine, Sunnybrook Health Sciences Centre, Toronto, ON, Canada
[b] Faculty of Medicine, University of Toronto, Toronto, ON, Canada
[c] Faculty of Medicine and Centre for Patient Safety, University of Toronto, Toronto, ON, Canada
* Corresponding author. Thromboembolism Service, Sunnybrook Health Sciences Centre, D-677 2075 Bayview Avenue, Toronto, ON M4N 3M5, Canada.
E-mail address: anne.mcleod@sunnybrook.ca.

VTE RATES IN CRITICALLY ILL PATIENTS WITHOUT ROUTINE THROMBOPROPHYLAXIS

Because clinical practice guidelines have recommended the routine use of thromboprophylaxis in critical care patients for more than 20 years, we review historical studies to understand the risk of VTE in patients not receiving pharmacologic or mechanical thromboprophylaxis.[4] Autopsies in 436 critically ill patients in six studies detected PE in 7% to 27% of patients (mean 13%), and PE that caused or contributed to death was found in 0% to 12% (mean 3%) of these patients (**Table 1**).[5–10] In the majority of patients with proven or fatal PE, there was no clinical suspicion of PE before death.

In an observational study of 100 critically ill medical patients, leg Doppler ultrasounds (DUS) were performed twice weekly during ICU admission and at 1 week after ICU discharge.[11] Proximal DVT was detected in 32% of patients receiving no prophylaxis, 40% of patients receiving low-dose unfractionated heparin (LDUH), and 33% of those receiving mechanical prophylaxis. Only four prospective studies have assessed the incidence of DVT in critically ill patients who did not receive thromboprophylaxis (**Table 2**).[6,12–14] In a study of 23 patients admitted to ICU with respiratory failure, Moser and coworkers[6] found that 13% had DVT detected by fibrinogen leg scanning. Cade and colleagues[12] detected DVT by fibrinogen leg scanning in 29% of patients in the placebo arm of a trial of 119 general ICU patients. Both studies are problematic because of poor characterization of patients, lack of follow-up, and the use of fibrinogen scanning for diagnosis. A study reported by Kapoor and colleagues in abstract form[13] evaluated 390 medical ICU patients for DVT using DUS examinations every 3 days during their ICU admission. DVT was detected in 31% of patients not receiving thromboprophylaxis. The only ICU study to use routine contrast venography was conducted in mechanically ventilated patients treated for exacerbation of chronic pulmonary disease.[14] DVT was diagnosed in 28% of patients in the placebo arm of this randomized trial; most of these were distal thrombi, with proximal DVT found in 8% of patients. In summary, screening of asymptomatic patients detected a prevalence of DVT in medical–surgical ICU patients not receiving thromboprophylaxis ranging from 13% to 31%. The clinical consequences of asymptomatic DVT detected by routine screening using any diagnostic method remain unclear. The presence of DVT, however, does significantly increase the risk of subsequent PE and it seems likely that this could contribute to adverse outcomes in patients with already compromised cardiorespiratory reserve.[15,16]

PREVALENCE OF VTE IN CRITICALLY ILL PATIENTS ON ADMISSION TO ICU

Some patients newly admitted to a critical care unit will already have unsuspected DVT. Among six case series, including 1164 patients who were screened for asymptomatic DVT on admission to ICU, DVT was found in 6.3%.[4] The recently published PROTECT study identified proximal DVT on the initial DUS, performed within 2 days after admission, in 3.5% of patients.[17] Clinicians should be aware that many patients admitted to ICU will have been exposed to high-risk situations for the development of VTE such as immobilization, surgery, cancer, and chronic illness and may arrive with thrombosis already present.

CLINICALLY SILENT VTE IN CRITICALLY ILL PATIENTS

Critically ill patients commonly have asymptomatic thromboembolic events. For example, in a study of 90 trauma patients with no clinical suspicion of PE, routine

Table 1
Autopsy studies of pulmonary embolism in critically ill patients

Author (year)	ICU Setting	Admissions to ICU	Deaths, n (% ICU admissions)	Autopsies, n (% deaths)	PE, n (% autopsies)	Fatal PE,[a] n (% autopsies)
Neuhaus et al (1978)[5]	Medical/surgical	617	102 (17)	66 (65)	18 (27)	8 (12)
Moser et al (1981)[6]	Respiratory	34	16 (47)	10 (63)	2 (20)	0
Pingleton et al (1981)[7]	Respiratory	197	56 (28)	40 (71)	19 (23)	NR
Cullen and Nemeskal (1986)[8]	Surgical	NR	Approx. 760	152 (23)	15 (10)	2 (1)
Blosser et al (1998)[9]	Medical–coronary	NR	132 (NR)	41 (31)	3 (7)	1 (2)
Willemsen et al (2000)[10]	Surgical	2,969	384 (13)	127 (33)	10 (8)	4 (3)

[a] Pulmonary embolism causing or contributing to death.
Abbreviation: NR, not reported.
From Geerts W, Cook D, Selby R, et al. Venous thromboembolism and its prevention in critical care. J Crit Care 2002;17:95–104; with permission.

Table 2
Prospective studies evaluating the rates of DVT in unprophylaxed critical care patients

Study Quality Features

Author (year)	ICU Setting	DVT Screening Test	Design	Recruitment of Consecutive Patients	Blinded Outcome Assessment	Noninvasive Test Confirmed by Venography	Follow-up for Negative Tests	No. of Patients	DVT (%)
Moser et al[6] (1981)	Respiratory ICU	Fg LS for 3–6 days	Prospective cohort	NR	No	No	No	23	13
Cade[12] (1982)	General ICU	Fg LS for 4–10 days	Blinded RCT	NR	Yes	No	No	Approx. 60	29
Kapoor et al[13] (1999)	Medical ICU	Serial DUS	Blinded RCT	Yes	Yes	No	NR	390	31
Fraisse et al[14] (2000)	Ventilated COPD	Contrast venography	Blinded multicenter RCT	Yes	Yes	All patients had venography	—	85	28

Note. Includes studies in which no prophylaxis was given and routine screening with an objective diagnostic test for DVT was used.

Abbreviations: COPD, chronic obstructive pulmonary disease; DUS, Doppler ultrasound; Fg LS, ^{125}I fibrinogen leg scanning; NR, not reported; RCT, randomized clinical trial.

Reprinted from Geerts W, Cook D, Selby R, et al. Venous thromboembolism and its prevention in critical care. J Crit Care 2002;17:95–104; with permission.

screening contrast CT detected PE in 24%.[18] Further, ICU patients are often unable to report symptoms because of sedation and mechanical ventilation. They are also immobilized and recumbent, making leg swelling and pain less likely to be apparent. Although clinical predictive models to assess the probability of DVT and PE have been well validated in outpatient populations, the reliability of physical examination in critically ill patients has not been found to be helpful in detecting lower limb DVT.[2] In the PROTECT trial, 8.6% of patients receiving LDUH or LMWH thromboprophylaxis developed DVT detected by DUS and none of these events were identified as a result of a clinical suspicion of DVT.[17]

Given that critically ill patients may develop asymptomatic VTE and that routine screening is both time consuming and costly, a predictive laboratory test for VTE in these patients might be of considerable value. A prospective cohort study was conducted to evaluate the utility of using D-dimer and tests of molecular hyperco-agulability as predictors of DVT in critically ill patients.[19] Neither D-dimer testing, performed serially during ICU admission, nor tests of hypercoagulablilty (activated protein C resistance, prothrombin mutation, protein C, protein S, antithrombin, IgG anticardiolipin antibody, and lupus anticoagulant) were able to predict patients who had DVT detected by routine DUS.

CLINICAL IMPACT OF VTE IN CRITICALLY ILL PATIENTS

The presence of DVT or PE adversely affects morbidity and mortality in critically ill patients. In a prospective cohort study, a diagnosis of DVT was associated with longer duration of mechanical ventilation (median 9 vs 6 days, $P = .03$), longer duration of ICU stay (median 17.5 vs 9 days, $P = .005$), and longer duration of hospital stay (median 51 vs 23 days, $P<.001$) compared with ICU patients without DVT.[1] Although less is known about the impact of PE in this population, it seems likely, given the negative impact of PE on outcomes in other patient groups, that this would also be true for critically ill patients.

RISK FACTORS FOR VTE IN CRITICALLY ILL PATIENTS

Although the spectrum of diagnoses that result in admission to an ICU is wide, all critically ill patients are at increased risk of VTE. The vast majority will have at least one major risk factor for VTE and many will have multiple risk factors. These risk factors can be categorized into those that are present before admission to a critical care unit and those acquired during the ICU admission (**Box 1**).[1,4] The relative contribution of each of these risk factors is unknown, but consideration of these risks is important in designating patients as moderate or high risk for VTE.

A number of studies have identified factors that were reported to predict an increased risk of VTE associated with an ICU admission, including increased age, APACHE (acute physiology and chronic health evaluation) score, recent surgery, sepsis, previous VTE, malignancy, major trauma, prolonged hospital stay preceding the ICU transfer, mechanical ventilation, use of paralytic drugs, insertion of a femoral vein catheter, and failure to use thromboprophylaxis.[4,11,20-27] However, these studies were underpowered to determine independent predictors for thrombosis in ICU patients.

Cook and coworkers[1] prospectively followed 261 medical–surgical ICU patients to determine the prevalence, incidence, and independent risk factors for proximal lower extremity DVT. Thromboprophylaxis was protocol driven and administered to all patients. The study found four independent DVT risk factors in the multivariable analysis. The two risk factors that were acquired before critical care admission were

> **Box 1**
> **Risk factors for critically ill patients**
>
> Present Before the ICU Admission
>
> - Increased age
> - Previous VTE
> - Trauma
> - Surgery
> - Malignancy
> - Sepsis
> - Immobilization: spinal cord injury, bedrest, stroke
> - Estrogen: pregnancy, puerperium
> - Cardiac or respiratory failure
>
> Acquired During the ICU Admission
>
> - Pharmacologic paralysis
> - Mechanical ventilation
> - Central venous lines, especially femoral vein catheters
> - Surgical procedures
> - Sepsis
> - Renal dialysis
> - Vasopressor use
> - Platelet transfusion
> - Use of recombinant factor VIIa
>
> *Data from* Geerts W, Cook D, Selby R, et al. Venous thromboembolism and its prevention in critical care. J Crit Care 2002;17:95–104.

personal or family history of DVT (hazard ratio 4.0; 95% confidence interval (CI) 1.5–10.3) and dialysis-dependent renal failure (hazard ratio 3.7; 95% CI 1.2–11.1). The ICU-acquired risk factors were platelet transfusion (hazard ratio 3.2; 95% CI 1.2–8.4) and vasopressor administration (hazard ratio 2.8; CI 1.1–7.2; **Table 3**).[1] Other studies have demonstrated that ICU patients who receive both LMWH and vasopressors have significantly lower anti-factor Xa activity than patients given the same dose of LWMH without vasopressors.[28] It is proposed that vasopressor use contributes to poor efficacy of subcutaneous LMWH as a result of impaired peripheral perfusion and subsequent inadequate systemic bioavailablity of the anticoagulant.

Several studies have identified central venous catheters, specifically femoral vein catheters, as significant risk factors for the development of VTE.[22–26,29] Cook and colleagues[1] also found that femoral vein catheterization was associated with lower extremity DVT but it was not an independent risk factor in the multivariable analysis. A small, unblinded randomized study of ultrasound-guided "low approach" femoral vein catheterization (10–15 cm below the inguinal ligament) in critical care patients, showed a significantly higher rate of DVT (13/40 vs 4/40; P<.001) with this approach compared to the classic insertion approach.[30] In the PROTECT trial, catheter-related thrombosis occurred in 2.2% of patients receiving LMWH or LDUH.[17]

Table 3
Risk factors for ICU-acquired lower extremity DVT

Risk Factor	Patients with DVT (%)	Patients without DVT (%)	Univariate Hazard Ratio (95% CI)	p Value	Multivariate Hazard Ratio (95% CI)	P Value
Personal or family history of VTE	28.0	6.0	3.7 (1.4–9.3)	0.007	4.0 (1.5–10.3)	0.004
Thrombophilic disorder	12.0	2.8	3.8 (1.1–12.8)	0.03	—	
Chronic hemodialysis	16.0	6.0	3.3 (1.1–9.9)	0.03	3.7 (1.2–11.1)	0.02
Femoral venous catheter	56.0	38.4	2.0 (0.9, 4.6)	0.09	—	
Surgery	32.0	17.6	2.9 (1.1–7.8)	0.04	—	
Platelet transfusion	24.0	10.6	3.1 (1.2–7.9)	0.02	3.2 (1.2–8.4)	0.02
Vasopressor administration	36.0	19.9	3.0 (1.2–7.4)	0.02	2.8 (1.1–7.2)	0.03

Reprinted from Cook DJ, Crowther M, Meade M, et al. Deep venous thrombosis in medical-surgical critically ill patients: prevalence, incidence, and risk factors. Crit Care Med 2005;33: 1565–71; with permission.

Risk factors for venous thrombosis in critically ill patients are many and varied. It is essential, however, to consider all critically ill patients to be at significant risk for VTE and to provide thromboprophylaxis routinely. Further studies are needed to help identify risk factors for the development of VTE despite the use of current thromboprophylaxis.

PHARMACOLOGIC THROMBOPROPHYLAXIS STUDIES IN CRITICAL CARE

Four randomized clinical trials of thromboprophylaxis in medical–surgical ICU patients have been completed using objective screening for DVT (**Table 4**).[12–14,17] In 1982, Cade and coworkers[12] randomized 119 general ICU patients to receive placebo or LDUH 5000 U subcutaneously twice daily. DVT, detected using fibrinogen leg scanning, was identified in 29% of patients in the placebo group and 13% of the treatment group, a relative risk reduction of 55% ($P<.05$). Bleeding rates in this study were not reported. Fraisse and colleagues[14] compared the LMWH nadroparin to placebo in 223 patients requiring mechanical ventilation for chronic obstructive pulmonary disease (COPD) exacerbations; DVT was detected by routine venography in 28% of patients receiving placebo and 15% of LMWH recipients for a relative risk reduction of 45% ($P = .045$). No significant difference in bleeding was reported (3% and 6% in the placebo and nadroparin arms, respectively). Kapoor and coworkers[13] reported, in abstract form only, a study of 791 medical ICU patients randomized to placebo or LDUH. Patients were screened for DVT using serial DUS; DVT was detected in 31% of patients receiving placebo and 11% of LDUH recipients ($P = .01$). Bleeding rates were not reported.

PROTECT is the only study to compare the effects of LMWH and LDUH for the prevention of VTE in medical–surgical ICU patients.[17] It is important to be aware that trauma, orthopedic, and neurosurgery patients were not included in this trial. The investigators randomized 3764 patients in 67 centers in 6 countries to receive either

Table 4
Thromboprophylaxis trials in critically ill patients

Author (year)	Method of Diagnosis	Intervention		DVT, n/N (%)	
		Control	Experimental	Control	Experimental
Cade[12] (1982)	Fibrinogen leg scan daily for 4–10 days	Placebo	LDUH, 5000 U SC bid	NR/NR (29)	NR/NR (13) P<.05
Kapoor[13] (1999)	DUS on admission and every 3 days	Placebo	LDUH, 5000 U SC bid	122/390 (31)	44/401 (11) P = .001
Fraisse[14] (2000)	Weekly DUS and venography at day 21	Placebo	Nadroparin, Approx. 65 U/kg SC qd	24/85 (28)	13/84 (15) P<.05
PROTECT[17] (2011)	DUS on admission and twice weekly	UFH 5000 U SC bid	Dalteparin, 5000 IU SC qd	109[a]/1873 (5.8)	96[a]/1873 (5.1) P = .57

Note. Results of randomized trials in which routine screening with an objective diagnostic test for DVT was used.
[a] Proximal DVT.
Abbreviations: DUS, Doppler ultrasound; NR, not reported.
Adapted from Geerts W, Cook D, Selby R, et al. Venous thromboembolism and its prevention in critical care. J Crit Care 2002;17:95–104; with permission.

dalteparin 5000 IU once daily plus placebo once daily or LDUH 5000 U twice daily. Study prophylaxis was continued for the duration of the ICU admission. Screening for proximal DVT was conducted using DUS performed within 2 days of admission, twice weekly during the ICU stay, and as clinically indicated. Investigations for PE were also performed as clinically indicated. Prevalent DVT was identified at initial screening in 3.5% of the study patients. The two patient groups were well balanced; 76% of admissions were medical and 90% of patients required mechanical ventilation. APACHE II scores were 21 in both groups. Overall, 5.1% of patients receiving dalteparin and 5.8% of patients receiving LDUH developed proximal DVT ($P = .57$). Fewer patients developed the prespecified secondary outcome, PE, in the dalteparin group (1.3% vs 2.3%; $P = .01$), but hospital death did not significantly differ in the two groups. Major bleeding occurred in 5.5% of patients receiving dalteparin and 5.6% of those receiving LDUH. There were 50% fewer cases of heparin-induced thrombocytopenia in the dalteparin group. In this large trial, 5% of patients developed proximal leg DVT and 9% developed venous thrombosis in any location despite the use of thromboprophylaxis.

There are a number of reasons that LMWH should replace LDUH as routine anticoagulant thromboprophylaxis in critical care and other patient populations. Although LMWH and LDUH have similar efficacy in some patient groups, including general surgical and medical patients, LMWH is superior to LDUH in other patient groups (major trauma, orthopedic surgery, ischemic stroke).[4] There are no significant differences in bleeding between these options while LMWH is associated with a 30-fold lower rate of heparin-induced thrombocytopenia compared with LDUH.[31] As a result, no routine platelet count monitoring is required when patients receive LMWH. LDUH must be administered two or three times daily but most patients can be given LMWH once daily. As the cost of unfractionated heparin has increased substantially in recent years, there is no longer a major difference in cost between these agents. Finally, because LMWH can be used as thromboprophylaxis for almost all patients, the use of a single agent allows for standardization of prophylaxis across the hospital that should be associated with greater institution-wide adherence.

MECHANICAL THROMBOPROPHYLAXIS STUDIES IN CRITICAL CARE

Evidence is lacking to guide clinicians in the use of mechanical thromboprophylaxis for most patient populations, and there are no studies of mechanical thromboprophylaxis in the ICU setting.[4,32] In some patient groups, mechanical prophylaxis is less effective than anticoagulant prophylaxis.[4,33] The use of graduated compression stockings (GCS) or intermittent pneumatic compression (IPC) or both is recommended for use in patients with a contraindication to anticoagulant prophylaxis.[4] Compliance with proper use of mechanical thromboprophylaxis is often poor, depriving patients of the protection this modality provides. A study of 137 patients who were prescribed either GCS or IPC found adherence in only 26% of the stocking patients and only 19% of the IPC patients.[34]

Despite the use of inferior vena cava (IVC) filters as primary prophylaxis in many centers, there is no direct evidence of their effectiveness in this capacity.[35] The only randomized trial of IVC filters was conducted in patients who were being treated for acute DVT. Patients who had filters inserted along with anticoagulation had fewer, mostly asymptomatic, PE but there was no reduction in death and there were significantly more recurrent DVTs than those who were anticoagulated alone.[36] Of additional concern, in 2010, the FDA reported that they had received 921 reports of complications associated with IVC filters since 2005.[37] The 8th ACCP Antithrombotic Guidelines recommend against the use of IVC filters for primary thromboprophylaxis in any patient group.[4] Until further evidence is available, we believe that IVC filters should be limited to patients with acute proximal DVT and an absolute contraindication to therapeutic anticoagulation. In this context, only retrievable filters should be inserted, therapeutic anticoagulation should be started as soon as it is safe to do so, and the filter should be removed shortly after the patient starts treatment for their DVT. We do not believe that IVC filters should be used as primary prophylaxis or as an adjunct to anticoagulation in patients with VTE.

ANTICOAGULANT THROMBOPROPHYLAXIS IN CRITICALLY ILL PATIENTS WITH RENAL INSUFFICIENCY

Approximately one third of medical–surgical patients admitted to ICU have severe renal failure as defined by a calculated creatinine clearance of less than 30 mL/min.[1,38,39] These patients are known to be at increased risk of VTE; however, because LMWH is dependent on renal clearance, there has been concern about bioaccumulation of this class of anticoagulants in patients with renal insufficiency. The DIRECT Study was conducted to assess the safety and pharmacodynamics of prophylactic dalteparin in patients with severe renal insufficiency.[40] This multicenter trial assessed the bioaccumulation of dalteparin 5000 IU once daily, by measuring trough anti-factor Xa levels twice weekly and serial anti-factor Xa levels at 0, 1, 2, 4, 8, 12, 20, and 24 hours on days 3, 10, and 17 of ICU admission. No patient developed bioaccumulation as defined by an anti-factor Xa trough level of greater than 0.4 IU/mL over the course of his or her ICU stay. Major bleeding occurred in 10 of 138 patients (7.2%; 95%CI, 4.0%–12.8%). Because trough anti-factor Xa levels in these patients were 0.18 IU/mL or lower, it is unlikely that bioaccumulation of dalteparin contributed to bleeding. In addition, peak levels were 0.2 to 0.40 IU/mL, reflecting appropriate thromboprophylaxis levels. This study provides strong evidence that prophylactic dosing of dalteparin in patients with severe renal insufficiency is not associated with bioaccumulation and establishes that there is no indication for dose adjustment or anti-factor Xa levels routinely in these patients. The impact of renal insufficiency on prophylactic doses of LMWHs other than dalteparin is unclear and further studies are needed to clarify the need for dose reduction in the management of patients on these medications.

SCREENING FOR ASYMPTOMATIC DVT IN CRITICALLY ILL PATIENTS

As a result of the poor correlation between symptoms and signs of VTE in critically ill patients and the high rate of VTE, a number of studies, including PROTECT, have used serial DUS screening of asymptomatic patients to assess for DVT.[17] This raises the question of whether this method should be used to screen all or a high-risk subset of critically ill patients for DVT. However, DUS is costly and time consuming, and the clinical importance of DVT detected by asymptomatic screening is unclear. Further, screening for asymptomatic DVT has not been shown to be effective in trauma or major orthopedic surgery patients and may cause harm because of possible false-positive results and due to resultant therapeutic anticoagulant therapy in the patients found to be positive.[4] We believe that a randomized trial of the addition of routine screening DUS to an optimal prophylaxis regimen would be important, feasible, and ethical. In the meantime, long-term follow-up studies to assess the clinical impact of screening and economic analyses with modeling of reasonable outcomes may help guide this decision. Currently, we recommend that DUS screening be limited to patients at very high risk for thrombosis who cannot be reasonably prophylaxed (eg, patients with combined intracranial bleeding and leg injuries that preclude the use of both anticoagulant and mechanical prophylaxis).[4,41]

SPECIAL CONSIDERATIONS FOR LMWH USE IN CRITICALLY ILL PATIENTS

Several studies have reported a lower plasma anti-factor Xa activity after LMWH administration in patients receiving vasopressors.[28,42] In a small study of ICU patients with normal renal function and not receiving vasopressors, anti-factor Xa levels were measured after administration of dalteparin 2500 IU, subcutaneously daily in seven patients with peripheral edema and seven patients without.[43] No significant differences were found. However, another small study documented lower anti-factor Xa activity in edematous compared to nonedematous trauma patients.[44] The number of patients in each of these studies is small and further investigations are needed.

In summary, critical illness, vasopressor use, and generalized edema may cause a reduction in anti-factor Xa levels in patients being prophylaxed with LMWH. However, the relationship between anti-factor Xa levels and the clinical effectiveness of LMWH remains uncertain. In a recent pharmacokinetic study, 72 ICU patients were randomized to a single dose of enoxaparin 40 mg, 50 mg, 60 mg, or 70 mg.[45] Although anti-factor Xa levels correlated with the enoxaparin dose there was wide variability in the levels within each dose group. Further, 28% of the enoxaparin 40 mg, patients had no increase in their level compared with the pre-enoxaparin baseline. Another study demonstrated that peak anti-factor Xa levels below 0.2 U/ml, seen in half of the 54 ICU patients who were given enoxaparin 30 mg SC twice a day, were associated with more than three times higher DVT rate (37% vs 11%) than in the patients with higher peak levels.[46] These studies, therefore, raises concerns about the appropriate LMWH dose in critically ill patients.

PRACTICAL RECOMMENDATIONS

Practical recommendations for the management of thromboprophylaxis in critical care patients are outlined in **Fig. 1**. All patients should be assessed on admission to the ICU and daily for their individual thrombosis and bleeding risks. Patients with active or high risk of clinically important bleeding should receive mechanical thromboprophylaxis with graduated compression stockings or intermittent pneumatic compression until their bleeding risk is reduced and anticoagulant thromboprophylaxis can be started. If mechanical devices are used, they must be properly fitted, applied to both legs and used continuously for almost 24 hours per day.

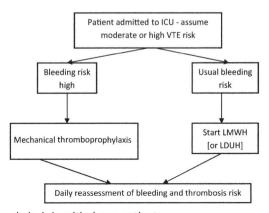

Fig. 1. Thromboprophylaxis in critical care patients.

Many patients in ICU are considered to be at increased risk for bleeding because of oozing from IV sites, around urinary catheters, or with minor gastrointestinal bleeding. For most patients, minor bleeding is not a contraindication to anticoagulant thromboprophylaxis, which can be safely initiated. Anticoagulant thromboprophylaxis is unlikely to contribute to clinically significant bleeding, as has been demonstrated in several bleeding risk factor analyses.[1,47,48] Even in patients with traumatic intracranial hemorrhage, there is evidence that early initiation of LMWH is not associated with an increased risk of rebleeding. For example, among 669 patients with traumatic intracranial hemorrhages, progression of the bleed was seen in 1.5% of patients who started LMWH within 72 hours with the same rate observed in patients who started after 72 hours.[49]

There is evidence that the effectiveness of thromboprophylaxis decreases if its initiation is delayed. For example, in a study of pelvic trauma patients, delaying the start of LMWH prophylaxis for more than 24 hours after injury was associated with a sevenfold increase in DVT rate compared with starting within 24 hours.[50] For most patients, LMWH can be started at the first dosing time after admission. If there is uncertainty about the patient's bleeding risk on admission, mechanical prophylaxis can be started at this time or a brief period of observation can ensue. In both situations, the patient should be reassessed within the next 24 hours for anticoagulant prophylaxis or mechanical prophylaxis if bleeding concerns persist. Because the risk of both thrombosis and bleeding can change frequently in ICU patients, the use of thromboprophylaxis should be reviewed by the critical care team on a daily basis.

For patients at very high risk for VTE and in whom pharmacologic thromboprophylaxis cannot be used for at least several days, screening with bilateral proximal DUS may be considered although there is no direct evidence to support this approach and it might cause overall harm. Prophylactic IVC filters are not recommended in this (or any) patient population. Thromboprophylaxis should always be included as part of the ICU transfer orders.

Many critical care units admit a spectrum of patients including major trauma, neurosurgical, major orthopedic surgery, and cancer surgery patients in addition to general medical–surgical patients. **Table 5** gives recommendations for thromboprophylaxis that include all of these patient groups. Patients deemed to be at usual or low risk for bleeding should be classified as moderate or high thrombotic risk based on the risk factors discussed previously such as personal or family history of VTE and end-stage renal disease. Patients with major trauma, spinal cord injury, major orthopedic surgery, or malignancy should be considered high risk and should receive LMWH and not LDUH.[4]

Table 5		
Thromboprophylaxis recommendations in critically ill patients		
Bleeding Risk	**Thrombosis Risk[a]**	**Prophylaxis Recommendations**
Low	Moderate	LMWH 4000–6000 anti-factor Xa U SC qd (or LDUH 5000 U SC bid]
Low	High[a]	LMWH 4000–6000 anti-factor Xa U SC qd
High	Moderate or high[a]	GCS or IPC; convert to LMWH when bleeding risk decreases

[a] High-risk patients include those who have had major trauma or spinal cord injury, major orthopedic surgery, or major surgery for cancer.

Adapted from Geerts W, Cook D, Selby R, et al. Venous thromboembolism and its prevention in critical care. J Crit Care 2002;17:95–104; with permission.

Box 2
General recommendations for thromboprophylaxis in critical care patients

- Develop local evidence-based thromboprophylaxis policy and guidelines.
- Update guidelines as new evidence emerges.
- Consider *all* ICU patients to be at risk for VTE.
- Use thromboprophylaxis in *all* ICU patients.
- Individualize prophylaxis but select from a small number of options according to the local policy.
- Start thromboprophylaxis as soon as possible.
- Embed thromboprophylaxis into preprinted or computer order sets.
- Review thromboprophylaxis daily.
- Do not interrupt for procedures or surgery (qhs dosing).
- Consider a daily checklist of key ICU patient safety strategies (including thromboprophylaxis).
- Include in ICU transfer orders.
- Monitor and evaluate compliance with regular audits and provide feedback.
- Empower all health care professionals to play a role in thromboprophylaxis.

For critical care units to consistently provide appropriate thromboprophylaxis, a formal policy, guideline or care map that is specific to the hospital is essential. The principles outlined in **Box 2** can serve as a guide for such a policy. All ICU patients should be considered at risk for VTE and all patients should be provided anticoagulant or mechanical prophylaxis depending on bleeding risk. Consideration of specific prophylaxis should be individualized to each patient's thrombotic and bleeding risks and this requires assessment on admission as well as daily reassessment. Mechanical prophylaxis should generally be restricted to patients with or at high risk for clinically important bleeding. Prophylaxis should generally not be interrupted for procedures or surgery. One strategy to reduce the temptation to hold anticoagulant prophylaxis for procedures is to provide the anticoagulant (usually a LMWH) in the evening; this will safely allow surgery or other procedures to be done the next morning without missing any doses. Prophylaxis should be included in postoperative and ICU transfer orders. Adherence to local prophylaxis guidelines should be supported with regular interactive education, preprinted order sets, reminders, and computer decision support systems.[51–53] Compliance with thromboprophylaxis also requires periodic audits of adherence to the unit policy with feedback to frontline ICU staff. Unless optimal thromboprophylaxis is consistently at 100%, the audit results should be used for local quality improvement interventions. It is essential that all members of the critical care team (physicians, nurses, pharmacists, physiotherapists, respiratory therapists, and other health care professionals) be encouraged to take an active role in the implementation and daily assessment of VTE prevention and other key patient safety strategies.

SUMMARY

Considerable progress has been made in our understanding of VTE epidemiology, risk factors, and appropriate thromboprophylaxis in this challenging patient population. The use of anticoagulant thromboprophylaxis significantly decreases the risk of VTE in ICU patients. Prophylactic LMWH (or LDUH) can be safely administered to the majority of critically ill patients while those at high risk for clinically important bleeding should receive mechanical thromboprophylaxis until the bleeding risk decreases. Renal insufficiency is not a contraindication to the use of LMWH or LDUH. Despite appropriate thromboprophylaxis, proximal DVT still occurs in approximately 5% of ICU patients prophylaxed with LMWH or LDUH. Studies to identify risk factors for patients who fail appropriate thromboprophylaxis and ways to manage patients at high risk of bleeding and thrombosis are needed. The Agency for Healthcare Research and Quality (AHRQ) has ranked "the appropriate use of prophylaxis to prevent venous thromboembolism in patients at risk" the number one safety practice for hospitals.[54] For health care providers in critical care units, the prevention of VTE must also be a high priority and should be a routine, daily consideration for every critically ill patient.

REFERENCES

1. Cook DJ, Crowther M, Meade M, et al. Deep venous thrombosis in medical-surgical critically ill patients: prevalence, incidence, and risk factors. Crit Care Med 2005;33:1565–71.
2. Crowther MA, Cook DJ, Griffith LE, et al. Deep venous thrombosis: clinically silent in the intensive care unit. J Crit Care 2005;20:334–40.
3. Geerts W, Cook D, Selby R, et al. Venous thromboembolism and its prevention in critical care. J Crit Care 2002;17:95–104.
4. Geerts WH, Bergqvist D, Pineo GF, et al. Prevention of venous thromboembolism: American College of Chest Physicians evidence-based clinical practice guidelines. 8th edition. Chest 2008;133(Suppl):381S–453S.
5. Neuhaus A, Bentz RR, Weg JG. Pulmonary embolism in respiratory failure. Chest 1978;73:460–5.
6. Moser KM, LeMoine JR, Nachtwey FJ, et al. Deep venous thrombosis and pulmonary embolism. Frequency in a respiratory intensive care unit. JAMA 1981;246:1422–4.
7. Pingleton SK, Bone RC, Pingleton WW, et al. Prevention of pulmonary emboli in a respiratory intensive care unit. Efficacy of low-dose heparin. Chest 1981;79:647–50.
8. Cullen DJ, Nemeskal AR. The autopsy incidence of acute pulmonary embolism in critically ill surgical patients. Intensive Care Med 1986;12:339–403.
9. Blosser SA, Zimmerman HE, Stauffer JL. Do autopsies of critically ill patients reveal important findings that were clinically undetected? Crit Care Med 1998;26:1332–6.
10. Willemsen HW, Wester JP, van Hattum AH, et al. The incidence of pulmonary embolism in a surgical intensive care unit [abstract]. Intensive Care Med 2000;26(Suppl 3):S242.
11. Hirsch DR, Ingenito EP, Goldhaber SZ. Prevalence of deep venous thrombosis among patients in medical intensive care. JAMA 1995;274:335–7.
12. Cade JF. High risk of the critically ill for venous thromboembolism. Crit Care Med 1982;10:448–50.
13. Kapoor M, Kupfer YY, Tessler S. Subcutaneous heparin prophylaxis significantly reduces the incidence of venous thromboembolic events in the critically ill [abstract]. Crit Care Med 1999;27(Suppl):A69.
14. Fraisse F, Holzapfel L, Couland J-M, et al. Nadroparin in the prevention of deep vein thrombosis in acute decompensated COPD. Am J Respir Crit Care Med 2000;161:1109–14.
15. Baum GL, Fisher FD. The relationship of fatal pulmonary insufficiency with cor pulmonale, rightsided mural thrombi and pulmonary emboli: a preliminary report. Am J Med Sci 1960;240:609–12.
16. Greene R, Zapol WM, Snider MT, et al. Early bedside detection of pulmonary vascular occlusion during acute respiratory failure. Am Rev Respir Dis 1981;124:593–601.
17. The PROTECT Investigators. Dalteparin versus unfractionated heparin in critically ill patients. N Engl J Med 2011;364:1304–14.

18. Schultz DJ, Brasel KJ, Washington L, et al. Incidence of asymptomatic pulmonary embolism in moderately to severely injured trauma patients. J Trauma 2004;56: 727–33.
19. Crowther MA, Cook DJ, Griffith LE, et al. Neither baseline tests of molecular hyper-coagulability nor D-dimer levels predict deep venous thrombosis in critically ill medi-cal-surgical patients. Intensive Care Med 2005;31:48–55.
20. Harris LM, Curl GR, Booth FV, et al. Screening for asymptomatic deep vein throm-bosis in surgical intensive care patients. J Vasc Surg 1997;26:764–9.
21. Wu C, Lee AY. Malignancy and venous thrombosis in the critical care patient. Crit Care Med 2010;38(2 Suppl):S64–S70.
22. Cook D, Attia J, Weaver B, et al. Venous thromboembolic disease: an observational study in medical-surgical intensive care unit patients. J Crit Care 2000:15;127–32.
23. Trottier SJ, Veremakis C, O'Brien J, et al. Femoral deep vein thrombosis associated with central venous catheterization: results from a prospective, randomized trial. Crit Care Med 1995;23:52–9.
24. Durbec O, Viviand X, Potie F, et al. A prospective evaluation of the use of femoral venous catheters in critically ill adults. Crit Care Med 1997;25:1986–9.
25. Timsit J-F, Farkas J-C, Boyer J-M, et al. Central vein catheter-related thrombosis in intensive care patients: incidence, risk factors, and relationship with catheter-related sepsis. Chest 1998;114:207–13.
26. Joynt GM, Kew J, Gomersall CD, et al. Deep venous thrombosis caused by femoral venous catheters in critically ill adult patients. Chest 2000;117:178–83.
27. Marik PE, Andrews L, Maini B. The incidence of deep venous thrombosis in ICU patients. Chest 1997;111:661–4.
28. Dorffler-Melly J, de Jonge E, de Pont A-C, et al. Bioavailability of subcutaneous low-molecular-weight heparin to patients on vasopressors. Lancet 2002;359: 849–50.
29. Merrer J, De Jonghe B, Golliot F, et al. Complications of femoral and subclavian venous catheterization in critically ill patients: a randomized controlled trial. JAMA 2001;286:700–7.
30. Karakitsos D, Saranteas T, Patrianakos AP, et al. Ultrasound-guided "low approach" femoral vein catheterization in critical care patients results in high incidence of deep vein thrombosis. Anesthesiology 2007;107:181–2.
31. Martel N, Lee J, Wells PS. Risk of heparin-induced thrombocytopenia with unfrac-tionated and low-molecular-weight heparin thromboprophylaxis: a meta-analysis. Blood 2005;106:2710–5.
32. Limpus A, Chaboyer W, McDonald E, et al. Mechanical thromboprophylaxis in critically ill patients: a systematic review and meta-analysis. Am J Crit Care 2006;15: 402–10.
33. Agnelli G, Piovella F, Buoncristiani P, et al. Enoxaparin plus compression stock-ings compared with compression stockings alone in the prevention of venous thromboembolism after elective neurosurgery. N Engl J Med 1998;339:80–5.
34. Brady D, Raingruber B, Peterson J, et al. The use of knee-length versus thigh-length compression stockings and sequential compression devices. Crit Care Nurs Q 2007;30:255–62.
35. Ingber S, Geerts WH. Vena caval filters: current knowledge, uncertainties and prac-tical approaches. Curr Opin Hematol 2009;16:402–6.
36. Decousus H, Leizorovicz A, Parent F, et al. A clinical trial of vena caval filters in the prevention of pulmonary embolism in patients with proximal deep-vein thrombosis. N Engl J Med 1998;338:409–15.

37. U.S. Food and Drug Administration. Removing retrievable inferior vena cava filters: initial communication. Available at: http://www.fda.gov/MedicalDevices/Safety/AlertsandNotices/ucm221676.htm. Accessed August 16, 2011.

38. Attia J, Ray JG, Cook DJ, et al. Deep vein thrombosis and its prevention in critically ill adults. Arch Intern Med 2001;161:1268–79.

39. Cook D, McMullin J, Hodder R, et al. Prevention and diagnosis of venous thromboembolism in critically ill patients: a Canadian survey. Crit Care 2001;5:336–42.

40. Douketis J, Cook D, Meade M, et al. Prophylaxis against deep vein thrombosis in critically ill patients with severe renal insufficiency with the low-molecular-weight heparin dalteparin: an assessment of safety and pharmacodynamics: The DIRECT Study. Arch Intern Med 2008;168:1805–12.

41. Crowther MA, Cook DJ. Thromboprophylaxis in medical-surgical critically ill patients. Curr Opin Crit Care 2008;14:520–3.

42. Priglinger U, Delle Karth G, Geppert A, et al. Prophylactic anticoagulation with enoxaparin: Is the subcutaneous route appropriate in the critically ill? Crit Care Med 2003;31:1405–9.

43. Rommers MK, Van Der Lely N, Egberts TC, et al. Anti-Xa activity after subcutaneous administration of dalteparin in ICU patients with and without subcutaneous oedema: a pilot study. Crit Care 2006;10:R93.

44. Haas CE, Nelsen JL, Raghavendran K, et al. Pharmacokinetics and pharmacodynamics of enoxaparin in multiple trauma patients. J Trauma 2005;59:1336–44.

45. Robinson S, Zincuk A, Strom T, et al. Enoxaparin, effective dosage for intensive care patients: double-blinded, randomised clinical trial. Crit Care 2010;14:R41.

46. Malinoski D, Jafari F, Ewing T, et al. Standard prophylactic enoxaparin dosing leads to inadequate anti-Xa levels and increased deep venous thrombosis rates in critically ill trauma and surgical patients. J Trauma 2010;68:874–80.

47. Arnold DM, Donahue L, Clarke FJ, et al. Bleeding during critical illness: a prospective cohort study using a new measurement tool. Clin Invest Med 2007;30:E93–E102.

48. Cook D, Douketis J, Meade M, et al. Venous thromboembolism and bleeding in critically ill patients with severe renal insufficiency receiving dalteparin thromboprophylaxis: prevalence, incidence and risk factors. Crit Care 2008;12:R32.

49. Koehler DM, Shipman J, Davidson MA, et al. Is early venous thromboembolism prophylaxis safe in trauma patients with intracranial hemorrhage. J Trauma 2011;70:324–9.

50. Steele N, Dodenhoff RM, Ward AJ, et al. Thromboprophylaxis in pelvic and acetabular surgery. The role of early treatment with low-molecular-weight heparin. J Bone Joint Surg 2005;87–B:209–12.

51. McMullin J, Cook D, Griffith L, et al. Minimizing errors of omission: *B*ehavioual *R*einforcement of *H*eparin to *A*vert *V*enous *E*mboli: the BEHAVE Study. Crit Care Med 2006;34:694–9.

52. Boddi M, Barbani F, Abbate R, et al. Reduction in deep vein thrombosis incidence in intensive care after a clinician education program. J Thromb Haemost 2010;8:121–8.

53. Scales DC, Dainty K, Hales B, et al. A multifaceted intervention for quality improvement in a network of intensive care units. JAMA 2011;305:363–72.

54. Shojana KG, Duncan BW, McDonald KM, et al. Making health care safer: a critical analysis of patient safety practices. Evidence Report/Technology Assessment No. 43 (prepared by the University of California at San Francisco-Stanford Evidence-Based Practice Center under Contract No. 290-97-0013). AHRQ Publication No. 01-E058. Rockville (MD): Agency for Healthcare Research and Quality. Available at: http://www.ahrq.gov/clinic/ptsafety/. Accessed August 16, 2011.

Vena Cava Interruption

Lindsay M. Fairfax, MD[a], Ronald F. Sing, DO, FCCM[a,b,]*

KEYWORDS
- Vena cava filter • Pulmonary embolus • Deep vein thrombosis
- Critical care • Anticoagulation

During the last decade, awareness over venous thromboembolic disease has risen markedly among health care professionals and the general public. The Surgical Care Improvement Project (SCIP) includes institution of venous thromboembolic prophylaxis within 24 hours of anesthesia end time as a core measure.[1] In 2008, the Joint Commission, National Quality Forum, and Centers for Medicare & Medicaid Services approved six inpatient quality measures. VTE-2 assesses the use of venous thromboembolic prophylaxis in intensive care unit patients and requires that prophylaxis is initiated or rationale to withhold prophylaxis is documented within 24 hours of ICU admission.[2] In addition, venous thromboembolism (VTE) was added as a "never event" following certain orthopaedic surgeries in 2008, and many fear this will be expanded to a larger patient population soon.[3]

Whether due to increased surveillance, increased risk, or both, prevalence of VTE increased 33% from 2002 to 2006, from 317 to 422 per 100,000 patients. Based on these data, the number of Americans with VTE is expected to increase to 1.82 million in 2050.[4] Systemic anticoagulation is the first line for prevention and treatment of VTE. However, there are many patient populations in whom this is contraindicated or fails.

The technique of vena caval interruption is not new. However, since the original Greenfield filter was introduced in 1973, technologic improvements have broadened the use of vena cava filters (VCFs). The filter evolved from a cutdown to a percutaneous technique and subsequently from permanent to retrievable. The current generation of optional filters, which can be retrieved when the indication for a VCF has subsided or left in place permanently if needed, has greatly expanded the use of VCFs.

Worldwide insertions of VCFs have increased exponentially, from 2000 in 1979 to 49,000 in 1999 and 140,000 in 2003.[5,6] With this increase in placement have come conflicting recommendations on the appropriate use of the VCF. Organizations such as the American College of Chest Physicians (ACCP), Eastern Association for the Surgery of Trauma (EAST), Society of Interventional Radiologists (SIR), Brain Trauma

Dr Sing has received grant support and is a speaker for CR Bard, Cook, Inc, and Angiotech.
[a] Department of Surgery, Carolinas Medical Center, Charlotte, NC 28232, USA
[b] Department of Surgery, University of North Carolina School of Medicine, Chapel Hill, NC 27599, USA
* Corresponding author. Department of Surgery, Carolinas Medical Center, Charlotte, NC 28232.
E-mail address: Ron.Sing@carolinashealthcare.org

Crit Care Clin 27 (2011) 781–804
doi:10.1016/j.ccc.2011.07.002
0749-0704/11/$ – see front matter © 2011 Elsevier Inc. All rights reserved.

Foundation (BTF), and the Consortium for Spinal Cord Medicine have all published guidelines and recommendations.[7–11] Importantly, many guidelines do not address specific patient factors, such as traumatic brain injury and comorbidities. Therefore, the indications for VCF insertion continue to vary between institutions and specialists.

INDICATIONS FOR INSERTION OF A VENA CAVA FILTER

The standard of care for treatment of venous thromboembolic disease is systemic anticoagulation. Patients diagnosed with deep venous thrombus (DVT) or pulmonary embolus (PE) are initially anticoagulated in the acute setting with therapeutic subcutaneous low molecular weight heparin or intravenous heparin drip. They are then transitioned to warfarin to undergo a minimum of 3 months of anticoagulation with a target international normalized ratio (INR) of 2.0 to 3.0. Patients at a high risk for recurrence are treated indefinitely. Risk factors for recurrence include male gender, advanced age, malignancy, and unprovoked PE. Even patients receiving a VCF for the indications discussed later should receive a course of anticoagulant therapy whenever possible (eg, when the previous contraindication is eliminated).[12]

The conventional indication for insertion of a VCF is a patient with documented VTE in whom anticoagulation is contraindicated or has failed. Level II and level III data have been used to add relative indications such as free-floating thrombus and severely reduced cardiopulmonary reserve. With advances in technology regarding insertion as well as retrieval of VCFs, the "prophylactic" insertion of optional filters skyrocketed. Despite this common nomenclature, all VCFs should be considered prophylactic, as they do not prevent or treat VTE; rather, they prevent, or prophylax against, an embolus traveling to the lungs. In the literature, however, most define a prophylactic VCF as one placed in a patient with no known active thromboembolic disease.

In 1998, Decousus and colleagues published the initial results of the PREPIC study, a randomized trial of "prophylactic" filter insertion. Four hundred patients at high risk for PE (195 of whom had established PE at inclusion) were randomized in a two-by-two design to VCF insertion or none as well as to receive enoxaparin or unfractionated heparin. At 12 days, the filter group demonstrated a significantly lower incidence of PE. However, at 2 years, there was no difference in symptomatic PE occurrence, although the filter group had significantly more recurrent DVT (20.8% vs 11.6%). There was no difference in mortality or major bleeding.[13] An 8-year follow-up of the same group showed a decrease in PE in the filter group. The incidence of DVT remained higher in this group, with no difference in post-thrombotic syndrome or mortality.[14] This lack of impact on mortality is often referenced by those opposing VCF insertion. However, given the low incidence of PE, an adequately powered trial to show mortality impact is essentially impossible.

Although, to our knowledge, the PREPIC trial is the only randomized controlled trial to date, the randomization of patients *already receiving anticoagulation* did not make it applicable to the majority of patients receiving prophylactic VCFs, and a mortality benefit would not be expected. In addition, this study was performed before widespread use of modern, optional devices. Therefore, the absolute indications for insertion of a VCF in patients without known VTE and unable to receive anticoagulation remain undefined.

As there has not been a randomized controlled trial to define high-risk patients who should receive a VCF, many groups have published recommendations. The American College of Chest Physicians (ACCP) recommends VCF insertion in patients with proximal vein thrombosis and an absolute contraindication to, or complication of, anticoagulation.[9] Similarly, the SIR produced a consensus document in 2005, summarized in the **Box 1**, stating absolute, relative, and prophylactic indications for VCFs.[10]

Box 1
Society of Interventional Radiology indications for VCF

Absolute (documented VTE and high risk for PE)

- Contraindication to or complication from anticoagulant therapy

Relative (documented VTE)

- High risk of significant PE despite primary therapy
  - Large free-floating proximal DVT
  - Iliocaval DVT with or without thrombolysis
  - Massive PE or chronic PE treated with thrombectomy, thrombolysis
- Increased risk of anticoagulation complications
- Noncompliant with medications
- Limited cardiopulmonary reserve

Prophylactic (no documented VTE)

- Unable to undergo pharmacologic prophylaxis and at high risk for PE as defined as the following patient groups:
  - Multisystem trauma (high-level evidence)
  - Critically ill with history of VTE
  - Perioperative with history of VTE
  - Bariatric surgery

Data from Kaufman JA, Kinney TB, Streiff MB, et al. Guidelines for the use of retrievable and convertible vena cava filters: report from the Society of Interventional Radiology multidisciplinary consensus conference. J Vasc Interv Radiol 2006;17:449–59.

Jacobs and coworkers reviewed these guidelines in depth in 2003.[15] Absolute contraindications to anticoagulation include ongoing significant traumatic brain injury, visceral or retroperitoneal hemorrhage, and the need for major surgery. Other relative contraindications are a subject of debate, including recent surgery, brain tumors, less severe traumatic brain injury, history of bleeding, uncontrolled hypertension, esophageal varices, and major trauma. Complications from anticoagulation include intracranial or retroperitoneal bleeding or requirement for hospitalization/transfusion. However, the risk of major bleeding in patients with an appropriate INR (range 2–3) is estimated at only 4%, making this a relatively uncommon indication for a VCF.[15] In addition, failure of anticoagulation is a rare event, with a 90% to 95% success rate provided appropriate anticoagulation is administered.

Patients with severe cardiopulmonary disease are presumed to have so little reserve that a PE of any size could be fatal, although there are no studies to support this assumption. In addition, the term severe cardiopulmonary disease is not well defined. VCF insertion in this population should be undertaken on a specific case basis, and systemic anticoagulation should still be continued.

Regarding free-floating thrombus, a study in 2007 found no difference in risk of clot migration between free-floating clot and occlusive thrombi.[16] However, before this, Norris and colleagues found a 60% risk of PE in patients with free-floating thrombus.[17] Systemic anticoagulation is recommended as first-line therapy for these patients. Another group with no clear guidelines is patients undergoing thrombolysis.

Animal studies of mechanical thrombosis showed reduction of PE with temporary VCFs.[18] However, in a retrospective review of both pharmacologic and pharmacomechanical lysis, no clear benefit was shown.[19] Given the conflicting evidence, VCFs should be considered in these patients on a case-by-case basis. The optional devices currently available offer a potential benefit in these patients given the ability to retrieve the filter post-thrombolysis.

VCF insertion in patients with no thromboembolic disease (often termed prophylactic) has skyrocketed. This is largely due to the ability to retrieve VCFs when they are no longer needed. Patients suffering multisystem trauma, patients with a history of VTE scheduled to undergo major surgery, and orthopaedic patients are most often included in this group. Other groups receiving such VCFs include bariatric patients and patients with significant total body surface burns.[20]

SPECIFIC PATIENT POPULATIONS

One of the greatest difficulties in defining guidelines for the use of VCFs in the critically ill is the wide variety of patient populations at risk for VTE. Although the ACCP is the most widely encompassing organization to define guidelines, the group still does not examine specific populations such as patients with traumatic brain injury. In addition, risk stratification for all groups is based predominantly on level II and level III evidence. All critically ill patients should be considered high risk for VTE and pharmacologic prophylaxis considered. Asymptomatic PE was found in 24% of critically ill trauma patients, 30% of whom were receiving pharmacologic prophylaxis.[21] In addition, many critically ill patients are unable to receive initial pharmacologic prophylaxis, and are therefore considered for "prophylactic" VCF insertion.

Spinal Cord Injury

Perhaps the most significant subset of critical care patients at risk for VTE are spinal cord injury (SCI) patients. Asymptomatic DVT has been reported in 60% to 100% of SCI patients.[22] In older studies, fatal PE has been shown to occur in 0.3% to 20% of trauma patients with SCI.[23–26] This high incidence has been attributed to not only venous stasis but also changes in fibrinolytic activity, catecholamine effects on platelet aggregation, high factor VIII concentrations, and increased acute phase reactants associated with the injury itself.[27,28] With improvements in the care of SCI patients resulting in longer life expectancy, late risk of VTE is now an even greater concern.

The incidence is low in the first 72 hours; however, DVT frequency is highest in the first 2 weeks after injury, with the majority of venous thromboembolic events occurring in the first 3 months.[29–31] However, some studies suggest the risk extends for years. Lamb and coworkers followed 287 SCI patients for a mean of 13.7 years. The incidence of VTE was 14%, with 83% of events occurring in the first 6 months after injury.[32]

Pulmonary embolism is the third leading cause of death in SCI patients in the first year after injury, with a reported incidence of 5%.[31] The relative risk of PE in SCI patients was 54 times higher than in the general trauma population, making this the highest of the high-risk groups studied by Rogers and colleagues.[33] This was confirmed in a meta-analysis by Velmahos and coworkers in 2000, which showed a twofold increase in VTE risk in patients with spinal fractures and a threefold increase in SCI patients.[34]

Rates of VTE in the nontraumatic SCI patient are also high at 8%. This lower risk compared with the trauma population may be due to a lower incidence of complete injury and therefore less neurologic impairment.[35]

The Consortium for Spinal Cord Medicine published clinical practice guideline regarding VTE prophylaxis in 1997. This guideline was largely based on case-control and expert opinion data, given the absence of level I data. It was emphasized that

---

Box 2
Consortium for Spinal Cord Medicine clinical practice guidelines

Absolute Indications for VCF Placement:

- Contraindication to anticoagulation such as active or potential bleeding sites not amenable to local control
- Failed anticoagulant prophylaxis

Consider VCF in patients with:

- Complete motor paralysis caused by lesions in the high cervical cord (C2 and C3)
- Poor cardiopulmonary reserve
- Thrombus in the IVC despite anticoagulant prophylaxis

Data from Consortium for Spinal Cord Medicine. Prevention of thromboembolism in spinal cord injury. J Spinal Cord Med 1997;20:259–83.

VCFs cannot substitute pharmacologic prophylaxis, which should be initiated as soon as feasible (**Box 2**).[7]

Multisystem Trauma

The incidence of VTE in trauma patients varies depending on screening modality, with rates from 17% to 58% for DVT using ultrasound or venography and 4% to 20% for PE on autopsy studies.[36–40] Several studies have examined independent risk factors for VTE in trauma (**Table 1**). Risk factors are additive. In one group, 77% of patients with both head injuries and lower extremity injuries were positive for VTE.[38] Winchell and colleagues found a 0.37% incidence of PE in 9721 trauma patients; however, 80% of patients with PE had received some form of prophylaxis (systemic anticoagulation or mechanical compression). No patients with VCF placement suffered PE. The authors estimated that a dramatic reduction in PE would have occurred had VCFs

Table 1
Analysis of risk factors for VTE in trauma

Geerts, et al, 1994[a]	Age (each 1-year increment with odds ratio of 1.05), blood transfusion, surgery, fracture of femur or tibia, spinal cord injury
Knudson, et al, 2004[b]	Age >40 years, lower extremity fracture, head injury, ventilator dependence, and major operative procedure
Winchell, et al, 1994[c]	Head injury plus spinal cord injury or long bone fracture or both, severe pelvic fracture plus long bone fracture, or multiple long bone fractures

[a] *Data from* Geerts WH, Code KI, Jay RM, et al. A prospective study of venous thromboembolism after major trauma. N Engl J Med 1994;331:1601–6.
[b] *Data from* Knudson MM, Ikossi DG, Khaw L, et al. Thromboembolism after trauma: an analysis of 1602 episodes from the American College of Surgeons National Trauma Data Bank. Ann Surg 2004;240:490–6 [discussion 496–8].
[c] *Data from* Winchell RJ, Hoyt DB, Walsh JC, et al. Risk factors associated with pulmonary embolism despite routine prophylaxis: implications for improved protection. J Trauma 1994;37:600–6.

Box 3
Eastern Association for the Surgery of Trauma guidelines for placement of VCF

Standard indications (level I evidence)	• Recurrent PE despite full anticoagulation • Proximal DVT and contraindications to full anticoagulation • Proximal DVT and major bleeding while on full anticoagulation • Progression of iliofemoral clot despite anticoagulation (rare)
Extended indications (level II evidence)	• Large free-floating thrombus in the iliac vein or the inferior vena cava • After massive PE in which recurrent emboli may prove fatal • During or after surgical embolectomy
Prophylactic indications (level III evidence)	Patients without a DVT/PE who cannot receive anticoagulation because of increased bleeding risk[a] *and* have one or more of the following injury patterns: • Severe closed head injury (Glasgow Coma Scale score <8) • Incomplete spinal cord injury with paraplegia or quadriplegia • Complex pelvic fractures with associated long-bone fractures • Multiple long-bone fractures

---

[a] Bleeding risk defined as intracranial hemorrhage, ocular injury with associated hemorrhage, solid intra-abdominal organ injury (ie, liver, spleen, kidney), or pelvic or retroperitoneal hematoma requiring transfusion. Other risk factors for bleeding include cirrhosis, active peptic ulcer disease, end-stage renal disease, and coagulopathy attributable to injury, medication, or congenital or hereditary conditions.
Data from Pasquale M, Fabian TC. Practice management guidelines for trauma from the Eastern Association for the Surgery of Trauma. J Trauma 1998;44:941–56.

been used in these patients. Based on this review, they recommended VCF insertion in patients with a PE risk of 2% to 5% despite primary prophylaxis.[41]

Given the high incidence and potentially devastating consequences of VTE, the Eastern Association for the Surgery of Trauma (EAST) produced a consensus document in 2002 (summarized in **Box 3**). High-risk patients include traumatic brain injury with Glasgow Coma Scale score less than 8, SCI, multiple long bone fractures, severe pelvic fracture plus long bone fracture, and head injury plus long bone fracture.[11] These recommendations are based on several retrospective and case series reports on the prophylactic use of VCFs.

In what some consider a landmark study, Rogers and coworkers in 1993 showed a significant decrease in PE compared with a historical control (1% vs 0.25%) after institution of a prophylactic VCF policy. The criteria for insertion were patients older than age 55 years with isolated long bone fractures, severe head injury/coma, multiple long bone fractures and pelvic fracture, and spinal cord injury with paraplegia or quadriplegia. DVT occurred in 18% of patients in which a VCF was placed.[33]

It is a common myth that VTE does not occur the first few days after injury. However, regarding the timing of PE after injury, Owings and colleagues reviewed 69 trauma patients with proven PE. Fifteen of these occurred in the first 4 days after injury, with four in the first 24 hours. Forty percent of patients who developed PE had no prophylaxis, while 33% had compression devices alone.[42] Our trauma service guideline calls for filter insertion within the 48 hours in patients who will be unable to receive pharmacologic prophylaxis (**Fig. 1**). All critically ill trauma patients automatically fall into the high-risk category for VTE risk according to the hospital algorithm, and therefore should receive subcutaneous low molecular weight heparin (LMWH), ie, enoxaparin, 30 mg every 12 hours. Contraindications to LMWH include unstable hemoglobin, solid organ injury (LMWH started when hemoglobin has dropped <1 gram in 24 hours), traumatic brain

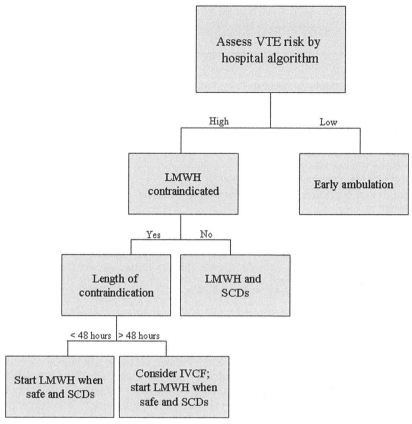

Fig. 1. Algorithm for initiation of anticoagulation and placement of vena caval filters in the multisystem trauma patient. (F. H. "Sammy" Ross Trauma Center, Carolinas Medical Center, Charlotte, NC.)

injury and spinal cord injury, and coagulopathy. The dose of LMWH is increased to 40 mg every 12 hours in patients weighing more than 150 kg. Patients with serum creatinine grater than 1.6 are started on subcutaneous heparin 5000 units every 8 hours.

Insertion of a VCF in patients unable to receive pharmacologic prophylaxis is generally accepted. However, further randomized, controlled trials to determine the effectiveness of prophylactic VCF insertion in the trauma patient despite primary prophylaxis are needed, which would be difficult to undertake given the relatively low incidence of PE.

Neurocritical Care

Blunt traumatic brain injury has been shown to be a significant risk factor for VTE; however, decisions on when it is "safe" to initiate pharmacologic prophylaxis are often based more on personal bias than on evidence. The Brain Trauma Foundation cites level III evidence supporting the use of pharmacologic prophylaxis but states that no reliable data can support a recommendation regarding when it is safe to begin.[8]

Norwood and coworkers found enoxaparin safe to use in neurotrauma patients in 2002 and then with a larger cohort in 2008.[21,43] However, even in the larger study,

---

Box 4
Default medical DVT prophylaxis timeframe in traumatic brain injury and spine fracture[a]

Type of Injury	Prophylaxis Initiation[b,c]
Subarachnoid hemorrhage (traumatic)	72 hours post injury or
Diffuse axonal injury	ICP monitor removal
Intraventricular hemorrhage (traumatic)	
Intracranial pressure monitor—post removal	
Ventriculostomy—post removal	
Vertebral body fractures without canal compromise (nonoperative)	
Contusion, intracerebral hemorrhage without mass effect	14 days
Postoperative shunt placement	
Craniotomy without mass effect	
Vertebral body fractures with canal compromise	
Contusion with mass effect,[d] subdural hematoma, or epidural hematoma	Individual case basis

[a] Timeframe for default initiation of DVT prophylaxis. Clinicians may agree to deviate for individual patients. CT obtained at 72 hours or greater to confirm stability of injury.
[b] Lovenox 30 mg SQ bid (if creatinine >1.6, heparin 5000 units SQ q8 hours).
[c] Consideration for IVCF placement should be made, and documented, within 72 hours for patients whose medical DVT prophylaxis will be delayed.
[d] Mass effect defined as effacement of ventricular system or cisterns, or midline shift.

---

almost 50% of eligible patients were excluded because of surgeon preference or unknown reasons. In the remaining patients enrolled, bleeding risk was shown to be 1.1%, compared with a cited risk of DVT at 18% and PE at 4.8% without prophylaxis.[43] Pharmacologic anticoagulation in elective neurosurgical patients has been shown to lower rates of DVT with no increased bleeding risk.[44,45] In conjunction with the neurosurgical group, the guideline in **Box 4** has been adopted for traumatic brain injury patients at our level I trauma center.

Boeer and colleagues randomized 68 patients with intracerebral hemorrhage to prophylactic heparin administration on day 2, 4, or 10. There was no increased rebleeding in any group; however, study size was small.[46] When it comes to patients with hemorrhagic stroke complicated by known VTE, opinions vary widely. In a survey of geriatricians, half reported using VCFs for such a scenario, and half gave therapeutic anticoagulation despite bleeding risk.[47] Therefore, decisions regarding prophylactic and therapeutic anticoagulation are still made on a case-by-case basis taking into account hemorrhage size and location. When the treating clinician decides against anticoagulation, VCF insertion is recommended for patients with known VTE.

Mechanical prophylaxis against VTE has been shown to be effective in elective surgical patients and is placed before starting the procedure.[48] However, medical patients, particularly those immobilized by stroke, are similar to trauma patients in that the insult cannot be predicted, and therefore prophylaxis cannot be started before immobilization. The CLOTS (clots in legs or stockings after stroke) trial sought to determine the effectiveness of graduated compression stocking for VTE prevention in stroke patients. CLOTS 1, published in 2009, showed no benefit of compression stockings, with 10% of patients in each group developing a proximal DVT, and a1% to 1.6% incidence of PE.[49] CLOTS 3 is currently in progress evaluating the effectiveness of intermittent pneumatic compression devices.[50]

Given the high risk of VTEs in this patient population in whom anticoagulation is commonly contraindicated, VCFs should be considered. Owing to the low incidence of PE, a trial examining PE prevention using VCFs in patients without known DVT would be difficult. Similar to the traumatic brain injury population, the availability of optional, retrievable filters and bedside insertion in the intensive care unit may shift the risk/benefit ratio toward the insertion of "prophylactic" VCFs in stroke patients.

Orthopaedics

In 2008, total hip and knee replacements became the first area in which VTE is a "never event."[3] This has led to a growing interest in VTE prevention for this group. The first study of prophylactic filter placement in orthopaedic patients was reported by Fullen and coworkers in 1973. It examined patients with traumatic fracture of the proximal femur and found a significant decrease of PE in the VCF group (32% vs 10%) and decreased mortality (24% vs 10%).[51] However, pharmacologic options have significantly increased since this study. In 2002, Molfetta and colleagues randomized 30 patients undergoing total hip arthroplasty to receive a temporary VCF; three patients developed filter thrombus, and two patients in the nonfilter group suffered PE.[52]

Pelvic fracture or lower extremity fracture has been shown in multiple studies to be independent risk factors for VTE.[38,53] Rogers and colleagues adopted a policy of prophylactic VCFs in all orthopaedic trauma patients having two or more high-risk criteria and reduced the incidence of PE from 1% to 0.2%.[54] Webb and coworkers placed VCFs in all patients undergoing surgery for acetabular fracture and having two or more risk factors for VTE. Using this approach, half the patients in the study received a VCF with no incidence of PE, and 2/27 patients without a VCF developed PE while receiving routine prophylaxis.[55]

Bariatrics

The American Society for Metabolic and Bariatric Surgery issued a statement in 2007 regarding VTE in bariatric surgery that "the possible role of vena cava filters, remain[s] controversial and recommendations . . . have not been established."[56(p1)] However, prophylactic VCF insertion in the morbidly obese before bariatric surgery is increasing.

An autopsy study following Roux-en-Y gastric bypass found 80% of patients to have evidence of PE.[57] Morbidly obese patients often have limited cardiopulmonary reserve, which increases the risk of death should a PE occur. Sugerman and colleagues identified venous stasis as an additional risk factor for PE in morbidly obese patients undergoing bariatric surgery.[58] In a larger study, Sapala and colleagues expanded independent risk factors to include sleep apnea/hypoventilation syndrome and body mass index greater than 60 with truncal obesity as well. This group recommended prophylactic VCF insertion in any patients meeting these criteria or with a history of VTE or hypercoagulability. Based on these criteria, VCFs were placed in 10% of patients.[59] Further studies are needed before adopting VCFs in the bariatric patient population as a standard of care.

VENA CAVA FILTER COMPLICATIONS

Mortality associated with VCFs is quite low. Becker and coworkers attributed three deaths in 2557 patients directly to filter complications.[60] Athanasoulis and colleagues found two periprocedural deaths in 1731 patients with the VCF insertion as a possible cause.[61] Infection is also infrequent; only one case has been documented with use of the modern VCF.[62]

As the indications for VCFs were broadened, concern arose over possible complications in patients with a fairly brief risk of VTE. Before 2003, all filters inserted were permanent devices. The PREPIC study published in 2005 showed a 35.7% incidence in late DVT in patients with a permanent VCF compared with 27.5% in patients with no filter. Both groups were treated for 3 months with therapeutic anticoagulation. However, the nonfilter group had a rate of symptomatic PE of 6%, compared with no PE in the patients with filters.[14]

Greenfield and Michna reviewed 12 years of experience with permanent VCFs in 1988. Recurrent PE occurred in 4% of patients, filter migration (although not clinically significant) in 8%, and inferior vena cava (IVC) patency in 96%.[63] Patton and coworkers found an early complication rate of 7% in 110 prophylactic, permanent filter placements, including 11 cases of postphlebitic syndrome, three filter misplacements, one significant migration, three insertion site thromboses, and one caval thrombus.[64] Athanasoulis and colleagues reviewed 1731 patients and found post filter, clinically significant PE in 5%; 30-day morbidity in 5%; and late complication in 6.2%. Complications included access site thrombus, caval thrombus, migration, and broken struts.[61]

The primary concern of implanting a permanent device, particularly in young trauma patients, was assuaged by the development of the temporary and then optional VCF. Temporary filters are inserted for 7 to 10 days and then removed. The filter remains in place tethered to a central venous line. These have largely fallen out of favor with the advent of the optional VCF, a device that can be removed when no longer needed; however; it does not *require* retrieval should the patient require permanent caval interruption. This is an improvement on strictly temporary filters, which become problematic when a filter full of thrombus must be removed.[65]

Even with the optional filter, other reported complications include filter misplacement/tilt, insertion site hematoma or thrombosis, arteriovenous fistula at the insertion site, filter migration, postphlebitic changes, and caval thrombosis. The incidence ranged from 0 to 36%.[66] Filter misplacement occurs in up to 5% of patients. This is more common with vascular anomalies such as IVC duplication, left-side IVC, and renal vein anamolies.[67] For this reason, preinsertion imaging is essential (discussed later in the article). Tilt can occur due to placement of a strut in a vessel opening or operator error during deployment. Rogers and coworkers found a higher incidence of PE with a filter tilt greater than 14°.[66] Therefore, it is recommended that a second filter be placed above the initial filter with a high degree of tilt.

Duperier and colleagues examined 133 patients with percutaneously placed VCFs. Fifty-eight of these patients had preinsertion and postinsertion lower extremity duplex, and 26% of these developed DVT. However, only four of these were located in the ipsilateral extremity.[68] Similarly, Sing and coworkers found two insertion site thrombi in a review of 158 patients. Six additional patients developed DVT elsewhere.[69]

Filter migration is more common in large vena cava. Most devices are approved only for use in caval diameters up to 28 mm. The overall reported incidence with the current generation of VCFs is 2.9% to 12%.[70,71] This could lead to filter embolus or, more often, occlusion of the renal veins.

Penetration of the cava by hooks or struts is believed to occur in 30% to 100% of patients in various series.[67,72,73] Despite this incidence, in a study of 1731 patients, none had symptomatic penetration.[61] Apparent penetration can be the result of an inflammatory response causing the appearance of struts outside of the contrast in a cavagram. Similarly, strut fracture, shown in 1.5% to 2.9% of patients, has unknown significance.[71,74,75] Rare cases of erosion into the duodenum and aorta have been reported.[76,77]

With regard to the concern of caval thrombus, this can alternatively be viewed as a life-saving event trapping an otherwise fatal large PE. To support this theory, the incidence of caval thrombus in Rogers' study was equivalent to the risk of PE in that patient population.[66] Athanasoulis and colleagues, in a 26-year review of 1765 filters, found a thrombosis incidence of 3.2%.[61] Specific filters have been shown to have variable occlusion rates, likely dependent on patient and physician variables as well. Treatment of symptomatic occlusion includes thrombectomy (open or endovascular), thrombolysis, or filter exclusion by endoluminal stent.[78] Filter occlusion is often managed by anticoagulation alone.[79-81]

Recurrent pulmonary emboli despite VCF insertion have been reported in 2.5% to 7.7% of patients.[71,82] This can occur with loss of contact between filter hooks and vessel wall, thrombus propagation above the filter, or upper extremity thrombus. Therefore, anticoagulation should be started as soon as possible in all patients at risk for VTE, regardless of the presence of a VCF.

TYPES OF FILTERS
Permanent

Greenfield and Michna reported the first use of the modern VCF.[63] Currently available designs include the Greenfield (Boston Scientific, Natick, MA, USA), Simon-Nitinol (Bard, Tempe, AZ, USA), TrapEase (Cordis, Miami, FL, USA), and Vena-Tech (R. Braun Medical, Evanston, IL, USA). The literature for these filters is based mainly on retrospective studies, case series, and single-center reports.[34,60,73,83-87] The Bird's Nest (Cook, Bloomington, IN, USA) is the only filter approved for caval diameters up to 40 mm, compared with other optional filters that are indicated in vena cava only up to 28 mm. This was the first percutaneous device and was released on a limited basis in 1983. This filter is made of four stainless steel wires, affixed to the cava by V-shaped struts with hook-like anchors. The original design had a high migration rate and was replaced with a filter having stiffer and wider struts. This filter has been associated with filament prolapse beyond the struts in up to 70% of patients; however, no clinical significance has been reported.[88] Post-filter PE occurred in 7% of 255 patients.[61]

Temporary

Temporary filters evolved as a result of the concern for placing permanent filters in young patients who were unable to undergo anticoagulation for only a short time because of operative procedures, traumatic brain injury, and other conditions. Temporary filters were originally recommended for removal after no more than 10 days and later up to 6 weeks. Benefits included use of the filter as a central venous line and ability to obtain a contrast cavagram using the in situ filter/catheter.[89] However, in a European study of the Protect catheter, 40% of patients were found to have clot present on repeat venography, necessitating thrombolysis or placement of a permanent VCF above the temporary device before removal.[90] For this reason, and with the development of the optional device, the use of temporary filters has diminished.

Optional

Several optional filters are currently available in the United States. All were initially approved for permanent use and were subsequently approved for removal. The first to be released was the Günther Tulip (Cook Inc, Bloomington, IL, USA) in October 2000 followed by the OptEase (Cordis Endovascular, Warren, NJ, USA) in December 2002. The Recovery (CR Bard Inc, Murray Hill, NJ, USA) was released in November of 2002, and replaced with the G2 in 2006. Other optional filters include the Cook Celect (Cook, Inc), SafeFlo (Rafael Medical Technologies Ltd), OptEase (Cordis Endovascular), Option (Medical Device Technologies, Inc; Angiotech Interventional) (**Fig. 2**). Overall, the successful retrieval of optional filters exceeds 90%.[5]

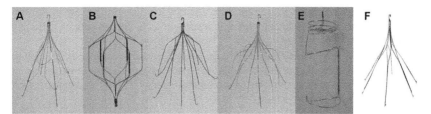

Fig. 2. Optional vena caval filters: (*A*) Günther Tulip. (*B*) OptEase. (*C*) G2. (*D*) Cook Celect. (*E*) SafeFlo. (*F*) Option.

In 2005, the Society of Interventional Radiology held a multidisciplinary conference regarding the VCF with a focus on optional filters. Key points of this consensus statement are summarized in **Box 5**. Again, the group emphasized the primary means of prophylaxis and therapy for VTE is pharmacologic and recommended the VCF for use when anticoagulation cannot be started, fails, or must be stopped. Even with a VCF in place, anticoagulation and other primary VTE prevention must still be instituted as early as possible (sequential compressions devices [SCDs], early ambulation).[10]

INSERTION OF THE VENA CAVA FILTER

Initially, permanent filters were placed in the operating room, originally using a cutdown technique. Percutaneous insertion led to an initial shift away from the surgeon to the interventional radiologist. A survey performed in 1997 of 210 US trauma centers determined that VCFs were placed by radiologists at 81% of centers, trauma surgeons at 34%, vascular surgeons at 33%, and general surgeons at 13%.[91] Insertion capabilities have also been expanded to properly trained medical intensivists, with a 2009 report of successful and safe insertions of VCFs in the medical ICU.[92]

Since the advent of percutaneous insertion in 1984, this procedure is now possible at the bedside. Transport of critically ill patients to the radiology suite carries significant risk; therefore, bedside placement of VCFs by general surgeons and

---

Box 5
Society of Interventional Radiology consensus statement key points

○ The primary means of therapy and prophylaxis for VTE are pharmacologic.

○ There are no unique indications for optional versus permanent vena cava filters.

○ Patients with filters in place should be managed with anticoagulation (prophylaxis or therapeutic) according to VTE risk as soon as possible.

○ There are no absolute indications for removal of the vena cava filter.

○ Vena cava filters should be removed only if the risk of clinically significant PE has been reduced to a level less than the risk of leaving the filter in place.

The quality of literature at this time is not sufficient to support evidence-based recommendations at this time.

Data from Kaufman JA, Kinney TB, Streiff MB, et al. Guidelines for the use of retrievable and convertible vena cava filters: report from the Society of Interventional Radiology multidisciplinary consensus conference. J Vasc Interv Radiol 2006;17:449–59.

surgical intensivists is increasingly common. A prospective matched cohort study by Hurst and colleagues of 100 transported patients showed a 66% incidence of physiologic deterioration related to travel.[93]

In critically ill patients, bedside insertion has been shown to be a safe and feasible alternative, avoiding the hazards associated with patient transport to the operating room or radiology suite.[94–97] Cost analysis at our institution in 1999 showed a savings of $1500 with bedside insertion compared with insertion in the radiology department or operating room.[96] Even when fluoroscopic procedures are performed in an open model intensive care unit, radiation exposure when using standard protective measures was shown to be minimal (<60 mrem per year, compared to an allowable <100 mrem per year in noncontrolled areas).[98]

Paton and coworkers reviewed a 9-year experience with bedside VCF insertions totaling 403 patients. Complication rates were similar to those for VCFs placed in the operating room or radiology suite. Though not screened routinely, 38 patients developed DVT, with 14 at the insertion site. There were seven caval occlusions and two post-VCF pulmonary emboli. Two filters were misplaced, and, before the use of CO_2 cavagram, two patients suffered renal failure. The most serious complication was right ventricular perforation by the dilator using the internal jugular approach.[95]

Technique

The technique of percutaneous insertion is similar whether performed in the operating room, angiography suite, or at the bedside. The right femoral approach is most often used, barring any contraindications such as thrombus. Sheath kinking occurs more often when using the left femoral or jugular approach.[72] The risk of pneumothorax is avoided using the femoral approach, which is also logisticallyeasier to access at the bedside. All catheters and sheaths are flushed with heparinized saline throughout the procedure. The vein is entered in the typical manner for central venous access procedures. A Newton J-wire is placed through the needle and the needle removed. A 5 French pigtail catheter is then placed over the wire just superior to the iliac veins and the wire removed. This procedure is generally performed under fluoroscopy, although alternate imaging techniques can be used. Cavagram is performed using contrast (30–60 mL injected through a pressure injector at a flow rate of 15–25 mL/s) or CO_2. This provides a roadmap to determine the location of the renal veins, caval diameter, and anomalies. The wire is replaced, the 5 French catheter removed, and the device-specific deployment sheath with dilator inserted over the wire. The dilator is removed, and the device is inserted. The device is deployed in an infrarenal position, generally at the level of the L2 vertebrae. The sheath is retracted slightly away from the filter so as not to engage the hooks. A completion cavagram is then performed to ensure adequate placement. The sheath is removed and pressure held for 5 to 7 minutes. After insertion of a VCF, it is essential to use straight wires or fluoroscopy for central line insertion to avoid entrapment in the filter. Therefore a sign is placed at the head of the patient's bed and on the patient's medical record.

Duplex Ultrasound

At our institution, patients who have been hospitalized longer than 48 to 72 hours undergo preoperative ultrasound on the lower extremities to rule out VTE, which may necessitate a jugular approach or alternate filter placement. Placement of a wire, sheath, or catheter through thrombus could result in PE. Deaths due to embolus during filter insertion have been reported.[99–101] In a 1999 review of 45 VCF insertions under ultrasound guidance, the lone technical complication was an incidence of thrombus above the filter on completion ultrasound, requiring transport to the operating room for insertion of a suprarenal VCF. Further ultrasound revealed a clinically occult DVT at the insertion site, which had not been imaged before the procedure.[102]

Caval Imaging

Caval imaging is required to define the anatomy of the IVC and the location of renal veins including anatomic variants, and to measure the cava itself to determine the appropriate filter to place. Savin and colleagues found a 43% rate of filter misplacement when a preinsertion cavagram was not performed compared with a rate of only 2.5% with imaging.[103] Based on these and other similar data, the Society of Cardiovascular and Interventional Radiology Standards of Practice committee stated in 2001 that the IVC should be assessed with imaging before insertion of a filter, and the current preferred imaging method is vena cavography.[104] Up to 11% of patients will be found to have an anomaly on preinsertion cavagram that will necessitate alternative placement.[105] Duplicate IVC occurs in fewer than 0.2% but could require placement of two VCFs or placement above the confluence.[106] Visualization of an IVC thrombus leads to insertion with a jugular approach at a level above the thrombus. In the large series by Athanasoulis and coworkers, a pre-procedure cavagram changed the position or number of filters required in 4% of procedures.[61] In 2.3% of patients, the caval diameter is greater than 28 mm, requiring a Bird's Nest filter (approved to 40 mm).[107]

Carbon Dioxide Cavagram

Iodinated contrast remains the gold standard for the essential preinsertion imaging of the vena cava. However, contrast agents carry risk of allergic reaction or nephrotoxicity. In the patient population at high risk for such complications, CO_2 is an alternative agent to determine caval anatomy. Medical-grade CO_2 is purged of room air and captured in a 60-mL syringe and is then hand injected through the 5 French pigtail catheter.

Sing and colleagues prospectively compared CO_2 with iodinated contrast in 23 patients. An IVC diameter measurement difference of a clinically insignificant 0.4 mm and no adverse effects were found with the use of CO_2.[108] The feasibility of performing CO_2 cavagrams was shown by Schmelzer and colleagues' review of 50 patients without complication. Forty-eight percent required only a single injection, 36% two injections, and 16% three injections to adequately determine anatomy. Two patients (4%) required iodinated contrast after failure of CO_2 imaging. Cost analysis in this study showed a minimal difference between the CO_2 and iodinated contrast cavagrams.[109] Of note, both of these studies involved insertion of filters at the bedside in critically ill patients.

Ultrasound

Attempts at filter insertion using transabdominal color-flow duplex ultrasound have shown a failure rate of 11% to 15%, most often due to inadequate visualization or VCF misplacement.[94,102,110] In addition, this still requires adequate interpretation, often by a radiologist or surgeon with specialized training. Kazmers and coworkers showed an accuracy of 98% and a sensitivity of 98% in determining an IVC diameter of 26 mm or less compared with contrast cavagraphy. However, this was in a subset of patients with adequate visualization of the IVC using the transabdominal approach.[111] In clinical practice, the IVC could not be visualized in 11% of attempts.[94,112]

Corriere and colleagues compared transabdominal ultrasound to contrast venography in a retrospective review in 2005. The procedure was feasible in 87% of patients screened and successful in 97.4%, compared with 99.7% of contrast venography patients. Failures in the ultrasound group included iliac vein deployment, tilt greater than 15°, incomplete opening, and inadvertent suprarenal placement. Post-procedure complication rates were not significantly different.[113]

Intravascular ultrasound (IVUS) is an attractive alternative to the transabdominal approach, avoiding the pitfalls of abdominal wounds, obesity, and poor visualization. Benefits include lack of contrast, lack of radiation exposure, and portable equipment. However, specialized training is required to interpret the results and not generally available to the intensivist.

Rosenthal and coworkers reported on bedside insertion of VCFs using IVUS in 94 patients. Three patients had filters deployed in iliac veins, retrieved, and replaced within 24 hours. Two groin hematomas were reported, and insertion site thrombus occurred in one patient. More recent data from Rosenthal showed 100 of 103 filters placed without complications.[114,115] Wellons and coworkers reported a 94% success rate using IVUS at the bedside, with one deployment in the iliac vein.[116] Despite these promising reports, IVUS has not been validated against the contrast cavagram. In addition, the high cost of the disposable probe ($600) makes this modality significantly more expensive than contrast or CO_2 cavagrams. In experienced hands, both of these techniques are feasible and demonstrate reasonable success rates. However, specialized training and equipment are required.

RETRIEVAL

For patients who have previously failed pharmacologic therapeutic anticoagulation, the VCF is a permanent device. However, a majority of VCFs are placed because of the patient's inability to receive anticoagulation. When this circumstance changes, for example, the risk of bleeding subsides or operative procedures are completed, these patients can be placed on anticoagulation and the filter removed.

Patients with new or progressive symptoms should undergo imaging to assess for additional or progressive VTE, which, if present, would delay retrieval. Patients without a known VTE should undergo duplex ultrasound of the lower extremities before retrieval. If DVT is found, retrieval is delayed and appropriate anticoagulation started. The vena cava is generally evaluated at the time of the procedure, although may be assessed up to 24 hours prior.[10] For patients requiring therapeutic anticoagulation, this should not be withheld for filter retrieval.[117,118] Given the continued risk for PE in these patients, therapeutic anticoagulation can and should be continued through the retrieval process.

Debate continues on the ideal timing of removal for prophylactic filters. If a filter is being used for prophylaxis against PE, the filter should be removed only when the patient is no longer at high risk. A study of four level-I trauma centers reviewed 146 cases of PE over 4 years. The mean time to PE after injury was 7.9 days; however, 24 patients suffered PE more than 15 days after injury, and 11% occurred after 21 days. Two of these were fatal emboli at day 21 and day 43.[119]

Several studies have examined the timing of VCF removal. Early reports had a mean implantation duration of 10 to 19 days.[42,114,119,120] These were based mainly on manufacturers' recommendations with little clinical criteria. The SIR examined this issue in their 2005 consensus statement, a summary of which is shown in **Box 6**.

Our practice is to remove filters at least 30 days after discharge or when patients are stable on anticoagulation for a minimum of 2 weeks. After implementation of this guideline, we reviewed filter retrievals over 16 months and observed successful

---

Box 6
Society of Interventional Radiology guidelines for VCF removal

VCF should be removed if:

- No indication for permanent filtration, with that indication defined as high risk of PE despite primary therapy or noncompliance
- Appropriate primary therapy or change in clinical status resulting in a low risk for PE
- No anticipated return to high-risk status, ie, no planned procedures/hospitalizations

In patients who meet the above criteria, the following conditions must also be present:

- Adequate life expectancy to benefit from VCF removal, defined as >6 months
- No contraindication to the retrieval procedure (eg, coagulopathy, renal insufficiency or contrast allergy, no sufficient venous access)
- VCF is suitable for removal (eg, no endotheliazation or trapped thrombus).

Data from Kaufman JA, Kinney TB, Streiff MB, et al. Guidelines for the use of retrievable and convertible vena cava filters: report from the Society of Interventional Radiology multidisciplinary consensus conference. J Vasc Interv Radiol 2006;17:449–59.

---

retrieval in 87% of attempts with no documented PE and a median duration of 142 days (range 17–475 days). Unsuccessful attempts were due to tilt with endothelialization in four cases, SVC thrombi in two, and one in which the force required to removed the filter was believed to be too great.[121]

Another concern in filter removal is trapped thrombus, which has a reported incidence of 0 to 25%.[5] The 2005 SIR consensus statement produced an algorithm for managing this issue (**Fig. 3**), with an emphasis on trapped thrombus being considered newly diagnosed VTE requiring therapeutic anticoagulation in patients with a VCF for prophylaxis.[10] At our institution, thrombus is managed with initiation of therapeutic anticoagulation (if not already receiving). The patient returns later for cavagram and retrieval of the filter when the thrombus has resolved.

Rarely, the filter itself may become a source of morbidity or malfunction. Examples include filter instability, dislodgement during other procedures, maldeployment, and pain related to perforation. In this case, a second filter may need to be placed following retrieval unless the patient meets the indications outlined previously.[10,72,103,122]

Filter retrieval is performed only in the operating room, as critically ill patients by definition are not candidates for removal. The patient is placed supine on the operating table and retrieval takes place under general anesthesia or sedation, depending on patient preference. A contrast cavagram is performed to determine the presence of luminal thrombus or potential filter tilt. If no contraindications are discovered on the cavagram, the filter can be removed and a completion cavagram performed to verify the absence of vascular leaks or defects. Minor abnormalities on completion cavagram have been followed expectantly or managed with anticoagulation.[10,123] Obstructive intimal flaps or thrombus often require additional intervention. Leak or retroperitoneal bleeding mandates admission with close observation, serial hemoglobin measurements, and possible computed tomography scan. In addition, the VCF must be inspected on removal. Retained fragments in a retroperitoneal or intrapulmonary location are rarely symptomatic and may be managed expectantly. Intracardiac fragments required cardiothoracic consultation.[10] Patients are generally observed for 2 hours in the post-anesthesia care unit and then discharged home.

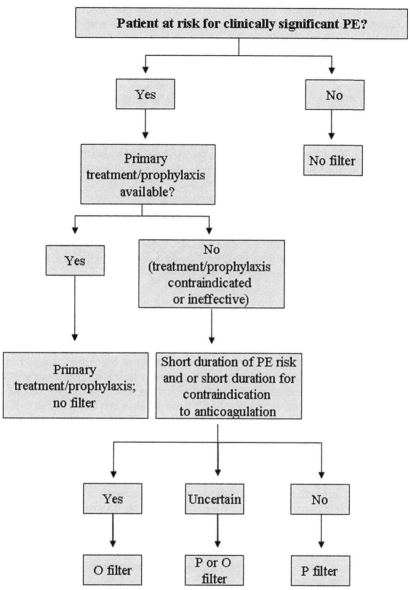

Fig. 3. The 2005 SIR consensus statement algorithm for managing removal of trapped thrombus. O, optional vena cava filter; P, permanent vena cava filter. (*Data from* Kaufman JA, Kinney TB, Streiff MB, et al. Guidelines for the use of retrievable and convertible vena cava filters: report from the Society of Interventional Radiology Multidisciplinary Consensus Conference. J Vasc Inter Rad 2006;17:452.)

FOLLOW-UP

In the 2005 SIR consensus document, the importance of tracking VCF patients was emphasized.[10] However, long-term follow-up of VCF patients is often difficult.

Establishment of a registry of filter patients is crucial for long-term follow-up of complications, as well as for determination of optimal retrieval time. Wojcik and coworkers created such a registry and were able to provide follow-up for 105 of 178 patients discharged with a VCF over 4 years. One patient had symptomatic caval occlusion, which resolved without thrombolysis, and one patient had VCF cephalad migration of 1 cm. Both were placed for "traditional" rather than prophylactic indications. Forty-four percent of patients with prophylactic VCF insertion had developed DVT while hospitalized. Only four patients were evaluated with post-discharge ultrasound, two of which revealed a DVT.[20]

Karmy-Jones reviewed 446 trauma patients with VCFs, 76% of which were prophylactic. Follow-up occurred in only 51%, and only 22% of VCFs were retrieved. Retrieval failure due to technical issues or thrombus occurred only in 25 patients, with the remaining non-retrieved filters lost to follow-up. They found a sixfold increase in patients lost to follow-up when the service placing the VCF was not directly responsible for the patient, for example, interventional radiologists placing a VCF in a trauma patient.[124] This again underscores the importance of a VCF registry.

At our institution, patients return for follow-up 1 month after discharge to determine eligibility for VCF removal. Duplex ultrasound is performed, and the presence of DVT leads to the filter being left as a permanent device.

SUMMARY

As the population ages and continued improvements to decrease mortality are made in the field of critical care, more and more patients will suffer thromboembolic events. The evolution of caval interruption from the original Greenfield filter placed using a cutdown technique to modern, percutaneous, retrievable filters has resulted in an explosion in their use. This has led to an increase in so-called "prophylactic" VCF placement, insertion in patients without known thromboembolic disease who are simply at high risk for such events. However, all VCFs are prophylactic in the sense that they provide no *treatment* for DVT or PE. Rather, vena caval interruption serves to significantly decrease the likelihood of emboli migrating to the pulmonary vasculature.

Despite the ease of VCF insertion, the importance of systemic anticoagulation to prevent DVT must be kept in mind. This must be started in patients at high risk for venous thromboembolic disease as soon as feasible. Vena caval interruption should be used as an adjunct to prophylaxis in high-risk patients who cannot receive appropriate systemic anticoagulation, regardless of the presence of known VTE. Although many risk factors for VTE have been studied, what constitutes a high-risk patient has not been clearly identified. Placement of a VCF outside of conventional indications, for example, active thromboembolic disease with a clear contraindication to anticoagulant or recurrent PE despite adequate anticoagulation, is a decision made based on risk assessment.

As the majority of VCF complications are related to long-term implantation, the optional device is able to reduce morbidity significantly while protecting patients during a high-risk period such as following multisystem trauma. Given the relatively low incidence of PE and the complexity of patient populations at risk, a definitive randomized controlled trial addressing the use of VCFs in patients at high risk for thromboembolic disease is unlikely to be achieved.

REFERENCES

1. National Quality Measures Clearinghouse. Agency for Healthcare Research and Quality; 2010. Available at: http://qualitymeasures.ahrq.gov/content.aspx?f=rss&id=16278. Accessed May 1, 2011.

2. Specifications Manual for National Hospital Inpatient Quality Measures Discharges. Available at: http://www.jointcommission.org/specifications_manual_for_national_hospital_inpatient_quality_measures. Accessed May 1, 2011.

3. Hospital-Acquired Conditions IPresent on Admission Indicator). Available at: http://www.cms.gov/HospitalAcqCond. Accessed May 1, 2011.

4. Deitelzweig SB, Johnson BH, Lin J, et al. Prevalence of clinical venous thromboembolism in the USA: current trends and future projections. Am J Hematol;86:217–20.

5. Sing RF, Rogers FB, Novitsky YW, et al. Optional vena cava filters for patients with high thromboembolic risk: questions to be answered. Surg Innov 2005;12:195–202.

6. Stein PD, Alnas M, Skaf E, et al. Outcome and complications of retrievable inferior vena cava filters. Am J Cardiol 2004;94:1090–3.

7. Prevention of thromboembolism in spinal cord injury. Consortium for Spinal Cord Medicine. J Spinal Cord Med 1997;20:259–83.

8. Bratton SL, Chestnut RM, Ghajar J, et al. Guidelines for the management of severe traumatic brain injury. V. Deep vein thrombosis prophylaxis. J Neurotrauma 2007; 24(Suppl 1):S32–6.

9. Buller HR, Agnelli G, Hull RD, et al. Antithrombotic therapy for venous thromboembolic disease: the Seventh ACCP Conference on Antithrombotic and Thrombolytic Therapy. Chest 2004;126:401S–28S.

10. Kaufman JA, Kinney TB, Streiff MB, et al. Guidelines for the use of retrievable and convertible vena cava filters: report from the Society of Interventional Radiology multidisciplinary consensus conference. J Vasc Interv Radiol 2006;17:449–59.

11. Pasquale M, Fabian TC. Practice management guidelines for trauma from the Eastern Association for the Surgery of Trauma. J Trauma 1998;44:941–56 [discussion: 56–7].

12. Agnelli G, Becattini C. Acute pulmonary embolism. N Engl J Med 2010;363:266–74.

13. Decousus H, Leizorovicz A, Parent F, et al. A clinical trial of vena caval filters in the prevention of pulmonary embolism in patients with proximal deep-vein thrombosis. Prevention du Risque d'Embolie Pulmonaire par Interruption Cave Study Group. N Engl J Med 1998;338:409–15.

14. Eight-year follow-up of patients with permanent vena cava filters in the prevention of pulmonary embolism: the PREPIC (Prevention du Risque d'Embolie Pulmonaire par Interruption Cave) randomized study. Circulation 2005;112:416–22.

15. Jacobs DG, Sing RF. The role of vena caval filters in the management of venous thromboembolism. Am Surg 2003;69:635–42.

16. Pacouret G, Alison D, Pottier JM, et al. Free-floating thrombus and embolic risk in patients with angiographically confirmed proximal deep venous thrombosis. A prospective study. Arch Intern Med 1997;157:305–8.

17. Norris CS, Greenfield LJ, Herrmann JB. Free-floating iliofemoral thrombus. A risk of pulmonary embolism. Arch Surg 1985;120:806–8.

18. Trerotola SO, McLennan MG, Eclavea AC, et al. Mechanical thombolysis of venous thrombosis in an animal model with use of temporary filtration. J Vasc Interv Radiol 2001;12:1075–85.

19. Protack CD, Bakken AM, Patel N, et al. Long-term outcomes of catheter directed thrombolysis for lower extremity deep venous thrombosis without prophylactic inferior vena cava filter placement. J Vasc Surg 2007;45:992–7 [discussion: 97].

20. Wojcik R, Cipolle MD, Fearen I, et al. Long-term follow-up of trauma patients with a vena caval filter. J Trauma 2000;49:839–43.

21. Schultz DJ, Brasel KJ, Washington L, et al. Incidence of asymptomatic pulmonary embolism in moderately to severely injured trauma patients. J Trauma 2004;56:727–31 [discussion: 31–3].

22. Geerts WH, Pineo GF, Heit JA, et al. Prevention of venous thromboembolism: the Seventh ACCP Conference on Antithrombotic and Thrombolytic Therapy. Chest 2004;126:338S–400S.

23. Black PM, Baker MF, Snook CP. Experience with external pneumatic calf compression in neurology and neurosurgery. Neurosurgery 1986;18:440–4.

24. Brach BB, Moser KM, Cedar L, et al. Venous thrombosis in acute spinal cord paralysis. J Trauma 1977;17:289–92.

25. Silver JR. The prophylactic use of anticoagulant therapy in the prevention of pulmonary emboli in one hundred consecutive spinal injury patients. Paraplegia 1974;12: 188–96.

26. Todd JW, Frisbie JH, Rossier AB, et al. Deep venous thrombosis in acute spinal cord injury: a comparison of 125I fibrinogen leg scanning, impedance plethysmography and venography. Paraplegia 1976;14:50–7.

27. Wilson JT, Rogers FB, Wald SL, et al. Prophylactic vena cava filter insertion in patients with traumatic spinal cord injury: preliminary results. Neurosurgery 1994;35: 234–9 [discussion: 39].

28. Winther K, Gleerup G, Snorrason K, et al. Platelet function and fibrinolytic activity in cervical spinal cord injured patients. Thromb Res 1992;65:469–74.

29. El Masri WS, Silver JR. Prophylactic anticoagulant therapy in patients with spinal cord injury. Paraplegia 1981;19:334–42.

30. Naso F. Pulmonary embolism in acute spinal cord injury. Arch Phys Med Rehabil 1974;55:275–8.

31. Kirshblum S. Rehabilitation of spinal cord injury. In: JA Delisa BG, editor. Rehabilitation medicine: principles and practice. 4th edition. Philadelphia: Lippincott Williams & Wilkins; 2005. p. 1715–51.

32. Lamb GC, Tomski MA, Kaufman J, et al. Is chronic spinal cord injury associated with increased risk of venous thromboembolism? J Am Paraplegia Soc 1993;16:153–6.

33. Rogers FB, Shackford SR, Wilson J, et al. Prophylactic vena cava filter insertion in severely injured trauma patients: indications and preliminary results. J Trauma 1993;35:637–41 [discussion: 41–2].

34. Velmahos GC, Kern J, Chan LS, et al. Prevention of venous thromboembolism after injury: an evidence-based report—part II: analysis of risk factors and evaluation of the role of vena caval filters. J Trauma 2000;49:140–4.

35. McKinley WO, Tewksbury MA, Godbout CJ. Comparison of medical complications following nontraumatic and traumatic spinal cord injury. J Spinal Cord Med 2002; 25:88–93.

36. Coon WW. Risk factors in pulmonary embolism. Surg Gynecol Obstet 1976;143: 385–90.

37. Freeark RJ, Boswick J, Fardin R. Posttraumatic venous thrombosis. Arch Surg 1967;95:567–75.

38. Geerts WH, Code KI, Jay RM, et al. A prospective study of venous thromboembolism after major trauma. N Engl J Med 1994;331:1601–6.

39. McCartney J. Pulmonary embolism following trauma. Am J Pathol 1934;10:709.

40. Headrick JR Jr, Barker DE, Pate LM, et al. The role of ultrasonography and inferior vena cava filter placement in high-risk trauma patients. Am Surg 1997;63:1–8.

41. Winchell RJ, Hoyt DB, Walsh JC, et al. Risk factors associated with pulmonary embolism despite routine prophylaxis: implications for improved protection. J Trauma 1994;37:600–6.

42. Owings JT, Kraut E, Battistella F, et al. Timing of the occurrence of pulmonary embolism in trauma patients. Arch Surg 1997;132:862–6 [discussion: 66–7].

43. Norwood SH, Berne JD, Rowe SA, et al. Early venous thromboembolism prophylaxis with enoxaparin in patients with blunt traumatic brain injury. J Trauma 2008;65: 1021–6 [discussion: 26–7].
44. Agnelli G, Piovella F, Buoncristiani P, et al. Enoxaparin plus compression stockings compared with compression stockings alone in the prevention of venous thrombo-embolism after elective neurosurgery. N Engl J Med 1998;339:80–5.
45. Nurmohamed MT, van Riel AM, Henkens CM, et al. Low molecular weight heparin and compression stockings in the prevention of venous thromboembolism in neu-rosurgery. Thromb Haemost 1996;75:233–8.
46. Boeer A, Voth E, Henze T, et al. Early heparin therapy in patients with spontaneous intracerebral haemorrhage. J Neurol Neurosurg Psychiatry 1991;54:466–7.
47. Cohen D. Treating thrombotic complications in patients with primary intracerebral haemorrhage. J Roy Coll Physicians. Lond 1998;5:417–9.
48. Roderick P, Ferris G, Wilson K, et al. Towards evidence-based guidelines for the prevention of venous thromboembolism: systematic reviews of mechanical meth-ods, oral anticoagulation, dextran and regional anaesthesia as thromboprophylaxis. Health Technol Assess 2005;9:iii-iv, ix-x, 1–78.
49. Dennis M, Sandercock PA, Reid J, et al. Effectiveness of thigh-length graduated compression stockings to reduce the risk of deep vein thrombosis after stroke (CLOTS trial 1): a multicentre, randomised controlled trial. Lancet 2009;373: 1958–65.
50. CLOTS Trial. Available at: http://www.dcn.ed.ac.uk/clots/. Accessed May 15, 2011.
51. Fullen WD, Miller EH, Steele WF, et al. Prophylactic vena caval interruption in hip fractures. J Trauma 1973;13:403–10.
52. Molfetta L PA, De Caro G, Pipino F. Temporary vena cava filters in the prevention of pulmonary embolism during total hop arthroplasty. J Orthop Trauma 2002;2:99–103.
53. Sevitt S, Gallagher N. Venous thrombosis and pulmonary embolism.A clinico-pathological study in injured and burned patients. Br J Surg 1961;48:475–89.
54. Rogers FB, Shackford SR, Ricci MA, et al. Prophylactic vena cava filter insertion in selected high-risk orthopaedic trauma patients. J Orthop Trauma 1997;11:267–72.
55. Webb LX, Rush PT, Fuller SB, et al. Greenfield filter prophylaxis of pulmonary embolism in patients undergoing surgery for acetabular fracture. J Orthop Trauma 1992;6:139–45.
56. ASMBS Position Statement on Prophylactic Measures to Reduce the Risk of Venous Thromboembolism in Bariatric Surgery Patients 2007. Available at: http://www.asbs.org/Newsite07/resources/vte_statement.pdf. Accessed May 1, 2011.
57. Melinek J, Livingston E, Cortina G, et al. Autopsy findings following gastric bypass surgery for morbid obesity. Arch Pathol Lab Med 2002;126:1091–5.
58. Sugerman HJ, Sugerman EL, Wolfe L, et al. Risks and benefits of gastric bypass in morbidly obese patients with severe venous stasis disease. Ann Surg 2001;234: 41–6.
59. Sapala JA, Wood MH, Schuhknecht MP, et al. Fatal pulmonary embolism after bariatric operations for morbid obesity: a 24-year retrospective analysis. Obes Surg 2003;13:819–25.
60. Becker DM, Philbrick JT, Selby JB. Inferior vena cava filters. Indications, safety, effectiveness. Arch Intern Med 1992;152:1985–94.
61. Athanasoulis CA, Kaufman JA, Halpern EF, et al. Inferior vena caval filters: review of a 26-year single-center clinical experience. Radiology 2000;216:54–66.
62. Millward SF, Peterson RA, Moher D, et al. LGM (Vena Tech) vena caval filter: experience at a single institution. J Vasc Interv Radiol 1994;5:351–6.

63. Greenfield LJ, Michna BA. Twelve-year clinical experience with the Greenfield vena caval filter. Surgery 1988;104:706–12.
64. Patton JH Jr, Fabian TC, Croce MA, et al. Prophylactic Greenfield filters: acute complications and long-term follow-up. J Trauma 1996;41:231–6 [discussion: 36–7].
65. Bovyn G, Gory P, Reynaud P, et al. The Tempofilter: a multicenter study of a new temporary caval filter implantable for up to six weeks. Ann Vasc Surg 1997;11: 520–8.
66. Rogers FB, Strindberg G, Shackford SR, et al. Five-year follow-up of prophylactic vena cava filters in high-risk trauma patients. Arch Surg 1998;133:406–11 [discussion: 12].
67. Joels CS, Sing RF, Heniford BT. Complications of inferior vena cava filters. Am Surg 2003;69:654–9.
68. Duperier T, Mosenthal A, Swan KG, et al. Acute complications associated with greenfield filter insertion in high-risk trauma patients. J Trauma 2003;54:545–9.
69. Sing RF, Jacobs DG, Heniford BT. Bedside insertion of inferior vena cava filters in the intensive care unit. J Am Coll Surg 2001;192:570–5 [discussion: 75–6].
70. Murphy TP, Dorfman GS, Yedlicka JW, et al. LGM vena cava filter: objective evaluation of early results. J Vasc Interv Radiol 1991;2:107–15.
71. Wolf F, Thurnher S, Lammer J. [Simon nitinol vena cava filters: effectiveness and complications]. Rofo 2001;173:924–30.
72. Ray CE Jr, Kaufman JA. Complications of inferior vena cava filters. Abdom Imaging 1996;21:368–74.
73. Streiff MB. Vena caval filters: a comprehensive review. Blood 2000;95:3669–77.
74. Babuty D, Quilliet L, Charbonnier B, et al. [Partial interruption of the inferior vena cava using a percutaneous endovenous filter]. Arch Mal Coeur Vaiss 1990;83:1389–96.
75. Ferris EJ, McCowan TC, Carver DK, et al. Percutaneous inferior vena caval filters: follow-up of seven designs in 320 patients. Radiology 1993;188:851–6.
76. al Zahrani HA. Bird's nest inferior vena caval filter migration into the duodenum: a rare cause of upper gastrointestinal bleeding. J Endovasc Surg 1995;2:372–5.
77. Feezor RJ, Huber TS, Welborn MB 3rd, et al. Duodenal perforation with an inferior vena cava filter: an unusual cause of abdominal pain. J Vasc Surg 2002;35:1010–2.
78. Joshi A, Carr J, Chrisman H, et al. Filter-related, thrombotic occlusion of the inferior vena cava treated with a Gianturco stent. J Vasc Interv Radiol 2003;14:381–5.
79. Amano Y, Kumita S, Takahama K, et al. [RI venography for retroperitoneal hematoma following anticoagulant therapy for IVC filter thrombosis]. Kaku Igaku 1993;30: 423–7.
80. Angle JF, Matsumoto AH, Al Shammari M, et al. Transcatheter regional urokinase therapy in the management of inferior vena cava thrombosis. J Vasc Interv Radiol 1998;9:917–25.
81. Tardy B, Mismetti P, Page Y, et al. Symptomatic inferior vena cava filter thrombosis: clinical study of 30 consecutive cases. Eur Respir J 1996;9:2012–6.
82. Hajduk B, Tomkowski W, Fijalkowska A, et al. [LGM inferior vena cava filters–observation of 79 patients]. Pol Arch Med Wewn 2000;104:753–60.
83. Girard TD, Philbrick JT, Fritz Angle J, et al. Prophylactic vena cava filters for trauma patients: a systematic review of the literature. Thromb Res 2003;112:261–7.
84. Grassi CJ. Inferior vena caval filters: analysis of five currently available devices. AJR Am J Roentgenol 1991;156:813–21.
85. Kercher K, Sing RF. Overview of current inferior vena cava filters. Am Surg 2003;69: 643–8.
86. Kinney TB. Update on inferior vena cava filters. J Vasc Interv Radiol 2003;14:425–40.

87. Velmahos GC, Kern J, Chan LS, et al. Prevention of venous thromboembolism after injury: an evidence-based report—part I: analysis of risk factors and evaluation of the role of vena caval filters. J Trauma 2000;49:132–8 [discussion: 39].
88. Nicholson AA, Ettles DF, Paddon AJ, et al. Long-term follow-up of the Bird's Nest IVC Filter. Clin Radiol 1999;54:759–64.
89. Cera SM, Sing RF, Kercher KW, et al. Role of retrievable vena cava filter following placement for thromboembolic prophylaxis in a high-risk trauma patient questioned. J Am Osteopath Assoc 2002;102:643.
90. Stoneham GW, Burbridge BE, Millward SF. Temporary inferior vena cava filters: in vitro comparison with permanent IVC filters. J Vasc Interv Radiol 1995;6:731–6.
91. Quirke TE, Ritota PC, Swan KG. Inferior vena caval filter use in U.S. trauma centers: a practitioner survey. J Trauma 1997;43:333–7.
92. Haley M, Christmas B, Sing RF. Bedside insertion of inferior vena cava filters by a medical intensivist: preliminary results. J Intensive Care Med 2009;24:144–7.
93. Hurst JM, Davis K Jr, Johnson DJ, et al. Cost and complications during in-hospital transport of critically ill patients: a prospective cohort study. J Trauma 1992;33:582–5.
94. Nunn CR, Neuzil D, Naslund T, et al. Cost-effective method for bedside insertion of vena caval filters in trauma patients. J Trauma 1997;43:752–8.
95. Paton BL, Jacobs DG, Heniford BT, et al. Nine-year experience with insertion of vena cava filters in the intensive care unit. Am J Surg 2006;192:795–800.
96. Sing RF, Cicci CK, Smith CH, et al. Bedside insertion of inferior vena cava filters in the intensive care unit. J Trauma 1999;47:1104–7.
97. Tola JC, Holtzman R, Lottenberg L. Bedside placement of inferior vena cava filters in the intensive care unit. Am Surg 1999;65:833–7 [discussion: 37–8].
98. Mostafa G, Sing RF, McKeown R, et al. The hazard of scattered radiation in a trauma intensive care unit. Crit Care Med 2002;30:574–6.
99. Fuochi C, Furlan F, Pellegrini M, et al. [Criteria for utilization and indications for use of permanent and short- and medium term temporary endocaval filters. Personal experience and review of the literature]. Radiol Med 1996;92:431–7.
100. Kinney TB, Rose SC, Lim GW, et al. Fatal paradoxic embolism occurring during IVC filter insertion in a patient with chronic pulmonary thromboembolic disease. J Vasc Interv Radiol 2001;12:770–2.
101. Ricco JB, Dubreuil F, Reynaud P, et al. The LGM Vena-Tech caval filter: results of a multicenter study. Ann Vasc Surg 1995;9(Suppl):S89-100.
102. Sato DT, Robinson KD, Gregory RT, et al. Duplex directed caval filter insertion in multi-trauma and critically ill patients. Ann Vasc Surg 1999;13:365–71.
103. Savin MA, Panicker HK, Sadiq S, et al. Placement of vena cava filters: factors affecting technical success and immediate complications. AJR Am J Roentgenol 2002;179:597–602.
104. Grassi CJ, Swan TL, Cardella JF, et al. Quality improvement guidelines for percutaneous permanent inferior vena cava filter placement for the prevention of pulmonary embolism. SCVIR Standards of Practice Committee. J Vasc Interv Radiol 2001;12:137–41.
105. Mejia EA, Saroyan RM, Balkin PW, et al. Analysis of inferior venacavography before Greenfield filter placement. Ann Vasc Surg 1989;3:232–5.
106. Cossu ML, Ruggiu M, Fais E, et al. [Congenital anomalies of the inferior vena cava]. Minerva Chir 2000;55:703–8.
107. Feed RA TG, Taylor FC, et al. Use of the Bird's Nest Filter in oversized inferior vena cavae. J Vasc Interv Radiol 1991;2:447–50.

108. Sing RF, Stackhouse DJ, Jacobs DG, et al. Safety and accuracy of bedside carbon dioxide cavography for insertion of inferior vena cava filters in the intensive care unit. J Am Coll Surg 2001;192:168–71.
109. Schmelzer TM, Christmas AB, Jacobs DG, et al. Imaging of the vena cava in the intensive care unit prior to vena cava filter insertion: carbon dioxide as an alternative to iodinated contrast. Am Surg 2008;74:141–5.
110. Van Natta TL, Morris JA Jr, Eddy VA, et al. Elective bedside surgery in critically injured patients is safe and cost-effective. Ann Surg 1998;227:618–24 [discussion: 24–6].
111. Kazmers A, Groehn H, Meeker C. Duplex examination of the inferior vena cava. Am Surg 2000;66:986–9.
112. Friedland M, Kazmers A, Kline R, et al. Vena cava duplex imaging before caval interruption. J Vasc Surg 1996;24:608–12 [discussion: 12–3].
113. Corriere MA, Passman MA, Guzman RJ, et al. Comparison of bedside transabdominal duplex ultrasound versus contrast venography for inferior vena cava filter placement: what is the best imaging modality? Ann Vasc Surg 2005;19:229–34.
114. Rosenthal D, Wellons ED, Levitt AB, et al. Role of prophylactic temporary inferior vena cava filters placed at the ICU bedside under intravascular ultrasound guidance in patients with multiple trauma. J Vasc Surg 2004;40:958–64.
115. Rosenthal D, Wellons ED, Lai KM, et al. Retrievable inferior vena cava filters: early clinical experience. J Cardiovasc Surg (Torino) 2005;46:163–9.
116. Wellons ED, Matsuura JH, Shuler FW, et al. Bedside intravascular ultrasound-guided vena cava filter placement. J Vasc Surg 2003;38:455–7 [discussion: 57–8].
117. Hoppe H, Kaufman JA, Barton RE, et al. Safety of inferior vena cava filter retrieval in anticoagulated patients. Chest 2007;132:31–6.
118. Schmelzer TM, Christmas AB, Taylor DA, et al. Vena cava filter retrieval in therapeutically anticoagulated patients. Am J Surg 2008;196:944–6 [discussion: 46–7].
119. Sing RF, Camp SM, Heniford BT, et al. Timing of pulmonary emboli after trauma: implications for retrievable vena cava filters. J Trauma 2006;60:732–4 [discussion: 34–5].
120. Hoff WS, Hoey BA, Wainwright GA, et al. Early experience with retrievable inferior vena cava filters in high-risk trauma patients. J Am Coll Surg 2004;199:869–74.
121. Stefanidis D, Paton BL, Jacobs DG, et al. Extended interval for retrieval of vena cava filters is safe and may maximize protection against pulmonary embolism. Am J Surg 2006;192:789–94.
122. Kaufman JA, Geller SC, Rivitz SM, et al. Operator errors during percutaneous placement of vena cava filters. AJR Am J Roentgenol 1995;165:1281–7.
123. Binkert CA, Bansal A, Gates JD. Inferior vena cava filter removal after 317-day implantation. J Vasc Interv Radiol 2005;16:395–8.
124. Karmy-Jones R, Jurkovich GJ, Velmahos GC, et al. Practice patterns and outcomes of retrievable vena cava filters in trauma patients: an AAST multicenter study. J Trauma 2007;62:17–24 [discussion: 24–5].

Heparin-Induced Thrombocytopenia in Critically Ill Patients

Theodore E. Warkentin, MD[a,b,c,d],*

KEYWORDS

- Heparin-induced thrombocytopenia • Intensive care unit
- Low molecular weight heparin • Dalteparin
- PF4-dependent enzyme immunoassay

Why should a *Critical Care Clinics* issue, "Venous Thromboembolism in the ICU," include the topic, "Heparin-induced thrombocytopenia in critically ill patients"? First, there is increasing focus on the prevention of venous thromboembolism (VTE) in critically ill patients, most widely through use of heparin, either unfractionated or low molecular weight. Immune heparin-induced thrombocytopenia (HIT) represents one of the complications of such prophylaxis. Ironically, since HIT is strongly associated with thrombosis—particularly deep-vein thrombosis (DVT) and pulmonary embolism (PE)—VTE can result through the very effort to prevent its occurrence! Second, HIT can be the reason for admission into the intensive care unit (ICU), either because of life-threatening thrombosis, adrenal failure, or anaphylactoid reaction. Third, thrombocytopenia of diverse etiology is common in critically-ill patients, either at the time of entry into the ICU ("prevalent") or which develops in the ICU ("incident"). The development of thrombocytopenia—particularly when it raises the specter of HIT—may trigger crucial treatment decisions, such as interruption or cessation of heparin, use of non-heparin anticoagulants, and so forth. However, given that HIT explains only a very small fraction of thrombocytopenia in the critically-ill, management consequences of HIT "overdiagnosis" could pose greater danger than does "true" HIT.

This article first discusses in general the significance of thrombocytopenia in the ICU. The clinical and laboratory features of HIT will be highlighted, emphasizing the

---

[a] Department of Pathology and Molecular Medicine, McMaster University, Hamilton, ON, Canada
[b] Department of Medicine, McMaster University, Hamilton, ON, Canada
[c] Hamilton Regional Laboratory Medicine Program, Hamilton Health Sciences, Hamilton, ON, Canada
[d] Division of Clinical Hematology, Department of Medicine, Hamilton Health Sciences, Hamilton, ON, Canada
* Hamilton Regional Laboratory Medicine Program, Room 1-270B, Hamilton Health Sciences (General Site), 237 Barton Street East, Hamilton, ON L8L 2X2, Canada.
E-mail address: twarken@mcmaster.ca

Crit Care Clin 27 (2011) 805–823
doi:10.1016/j.ccc.2011.08.001
0749-0704/11/$ – see front matter © 2011 Elsevier Inc. All rights reserved.

key role of platelet-activating antibodies in HIT pathogenesis, and the importance of detecting these antibodies directly using platelet activation assays. Problems with HIT diagnosis, and its overdiagnosis in the ICU, are also examined. The issue of early-onset and persisting thrombocytopenia is discussed, including the recognition that these patients usually do not have HIT even when heparin-dependent antibodies are detectable.

Finally, management issues are reviewed. Problems of anticoagulant choice and dosing will be addressed, focusing on the problem of dose-confounding by coagulopathies. Indeed, heparin—as the "approved" drug for disseminated intravascular coagulation (DIC)—may well be the drug of choice even when HIT is a diagnostic possibility. Finally, the issue of HIT prevention in the ICU through the use of low molecular weight heparin (LMWH) is presented.

CLINICAL SIGNIFICANCE OF THROMBOCYTOPENIA IN THE CRITICALLY ILL

Hui and colleagues[1] recently performed a systematic review that examined the frequency and clinical significance of thrombocytopenia complicating critical illness. They identified 24 studies (12 prospective) that enrolled 6894 patients from medical, surgical, mixed, or trauma ICUs. Both "prevalent" and "incident" thrombocytopenia were commonly reported. An association between thrombocytopenia and mortality (by multivariate analysis) was observed in six of eight studies[2–7]: reported odds ratios (OR) ranged from approximately 2.0 to 4.0. Moreover, one study examining serial platelet counts in critically ill patients found that a 10% or greater decline in platelet count on day 4 (compared with admission baseline) was associated with increased mortality,[8] whereas another reported that platelet count recovery occurred faster in ICU survivors than in nonsurvivors.[9]

Two studies[10,11] that evaluated heparin use did not find it to be an independent risk factor for development of thrombocytopenia. However, this is not surprising, given that heparin administration is nearly ubiquitous in this patient population and that HIT explains few episodes of ICU thrombocytopenia.

PATHOGENESIS OF HIT

HIT is caused by antibodies of immunoglobulin G (IgG) class that lead to activation of platelets,[12] coagulation,[13] monocytes,[14] and, possibly, endothelium.[15] The result is a prothrombotic state: the observed OR for thrombosis in HIT ranges from about 20 to 40.[16] The HIT antigen(s) do not reside on heparin itself, but rather on neoepitopes formed on (positive-charged) platelet factor 4 (PF4) when it is complexed with (negatively charged) heparin,[17] possibly through close apposition of two PF4 tetramers that would normally repel one another.[18] (PF4 monomer is a 70-amino-acid, 7.8-kDa member of the C-X-C subfamily of chemokines that self-associates to form ~30-kDa tetramers.) Platelet activation results from cross-linking of IgG platelet Fc receptors (FcγIIa), which occurs when PF4/heparin–IgG immune complexes are formed on platelet surfaces.[12] "Strong" platelet activation results, which results in release of intracellular granules and formation of procoagulant, platelet-derived microparticles.[19]

Only a small minority of antibodies triggered by heparin administration are able to activate platelets and hence potentially to cause HIT.[20–22] **Fig. 1** illustrates this "iceberg" phenomenon of HIT. As this model infers, detection of platelet-activating antibodies using platelet activation assays, such as the platelet serotonin-release assay (SRA),[23,24] has a high sensitivity for clinical HIT similar to that of the PF4-dependent enzyme immunoassays (EIAs), but with much greater diagnostic

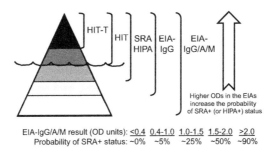

EIA-IgG/A/M result (OD units): ≤0.4 0.4-1.0 1.0-1.5 1.5-2.0 >2.0
Probability of SRA+ status: ~0%   ~5%   ~25%   ~50%   ~90%

Fig. 1. "Iceberg model" of HIT. Clinical HIT, ie, comprising HIT with (HITT) or without thrombosis, is represented by the portion of the iceberg above the waterline; the portion below the waterline represents subclinical anti-PF4/heparin seroconversion. Three types of assays—the washed platelet activation assays (SRA, heparin-induced platelet activation [HIPA] test), the IgG-specific PF4-dependent EIAs (EIA-IgG), and the polyspecific EIAs that detects anti-PF4/heparin antibodies of the three major immunoglobulin classes (EIA-IgG/A/M)—are highly sensitive for the diagnosis of HIT. In contrast, diagnostic specificity varies greatly among these assays: It is highest for the platelet activation assays (SRA, HIPA), but lowest for the EIA-IgG/A/M because the EIA-IgG/A/M is most likely to detect clinically irrelevant non–platelet-activating anti-PF4/heparin antibodies. The approximate probability of a positive SRA (SRA+) status in relation to a given EIA result, expressed in OD units, is obtained from the literature. (*Reprinted from* Warkentin TE. How I diagnose and manage HIT. Hematology Am Soc Hematol Educ Program 2011; in press; with permission.)

specificity.[20,25,26] However, even patients who form platelet-activating antibodies do not necessarily develop clinical HIT, suggesting that other patient-dependent factors are relevant. As discussed later, the magnitude of a positive EIA—measured in optical density (OD) units—is a strong predictor of a positive SRA and hence of HIT[22] (see **Fig. 1**).

LABORATORY DETECTION OF PATHOGENIC HIT ANTIBODIES

Pathogenic HIT antibodies are platelet-activating, and the optimal way to detect them is by using a "washed" platelet activation assay, such as the SRA. Most often, however, the potential presence of platelet-activating antibodies is inferred, rather than proven, using a PF4-dependent EIA. This approach, however, leads to HIT "overdiagnosis" because at most 50% of patients with a positive EIA also have a positive SRA.[22,25,27] Indeed, in certain clinical settings, such as the ICU, the probability of EIA+ status indicating the presence of platelet-activating antibodies—and hence the possibility of HIT—is only approximately 10% to 20%.[28]

HIT antibodies have a characteristic reaction profile: strong platelet activation (usually >80% serotonin release) is triggered by HIT serum or plasma at pharmacologic unfractionated heparin (UFH) concentrations (0.1–0.3 IU/mL), whereas background activation (<20% serotonin release) is seen at high (100 IU/mL) concentrations.[24] Platelet activation assays are optimal when normal donor platelets are "washed" and resuspended in cation-containing buffer, and when platelet donors are selected based on the ability of their platelets to be readily activated by HIT sera.[24] Moreover, an important quality control step is the inclusion of a "weak" positive HIT control, to ensure that the assay can readily detect HIT antibodies.[24] It is also important to test acute serum (obtained during or soon after resolution of thrombocytopenia) because HIT antibodies are transient.[29] The SRA is technically demanding, and performed only in a few reference laboratories. Nevertheless, physicians can refer patient serum or plasma for SRA testing, much like certain other specialized immunohematology assays (eg, testing for platelet-reactive alloantibodies to diagnose posttransfusion purpura).

The SRA is much more specific for HIT than the PF4-dependent EIAs, particularly the "polyspecific" EIAs that detect antibodies of IgG, IgM, and IgA class (only IgG class antibodies can activate platelets via platelet IgG Fc receptors[12,25]). In a review of three studies that compared predictivity for thrombocytopenia among SRA+/EIA+ patients in comparison with EIA+/SRA– patients, it was found that approximately 50% (20/39) of SRA+ patients exposed to heparin developed thrombocytopenia, whereas none of 225 EIA+/SRA– patients did.[21]

Another study[27] compared SRA+ versus SRA– status among EIA+ patients who were investigated because of thrombocytopenia: an additional comparison group comprised 68 patients who tested negative in both assays (EIA–/SRA–). This study found that only SRA+/EIA+ status correlated strongly with thrombosis; in contrast, SRA– patients (whether EIA+ or EIA–) had a high 30-day morality (~25%) exceeding that of SRA+ patients. This is consistent with the adverse prognosis of thrombocytopenia discussed earlier, and suggests that mortality is higher in patients investigated serologically for HIT who turn out not to have this diagnosis.

Commercial PF4-dependent EIAs are commonly performed to investigate HIT.[30] Both IgG-specific and polyspecific assays are used, with antigen targets being PF4/heparin or PF4/polyvinylsulfonate.[31,32] As only IgG antibodies are pathogenic,[24] IgG-specific assays have greater diagnostic specificity than do polyspecific assays.[25,32] A negative EIA essentially rules out HIT (SRA+ status <1%). On the other hand, the predictivity for platelet-activating antibodies ranges enormously, depending on the strength of a positive EIA.[22] For example, for a "weak" positive EIA (0.4–1.0 OD units), the probability of a positive SRA is approximately 5%; in contrast, for an EIA greater than 2.0 OD units, the probability is approximately 90%. Even for an OD result from 1.0 to 1.5, the probability of a positive SRA is only 20% to 25%. *Thus, in a thrombocytopenic ICU patient, an OD less than 1.50 units in a PF4-dependent EIA suggests that the patient is more likely to have a non-HIT diagnosis.*

CLINICAL PRESENTATION OF HIT

The classic presentation of HIT is a large-magnitude platelet count fall—usually 50% or more—that begins 5 to 10 days after a proximate immunizing exposure to heparin, often accompanied by venous or arterial thrombosis, and without another clinical explanation.[29,33–35] These features comprise a pretest probability scoring system, the "4 T's": *T*hrombocytopenia, *T*iming (of thrombocytopenia or thrombosis), *T*hrombosis (or other clinical sequelae of HIT), and no o*T*her explanation for thrombocytopenia[35–37] (**Table 1**). Platelet-activating HIT antibodies are unlikely (<2%) when a low score (≤3 points) is obtained, but relatively probable (~50%) with a high score (≥6 points).[37] An intermediate score (4 or 5 points) indicates a clinical profile compatible with HIT but also with another plausible explanation, such as sepsis; here the frequency of SRA+ status is still only approximately 10% to 20%.

Thrombocytopenic patients in the ICU usually have a low 4 T's score because the onset of thrombocytopenia is usually earlier than is seen in HIT, and there generally is at least one other non-HIT explanation for the thrombocytopenia (eg, postoperative hemodilution, sepsis, or multiorgan failure). It remains to be seen whether the 4 T's (or any other) scoring system proves useful in evaluating thrombocytopenic patients in an ICU setting.[38,39]

Table 1
Estimating the pretest probability of HIT: "4 T's" scoring system

	Points (0, 1, or 2 for each of four categories: maximum possible score = 8)		
	2	1	0
Thrombocytopenia (acute)	Platelet fall >50% (nadir, >20 × 10⁹/L) and no surgery within preceding 3 days	Nadir, 10–19 × 10⁹/L; or any 30%–50% fall; or >50% fall within 3 days of surgery	Nadir, <10 × 10⁹/L; or any <30% fall
Timing[a] of platelet count fall, thrombosis, or other sequelae	Clear onset between days 5–10; or <1 day (if heparin exposure within past 5–30 days)	Consistent with day 5–10 fall, but not clear (eg, missing platelet counts); or <1 day (heparin exposure within past 31–100 days); or platelet fall after day 10	Platelet count fall ≤4 days without recent heparin exposure
Thrombosis or other clinical sequelae	New proven thrombosis; skin necrosis[b]; anaphylactoid reaction after IV heparin bolus; adrenal hemorrhage	Progressive or recurrent thrombosis; erythematous skin lesions[b]; suspected thrombosis (awaiting confirmation with imaging)	None
OTher cause for thrombocytopenia not evident	No other explanation for platelet count fall is evident	Possible other cause is evident	Definite other cause is present
Pretest probability score: 6–8 = High; 4–5 = Intermediate; 0–3 = Low			

The scoring system shown here has undergone minor modifications from previously published scoring systems.[35,36,40]

[a] First day of immunizing heparin exposure considered day 0, usually heparin given during or soon after surgery (eg, UFH during heart surgery is more immunogenic than UFH given during preceding acute coronary syndrome or with heart catheterization); the day the platelet count *begins* to fall is considered the day of onset of thrombocytopenia.

[b] Skin lesions occurring at heparin injection sites.

From Warkentin TE. Clinical picture of heparin-induced thrombocytopenia. In: Warkentin TE, Greinacher A, editors. Heparin-induced thrombocytopenia. 4th edition. New York: Informa Healthcare USA; 2007. p. 21–66; with permission.

In some patients with severe HIT, evidence of inflammation, including leukocytosis and overt DIC (low fibrinogen levels, elevated international normalized ratio [INR]) can be seen.[40] This can make it difficult on clinical grounds to distinguish HIT from other non-HIT disorders in the ICU.

HIT IN THE ICU
HIT as an Explanation for Admission to the ICU

Three ways that HIT can trigger an ICU admission are summarized here: PE, adrenal failure, and acute anaphylactoid reaction. PE is strongly associated with HIT (OR, ~40).[33–35] In the author's experience, approximately 50% of patients with (SRA+) HIT develop symptomatic DVT; half of these have PE.[41]

An uncommon but important complication of HIT is adrenal hemorrhagic necrosis,[40,42,43] which results from adrenal vein *thrombosis*, with secondary hemorrhage. Acute adrenal crisis results when adrenal destruction is bilateral. Thus, corticosteroids are appropriate for a hypotensive patient in whom thrombocytopenia suggests the possibility of HIT, and may be life-saving. Later in the section, "Coagulopathy-Associated Confounding of PTT-Monitored DTI Therapy," a case of adrenal failure complicating HIT is presented.

Anaphylactoid reactions can be explained by HIT.[44–46] Here, the patient develops one or more of the following: acute hypertension, dyspnea, fever/chills, chest pain, tachycardia or flushing, 10 to 30 minutes after receiving an intravenous heparin bolus, or 30 to 90 minutes after a subcutaneous injection of heparin, accompanied by an abrupt drop in platelet count. Affected patients have also received heparin within the previous 5 to 100 days, which explains why antibodies are present at the time of repeat heparin exposure. When these reactions are accompanied by respiratory or cardiac arrest, the patient usually requires admission to the ICU. **Fig. 2** summarizes the case of patient with HIT-associated cardiorespiratory arrest, prompting ICU admission.[45]

Frequency of HIT in the ICU

Overall, the frequency of HIT with UFH exposure in hospitalized patients is estimated to be approximately 0.2%.[47] In some circumstances, for example, UFH given for more than 1 week after surgery, the frequency of HIT can exceed 1%.[33,34,48] Females are at greater risk of HIT than males, as are surgical compared with medical patients.[49] In one study, greater severity of trauma increased the risk of immunization and of HIT itself.[50]

Prospective studies indicate that the frequency of HIT in the ICU is approximately 0.3% to 0.5%.[49] This is only 1/100th of the overall frequency of thrombocytopenia among critically ill patients (30%–50%). Thus, when I consult on a thrombocytopenic patient in the ICU, I remind myself that the odds of a diagnosis of HIT are 100 to 1 against! Three studies are highlighted.

Community-based combined intensive and cardiac care unit

A study by Verma and colleagues[51] evaluated consecutive, heparin-treated patients older than the age of 18 who were admitted during a 2-year period to a combined intensive and coronary care unit within a 350-bed community-based hospital. Patients were excluded if they had thrombocytopenia (platelet count $<100 \times 10^9$/L) at admission or did not receive heparin. Patients were evaluated for HIT antibodies if their platelet count fell below 150×10^9/L, or by more than 33%, beginning 5 or more days after starting heparin; or if an earlier fall in platelet count meeting either criterion occurred in a patient with recent exposure to heparin within the preceding 8 weeks. The "gold standard" assay was the SRA. In addition, most patients with possible HIT

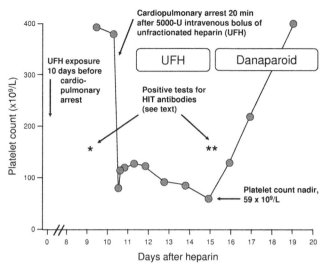

Fig. 2. A 53-year-old woman with HIT-associated anaphylactoid reaction (cardiopulmonary arrest) after an intravenous bolus of UFH. The patient had received UFH 10 days earlier at another hospital and was subsequently transferred for cardiac surgery. She had severe mitral stenosis and a large dense intra-atrial thrombus. While awaiting surgery, she therefore received a 5000-U bolus of UFH; within 20 minutes after bolus, the patient was found to have a "pulseless/electrical activity arrest." After cardiopulmonary resuscitation and administration of epinephrine and atropine, the circulation was restored. CT brain examination showed multiple cerebral infarcts consistent with a combination of anoxic and ischemic injury. The surgery was cancelled and intravenous UFH by infusion was commenced. The platelet count fell from 127 to 59×10^9/L over the next 4 days, at which time the diagnosis of HIT was first suspected and the presence of platelet-activating anti-PF4/heparin antibodies was confirmed by laboratory tests. In retrospect, the cardiac arrest after bolus UFH was recognized as being an "anaphylactoid" reaction secondary to acute HIT, based upon the abrupt 78% platelet count fall (from 376 to 81×10^9/L). This diagnosis was further supported by positive tests for HIT antibodies in a blood sample obtained 1 day before the cardiopulmonary arrest. Thus, it appeared that the UFH administered 10 days earlier at the referring hospital triggered the presence of HIT antibodies, which accounted for the acute anaphylactoid reaction triggered by bolus UFH administration. Results of HIT antibody tests (tests performed using patient serum: *(day 9) = 94% serotonin release at 0.3 IU/mL heparin (normal, <20% release); <10% release at 0 and 100 IU/mL heparin; commercial EIA from GTI Inc (Waukesha, WI, USA) = 0.85 units (normal, <0.40 units). **(day 15) = 93% serotonin release at 0.3 IU/mL heparin (normal, <20% release); <10% release at 0 and 100 IU/mL heparin. For all assays, the positive and negative controls reacted as expected. (*Reprinted from* Warkentin TE, Greinacher A. Heparin-induced anaphylactic and anaphylactoid reactions: two distinct but overlapping syndromes. Expert Opin Drug Saf 2009;8(2):129–44; with permission.)

also underwent testing with a commercial EIA. To evaluate test specificity, 91 patients who did not meet the clinical criteria for possible HIT also underwent testing using both the SRA and EIA.

Of the 748 patients who met the inclusion criteria, 267 were exposed to heparin for a sufficient length of time to be considered at risk for HIT. Forty of these 267 patients met the predefined clinical criteria for possible HIT, 32 of whom had available serum or plasma for HIT antibody testing. Only 1 of these 32 patients tested positive by both SRA and EIA (and the clinical picture was ambivalent as to whether the patient really had HIT). None of the remaining 31 patients tested SRA+, although 9 of 31 (29%) tested EIA+. Thus, the frequency of HIT among the 267 at-risk patients was found to be 0.4% (95% CI, 0.01%–2.1%). The results of this study also support the clinical "rule" that only approximately 1 or 2 in 10 patients with a positive PF4-dependent EIA in an ICU setting will also test positive in the SRA.

Tertiary care medical–surgical ICU

In another prospective cohort study aimed at determining the prevalence, incidence, and risk factors for lower extremity DVT among critically ill medical–surgical patients, consecutive patients 18 years of age or older expected to be in ICU for 72 or more hours were enrolled.[52] Bilateral lower extremity compression ultrasound was performed within 48 hours of ICU admission, twice weekly, and if VTE was clinically suspected. Most patients received thromboprophylaxis with UFH (5000 U twice a day by subcutaneous injection), although some received LMWH.

Among the 261 enrolled patients, thrombocytopenia was common: 62 patients (23.7%) had a platelet count of less than 150×10^9/L on admission into the ICU ("prevalent" thrombocytopenia), and among the remaining 199 patients, 59 (29.6%) developed "incident" thrombocytopenia while in the ICU; severe thrombocytopenia ($<50 \times 10^9$/L) was observed in 7 patients.

Among the original 261 patients, 33 (12.6%) underwent blood testing for HIT antibodies on at least one occasion using the SRA, with anti-PF4/heparin-IgG measured by EIA if the SRA gave an "indeterminate" result. Patients who underwent testing (in comparison with those who did not undergo testing) had lower platelet counts (median: 63×10^9/L vs 182×10^9/L; $P<.001$), but were similar with respect to age, sex, APACHE II score, and ICU mortality. A similar percent of those tested for HIT antibodies (compared to those who were not tested) had a prior heparin exposure (20.0% vs 25.5%, $P = .51$), and were just as likely to be receiving UFH (83.3% vs 85.7%, $P = .73$), and to be receiving LMWH (6.7% vs 7.4%, $P = .89$), but had a longer duration of ventilation (10 vs 6 days, $P = 0.03$) and ICU stay (15 vs 9 days, $P = .002$), although not a longer total duration of hospitalization (26.5 vs 25 days, $P = .73$). None of the 33 patients tested positive for HIT antibodies: 32 patients tested negative in the SRA, and 1 patient (with an indeterminate SRA) tested negative by EIA. Therefore, despite thromboprophylaxis of these medical–surgical ICU patients primarily with UFH, no patients with HIT were identified.

PROTECT

The PROphylaxis for ThromboEmbolism in Critical Care Trial (PROTECT) was a multicenter trial that randomized 3764 patients to receive either dalteparin (5000 IU once a day) or UFH (5000 IU twice a day) while they were in the ICU.[53] The primary outcome was proximal-leg DVT diagnosed by compression ultrasonography, performed twice weekly and as clinically indicated. Secondary end points included PE and HIT (confirmed by the SRA). By intention-to-treat analysis, 12 of 1873 (0.6%) patients randomized to receive UFH developed HIT, compared with 5 of 1873 (0.3%) patients randomized to receive dalteparin (hazard ratio, 0.47 [95% CI, 0.16–1.35]; $P = .16$. These reported frequencies of HIT are consistent with the expected 0.3% to 0.5% range reported observed for HIT in critically ill patients. It is interesting to note that by a prespecified per-protocol analysis, significantly fewer patients who received dalteparin developed HIT (hazard ratio, 0.27; 95% CI, 0.08–0.98; $P = 0.046$). Some perspective regarding the implications of the PROTECT trial vis-à-vis potential to reduce the risk of HIT are discussed further at the end of this article.

Conclusions from Prospective Studies of HIT In the ICU

These studies of HIT incidence in ICU patients indicate the following. First, only a small minority of thrombocytopenic patients receiving UFH or LMWH in the ICU have HIT. Second, testing with an EIA is much more likely to detect clinically irrelevant anti-PF4/heparin antibodies than the SRA, suggesting the potential for significant overdiagnosis of HIT in this patient population. Third, there is the potential to reduce the risk of HIT through use of LMWH in ICU patients.

EARLY-ONSET AND PERSISTING THROMBOCYTOPENIA

As discussed earlier, the typical picture of HIT is that of thrombocytopenia that begins between 5 and 10 days after an immunizing heparin exposure[29]; given that HIT usually occurs in postoperative patients,[49] and given that there invariably is an early postoperative platelet count decline that reaches its nadir most often between postoperative days 1 to 3, this means that HIT usually evinces as a *second* (pathologic) platelet count fall that follows the first (normal and expected) early postoperative decline.[33,34,54,55] However, what about the scenario—commonly seen in the ICU—where a patient develops "early-onset and persisting thrombocytopenia"? In theory, although the early thrombocytopenia would not indicate HIT, it is at least theoretically possible that persistence of thrombocytopenia beyond day 5 could be due to concomitant formation of HIT antibodies, as posited by Pouplard and colleagues.[54,55] Interestingly, although these French workers had observed such a patient profile attributable to HIT,[54] they failed to find any such patient with early-onset and persistent thrombocytopenia due to HIT in their later study.[55]

More recently, Selleng and colleagues corroborated these findings in a systematic study of 25 patients (identified among 581 prospectively studied subjects) who evinced early-onset and persisting thrombocytopenia after cardiac surgery.[56] They found the frequency of anti-PF4/heparin antibodies—including the subset with platelet-activating antibodies—to be similar to the "background" rate of antibody formation among "well" post-cardiac surgery patients and patients whose platelet counts recovered in the normal fashion. This indicates that the explanation for early-onset and persisting thrombocytopenia is usually *not* HIT, but rather a non-HIT complication that begins soon after surgery and that persists into the period when "incidental" anti-PF4/heparin seroconversion occurs. Note that approximately 1% of post-cardiac surgery patients will develop "true" HIT, and thus it remains likely that a similar (~1%) frequency of "true" HIT can develop among such patients with early-onset and persisting thrombocytopenia. Clues supporting a diagnosis of true HIT would include thrombosis (on or after postoperative day 5) and especially a new platelet count decline that is "superimposed" upon the prevailing thrombocytopenia. Indeed, this profile was reported by Selleng and colleagues in an earlier prospective study of HIT post-cardiac surgery.[57]

MANAGEMENT OF SUSPECTED HIT IN THE ICU

The management principles of strongly suspected (or confirmed) HIT include (**Table 2**)[58,59]: substituting heparin with a suitable non-heparin anticoagulant; avoiding/postponing warfarin (due to the substantial risk of precipitating warfarin-induced microthrombosis manifesting as venous limb gangrene[13]); testing for HIT antibodies; avoiding/minimizing platelet transfusions; and diagnostic imaging (eg, ultrasonography) for lower-limb DVT. Especially in ICU patients, strong consideration for confirming the diagnosis with a platelet activation assay should be made, even if this requires referral to an outside laboratory.

Table 2
Treatment principles of HIT: ICU considerations

Treatment Principle	ICU-Specific Considerations (NOTE: Only approximately 1% of thrombocytopenia in the ICU is attributable to HIT.)
1. Stop and avoid all heparin.	UFH is the preferred anticoagulant in critically ill patients due to its short half-life, availability of anti-factor Xa monitoring, antidote (protamine), and nonrenal clearance (dalteparin is another option for antithrombotic prophylaxis among renally impaired patients).
2. Give a non-heparin alternative anticoagulant (usually in therapeutic doses).	PTT-adjusted DTI therapy may be ineffective or even deleterious in coagulopathic ICU patients (confounding of PTT-adjusted therapy); therapeutic-dose anticoagulation with DTIs may pose high bleeding risk when non-HIT thrombocytopenia is the most likely diagnosis.
3. Avoid/postpone warfarin therapy.	This proscription against warfarin also applies more generally to critically ill patients with non-HIT thrombocytopenia.
4. Test for HIT antibodies.	The importance of high diagnostic specificity of platelet activation assays (eg, SRA) is especially important in the ICU, as only 10 to 20% of EIA+ patients in the ICU also test SRA+.
5. Image for (lower-limb) DVT.	Absence of DVT helps to justify avoidance of therapeutic-dose anticoagulation; asymptomatic upper-limb DVT at sites of central line insertion are common and do not point to high probability of HIT.
6. Avoid prophylactic platelet transfusions.	Platelet transfusions may be justified in critically ill patients where the diagnosis of HIT seems unlikely, bleeding risk appears high, and invasive procedures are required.

However, certain of these treatment principles should not be applied indiscriminately to the critically ill patient, for several reasons. First, thrombocytopenia in an ICU patient is caused by HIT in only 1% of patients, and thus the overwhelming probability is that the patient does *not* have HIT. Thus, the expected risk/benefit profile of therapeutic-dose, non-heparin anticoagulation in a patient believed to have "true" HIT (high thrombotic risk, low bleeding risk) does not necessarily apply in a non-HIT, critically ill patient, in whom bleeding risk is substantial and the safety and efficacy of direct thrombin inhibitor (DTI) therapy for non-HIT patients has not been established. Second, renal and hepatic dysfunction are common in critically ill patients, which can lead to drug accumulation. Third, coagulopathies are common in critically ill patients, which besides conferring greater bleeding risk, can also confound partial thromboplastin time (PTT)-adjusted DTI therapy (discussed subsequently in the section "Coagulopathy-Associated Confounding of PTT-Monitored DTI Therapy." Fourth, comorbidities within an ICU patient population, including gastritis, mechanical ventilation, and presence of invasive lines, predisposes to greater likelihood of bleeding during anticoagulant therapy.

The issue of substituting heparin with an alternative non-heparin anticoagulant is not straightforward. If very few thrombocytopenic ICU patients actually have HIT, this infers that switching from heparin to a non-heparin anticoagulant will occur predominantly in non-HIT patients. But heparin is a near-ideal anticoagulant for ICU-associated thrombocytopenia: it is cleared through non-renal, non-hepatic mechanisms, its levels can be directly quantitated through antifactor Xa levels, it is the only anticoagulant that is approved by the U.S. Food and Drug Administration (FDA) for the indication, "diagnosis and treatment of acute and chronic consumptive coagulopathies (disseminated intravascular coagulation)"[60]; its anticoagulant effects can be reversed quickly with an antidote (protamine); its pharmacologic properties are understood by many practitioners; and it is inexpensive. In contrast, the safety and efficacy of non-heparin anticoagulants are largely unknown and unproven in non-HIT settings.

Moreover, dosing and monitoring of DTIs can be problematic in critically ill patients. The standard (FDA-approved) dosing of lepirudin and argatroban is now recognized as being too high,[61-63] particularly in critically ill patients.[64-66] Moreover, coagulopathies—whether associated with HIT itself or with non-HIT illness (eg, liver dysfunction, sepsis-associated consumptive coagulopathy, nonspecific inhibitors)—can result in confounding of PTT-adjusted anticoagulant dosing (discussed subsequently).

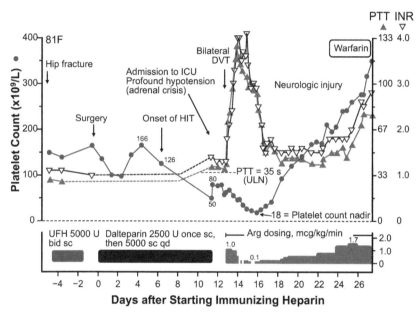

Fig. 3. HIT-associated consumptive coagulopathy: confounding of PTT monitoring. The patient developed HIT beginning 6 days after starting dalteparin thromboprophylaxis after hip fracture surgery. On day 11, the patient required admission to the ICU for severe hypotension secondary to adrenal failure (flat ACTH stimulation test; CT imaging: bilateral adrenal hemorrhagic infarction). HIT-associated bilateral lower-limb DVT was treated with argatroban begun at 1 μg/kg per minute). Despite stopping heparin, the platelet count fell over 4 days from 80 to 18×10⁹/L (nadir). Five PTT measurements before argatroban therapy were all elevated (range, 38–41 seconds; normal, 22–35 seconds). After initiation of argatroban, persisting supratherapeutic PTT values resulted in multiple argatroban dose reductions and interruptions; when HIT was most intense (as judged by platelet count nadir), argatroban dosing ranged from 0 to only 0.1 μg/kg per minute). The laboratory and clinical profile is consistent with intense HIT-associated consumptive coagulopathy, with confounding of PTT monitoring of argatroban therapy and associated underdosing despite supratherapeutic PTT values. *Abbreviations:* Arg, argatroban; bid, twice daily; DVT, deep-vein thrombosis; F, female; HIT, heparin-induced thrombocytopenia; ICU, intensive care unit; INR, international normalized ratio; qd, once daily; PTT, partial thromboplastin time; sc, subcutaneous; U, units; ULN, upper limit of normal. (*From* Linkins LA, Warkentin TE. Heparin-induced thrombocytopenia: real-world issues. Semin Thromb Hemost 2011;37(6):653–63; with permission.)

Coagulopathy-Associated Confounding of PTT-Monitored DTI Therapy

Two examples of PTT confounding of DTI are described, one associated with HIT and the other with non-HIT thrombocytopenia. **Fig. 3** illustrates a patient with SRA+ HIT[67]: here the patient required admission to ICU because of HIT-associated critical illness related to bilateral adrenal hemorrhagic necrosis, shock, progressive multiorgan failure, and severe HIT-associated consumptive coagulopathy. Initial argatroban dosing at 2 μg/kg per minute produced supratherapeutic PTT levels and multiple dose interruptions/reductions, ultimately leading to a period where no or little argatroban was given, with associated irreversible neurologic injury. The later requirement for much higher argatroban dosing suggested that the preceding period of underdosing was an artifact of PTT monitoring because of intense HIT-associated coagulopathy. Although this problem can in theory be avoided by measuring drug levels directly, this is infrequently available or performed, at least in North American hospital laboratories.

Fig. 4 presents a non-HIT patient case that also illustrates PTT confounding of DTI therapy. This critically ill patient developed fungal pneumonia, associated thrombocytopenia, acute ischemic hepatitis, DIC, and acquired natural anticoagulant deficiency (severe antithrombin [AT3] depletion). As HIT was initially suspected, the patient received argatroban (day 5): however, only a brief infusion was given, because subsequent serial PTT levels were supratherapeutic. By day 8, the patient developed multiple sites of central skin necrosis. Although the patient eventually seroconverted to a positive EIA, careful review of the data suggests that the patient did *not* have HIT: (1) the initial EIA test results ("borderline" and "negative") at a time of well-established thrombocytopenia rules out HIT as the explanation for the platelet count fall[68]; (2) the

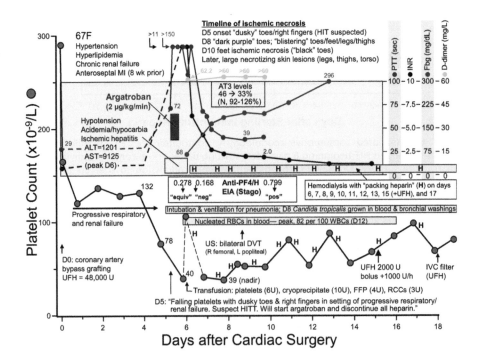

positive EIA of 0.799 OD units is a weak-positive result (indicating <5% probability of SRA+ status[22]); (3) fungal pneumonia is a better overall explanation for the clinical course; and (4) the multiple lesions of central skin necrosis—which are not a classic finding of HIT[40]—can be explained by sepsis-associated DIC, profound natural anticoagulant failure, and (perhaps) interference of protein C activation by the DTI, or post-DTI thrombin "rebound." In any event, this severe patient outcome—despite prompt initiation of argatroban—contradicts the notion that simple substitution of heparin with a DTI will avoid complications in coagulopathic critically ill patients.

←

Fig. 4. Non–HIT-associated thrombocytopenia and coagulopathy treated as HIT: confounding of PTT monitoring. A 67-year-old woman with recent myocardial infarction underwent coronary artery bypass grafting. The early postoperative course (day [D] 1–4) was characterized by progressive respiratory failure with pulmonary infiltrates (treated with bilevel positive airway pressure, antibiotics, corticosteroids, and high-dose intravenous gammaglobulin) and progressive renal failure (rise in serum creatinine from 1.9 to 3.1 mg/dL [normal, 0.6–1.3 mg/dL]); no postoperative heparin prophylaxis was given. On D5 the patient developed hypotension (treated with albumin, dopamine, and neosynephrine), acidemia/hypocarbia, and ischemic hepatitis (marked increase in alanine transaminase [ALT] and aspartate transaminase [AST]); the platelet count fell from 132 (D4) to 78 (D5) × 10⁹/L. Several hours later the toes and right fingers appeared "dusky" and HIT-associated thrombosis (HITT) was suspected (despite the patient not having received heparin since surgery). Argatroban (Arg) was started, but was stopped approximately 4 hours later when the PTT measured >150 seconds (target PTT range, 60–90 seconds). The next morning (D6), the platelet count had fallen further to 40; the PTT remained >150, the INR was >11 (normal, 0.9–1.1), and the fibrinogen (Fbg) measured only 68 mg/dL (normal, 200–450 mg/dL). The patient received platelets, cryoprecipitate, fresh-frozen plasma (FFP), and red cell concentrates (RCCs). The PF4-dependent EIA from Diagnostica Stago (Asnieres-sur-Seine, France) was reported as "equivocal" ("equiv") and a repeat test performed the next day was reported as "negative" ("neg"). Despite "therapeutic" (or greater) PTT and INR values, by D8, progression to ischemic necrosis of the toes was evident (despite Doppler-identifiable pulses), as well as blistering of numerous sites on the lower extremities; in addition, bilateral lower-limb DVT was documented by ultrasound (US), but anticoagulation was not restarted because of (minor) gastrointestinal bleeding. A repeat EIA measured "positive" ("pos") on D10. Ultimately, the patient developed numerous large, full-thickness, burn-like necrotic skin lesions involving feet, legs, thighs, buttocks, and torso. This patient case illustrates failure to prevent extensive acral limb and multiple central necrotizing skin lesions despite prompt institution of alternative non-heparin anticoagulation for clinically suspected HIT. In my opinion, despite the positive PF4-dependent EIA on D10, the patient almost certainly did not have HIT, based upon (1) equivocal/negative EIAs (D5, D6) despite established thrombocytopenia; (2) a clear alternative explanation for thrombocytopenia (fungemia); and (3) lack of platelet count fall when the patient inadvertently received unfractionated heparin (UFH) on D15 (during hemodialysis) and D18 (during insertion of inferior vena cava [IVC] filter); it is unlikely that "packing heparin" administered into the tubing immediately after dialysis (H) played any deleterious role. The dramatic multicentric skin necrosis probably resulted from a profound disturbance in procoagulant–anticoagulant balance, resulting from (1) disseminated intravascular DIC and (2) natural anticoagulant failure (marked AT3 depletion [note: protein C and protein S levels were not measured, but likely were also profoundly reduced]). On D7 and D8, the patient had the combination of high fibrin D–dimer levels (>60 mg/L [normal, <2.8 mg/L]) and profoundly low AT3 levels (D8 nadir, 33% of normal). The case also illustrates the issue of coagulopathy-associated confounding of PTT-adjusted argatroban therapy. The high baseline PTT (72 seconds immediately before argatroban)—likely reflecting both DIC and hepatic dysfunction—meant that subsequent (supra)therapeutic PTTs did not indicate truly "therapeutic" concentrations of argatroban.

Strategies for Managing Suspected HIT in the ICU

Given that most patients in the ICU with suspected HIT do not have HIT, this suggests that heparin is a reasonable choice for patients judged to have a low-probability of HIT, for example, a low 4 T's score of 3 or fewer points. However, there may be patients for whom *low-dose* strategies of non-heparin alternatives are appropriate. These include low-dose danaparoid (750 U SC three times a day), low-dose fondaparinux (2.5 mg SC once a day), and low-dose desirudin (15 mg SC twice a day). For patients with renal insufficiency, dosing can be reduced further: danaparoid (750 U SC twice a day); fondaparinux (2.5 mg every 2nd or 3rd day); desirudin (5 mg SC twice a day for patients with estimated creatinine clearance 31–60 mL/min/1.73 m^2 body surface area [BSA]; and 1.7 mg SC twice a day for <31 mL/min/1.73 m^2 BSA). All of these strategies represent "off-label" uses of these agents, but presumably no approval will be sought for any anticoagulant for the indication, "low likelihood of HIT but because of thrombocytopenia and the possibility of HIT we would prefer not to use UFH or LMWH."

For patients with strongly suspected (or confirmed) HIT, there are several options, including DTIs and the (AT-dependent) factor Xa inhibitors (danaparoid, fondaparinux). Although the DTIs lepirudin and argatroban are approved agents for treating HIT, there is some rational to use bivalirudin in critically ill patients, given that most of its excretion occurs through nonrenal mechanisms, primarily enzymic clearance.[69] Several reports have described its use in the critically ill patient population.[70,71] My own preference, however, is to use danaparoid (not available in the United States) in these patients because of longstanding experience in treatment of HIT, availability of antifactor Xa monitoring, and theoretical considerations discussed elsewhere.[72]

Table 3
PROTECT trial: main findings per "as-treated" analysis

Outcome	Dalteparin (N = 1827)	UFH (N = 1832)	Hazard Ratio (95% CI)	P
Proximal DVT	94 (5.1)	108 (5.9)	0.91 (0.68, 1.23)	0.54
PE (any)[a]	22 (1.2)	42 (2.3)	0.48 (0.27, 0.84)	0.01
Death (in-hospital)	396 (21.7)	446 (24.3)	0.90 (0.78, 1.04)	0.15
Bleeding (major)	100 (5.5)	105 (5.7)	0.98 (0.73, 1.31)	0.88
HIT	5 (0.3)	12 (0.7)	0.47 (0.16, 1.37)	0.17
HIT (per-protocol analysis[b])	3/1566 (0.2)	12/1561 (0.8)	0.27 (0.08, 0.98)	0.046

The as-treated protocol included all patients except those who had been excluded because consent was withdrawn, an incorrect randomization procedure was performed, or a study drug had not been administered.

[a] Includes any patient with PE classified either as "definite" (characteristic intraluminal filling defect on computed tomography of the chest, a high-probability ventilation-perfusion scan, or autopsy finding), "probable" (high clinical suspicion and either no test results or nondiagnostic results on noninvasive testing); or "possible" (clinical suspicion and nondiagnostic results on noninvasive testing).

[b] The per-protocol analysis included only patients who were not treated for a prevalent venous thromboembolism, received a study drug for at least 2 days, and had results on at least two tests for venous thromboembolism that were technically adequate.

Data from PROTECT Investigators for the Canadian Critical Care Trials Group and the Australian and New Zealand Intensive Care Society Clinical Trials Group; Cook D, Meade M, Guyatt G, et al. Dalteparin versus unfractionated heparin in critically ill patients. N Engl J Med 2011;364(14):1305–14.

PREVENTION OF HIT IN THE ICU WITH LMWH

It is widely accepted that the frequency of HIT is lower with LMWH than with UFH. However, this advantage of LMWH is well established only in surgical patients[49]; in medical patients it remains controversial whether HIT risk is similarly reduced.[73] Until recently, no data existed as to whether the reduced risk of HIT with LMWH might also be applicable to critically ill patients. Recently, the PROTECT Trial provided evidence that the frequency of HIT may be less with dalteparin than with UFH in critically ill patients.[53] The significant reduction in frequency of HIT was observed in a prespecified per-protocol analysis, which excluded patients with prevalent VTE (n = 38), or who underwent fewer than 2 ultrasound screens for DVT (n = 221), or who only received 1 day of study drug (n = 12). This analysis showed an approximate 73% relative risk reduction of HIT with dalteparin compared with UFH: 3/1566 (0.2%) versus 12/1561 (0.8%); hazard ratio, 0.27 (95% CI, 0.08–0.98); P = .046 (**Table 3**).

Although the absolute risk reduction of HIT was small (0.6%), this represents a potentially important benefit of the LMWH, dalteparin, in antithrombotic prophylaxis of critically ill patients. Further, the overall trial results (no significant reduction in proximal DVT, but a statistically significant ~50% relative risk reduction in PE [absolute risk reduction, ~1%] with dalteparin vs UFH [**Table 3**])—at comparable bleeding risk even in renally compromised patients—indicate that dalteparin use in critically ill patients likely reduces the risk of both PE and HIT, compared with UFH.

SUMMARY

Critically ill patients commonly evince thrombocytopenia, either already evident upon admission to the ICU or that develops during their ICU stay. HIT explains thrombocytopenia in only approximately 1 in 100 critically ill patients; also, for every 10 ICU patients with a positive PF4-dependent EIA, only 1 or 2 has "true" HIT. Thus, there is major potential for overdiagnosis of HIT in the ICU. A recent study showing that dalteparin is associated with a reduced frequency of HIT indicates that critically ill patients too can benefit from the HIT-reducing potential of this LMWH preparation.

ACKNOWLEDGEMENTS

Studies described in this article were supported by the Heart and Stroke Foundation of Ontario (grants A2449, T2967, B3763, T4502, T5207, NA6186, T6157, T6898, T6950).

REFERENCES

1. Hui P, Cook DJ, Lim W, et al. The frequency and clinical significance of thrombocytopenia complicating critical illness: a systematic review. Chest 2011;139(2):271–8.
2. Martin CM, Priestap F, Fisher H, et al. STAR Registry Investigators. A prospective, observational registry of patients with severe sepsis: the Canadian Sepsis Treatment and Response Registry. Crit Care Med 2009;37(1):81–8.
3. Brogly N, Devos P, Boussekey N, et al. Impact of thrombocytopenia on outcome of patients admitted to ICU for severe community-acquired pneumonia. J Infect 2007; 55(2):136–140.
4. Vanderschueren S, De Weerdt A, Malbrain M, et al. Thrombocytopenia and prognosis in intensive care. Crit Care Med 2000;28(6):1871–6.
5. Vandijck DM, Blot SI, De Waele JJ, et al. Thrombocytopenia and outcome in critically ill patients with bloodstream infection. Heart Lung 2010;39(1):21–26.

6. Caruso P, Perreira AC, Laurienzo CE, et al. Short- and long-term survival of patients with metastatic solid cancer admitted to the intensive care unit: prognostic factors. Eur J Cancer Care (Engl) 2010;19(2):260–6.

7. Stephan F, Montblanc JD, Cheffi A, et al. Thrombocytopenia in critically ill surgical patients: a case-control study evaluating attributable mortality and transfusion requirements. Crit Care 1999;3(6):151–8.

8. Moreau D, Timsit JF, Vesin A, et al. Platelet count decline: an early prognostic marker in critically ill patients with prolonged ICU stays. Chest 2007;131(6):1735–41.

9. Nijsten MWH, Nap R, Reis MD. Rate of change in platelet count is related with survival in surgical and medical ICU-patients in EURICUS-II study. Intensive Care Med 1999;25(Suppl 1):S26 [abstract 88].

10. Strauss R, Wehler M, Mehler K, et al. Thrombocytopenia in patients in the medical intensive care unit: bleeding prevalence, transfusion requirements, and outcome. Crit Care Med 2002;30(8):1765–71.

11. Shalansky SJ, Verma AK, Levine M, et al. Risk markers for thrombocytopenia in critically ill patients: a prospective analysis. Pharmacotherapy 2002;22(7):803–13.

12. Kelton JG, Sheridan D, Santos A, et al. Heparin-induced thrombocytopenia: laboratory studies. Blood 1988;72(3):925–30.

13. Warkentin TE, Elavathil LJ, Hayward CPM, et al. The pathogenesis of venous limb gangrene associated with heparin-induced thrombocytopenia. Ann Intern Med 1997; 127(9):804–12.

14. Arepally GM, Mayer IM. Antibodies from patients with heparin-induced thrombocytopenia stimulate monocytic cells to express cells to express tissue factor and secrete interleukin-8. Blood 2001;98(4):1252–4.

15. Warkentin TE. An overview of the heparin-induced thrombocytopenia syndrome. Semin Thromb Hemost 2004;30(3):273–83.

16. Warkentin TE. Management of heparin-induced thrombocytopenia: a critical comparison of lepirudin and argatroban. Thromb Res 2003;110(2/3):73–82.

17. Li ZQ, Liu W, Park KS, et al. Defining a second epitope for heparin-induced thrombocytopenia/thrombosis antibodies using KKO, a murine HIT-like monoclonal antibody. Blood 2002;99(4):1230–6.

18. Greinacher A, Gopinadhan M, Guenther JU, et al. Close approximation of two platelet factor 4 tetramers by charge neutralization forms the antigens recognized by HIT antibodies. Arterioscler Thromb Vasc Biol 2006;26(10):2386–93.

19. Warkentin TE, Hayward CPM, Boshkov LK, et al. Sera from patients with heparin-induced thrombocytopenia generate platelet-derived microparticles with procoagulant activity: an explanation for the thrombotic complications of heparin-induced thrombocytopenia. Blood 1994;84(11):3691–9.

20. Warkentin TE, Sheppard JI, Horsewood P, et al. Impact of the patient population on the risk for heparin-induced thrombocytopenia. Blood 2000;96(5):1703–8.

21. Warkentin TE. How I diagnose and manage HIT. Hematology Am Soc Hematol Educ Program 2011. [Epub ahead of print].

22. Warkentin TE, Sheppard JI, Moore JC, et al. Quantitative interpretation of optical density measurements using PF4-dependent enzyme-immunoassays. J Thromb Haemost 2008;6(8):1304–12.

23. Sheridan D, Carter C, Kelton JG. A diagnostic test for heparin-induced thrombocytopenia. Blood 1986;67(1):27–30.

24. Warkentin TE, Hayward CPM, Smith CA, et al. Determinants of donor platelet variability when testing for heparin-induced thrombocytopenia. J Lab Clin Med 1992;120(3):371–9.

25. Warkentin TE, Sheppard JI, Moore JC, et al. Laboratory testing for the antibodies that cause heparin-induced thrombocytopenia: how much class do we need? J Lab Clin Med 2005;146(6):341–6.
26. Warkentin TE, Davidson BL, Büller HR, et al. Prevalence and risk of preexisting heparin-induced thrombocytopenia antibodies in patients with acute VTE. Chest 2011; 140(2):366–73.
27. Lo GK, Sigouin CS, Warkentin TE. What is the potential for overdiagnosis of heparin-induced thrombocytopenia? Am J Hematol 2007;82(12):1037–43.
28. Levine RL, Hergenroeder GW, Francis JL, et al. Heparin-platelet factor 4 antibodies in intensive care unit patients: an observational seroprevalence study. J Thromb Thrombolysis 2010;30(2):142–8.
29. Warkentin TE, Kelton JG. Temporal aspects of heparin-induced thrombocytopenia. N Engl J Med 2001;344(17):1286–92.
30. Warkentin TE, Sheppard JI. Testing for heparin-induced thrombocytopenia antibodies. Transfus Med Rev 2006;20(4):259–72.
31. Visentin GP, Moghaddam M, Beery SE, et al. Heparin is not required for detection of antibodies associated with heparin-induced thrombocytopenia/thrombosis. J Lab Clin Med 2001;138(1):22–31.
32. Bakchoul T, Giptner A, Bein G, et al. Performance characteristics of two commercially available IgG-specific immunoassays in the assessment of heparin-induced thrombocytopenia (HIT). Thromb Res 2011;127(4):345–8.
33. Warkentin TE, Levine MN, Hirsh J, et al. Heparin-induced thrombocytopenia in patients treated with low-molecular-weight heparin or unfractionated heparin. N Engl J Med 1995;332(20):1330–5.
34. Warkentin TE, Roberts RS, Hirsh J, et al. An improved definition of immune heparin-induced thrombocytopenia in postoperative orthopedic patients. Arch Intern Med 2003;163(20):2518–24.
35. Lo GK, Juhl D, Warkentin TE, et al. Evaluation of pretest clinical score (4 T's) for the diagnosis of heparin-induced thrombocytopenia in two clinical settings. J Thromb Haemost 2006;4(4):759–65.
36. Warkentin TE, Linkins LA. Non-necrotizing heparin-induced skin lesions and the 4T's score. J Thromb Haemost 2010;8(7):1483–5.
37. Bakchoul T, Giptner A, Najaoui A, et al. Prospective evaluation of PF4/heparin immunoassays for the diagnosis of heparin-induced thrombocytopenia. J Thromb Haemost 2009;7(8):1260–5.
38. Crowther MA, Zytaruk N, Krolicki K, et al. Inter-rate reliability of the 4Ts scoring system for diagnosing heparin-induced thrombocytopenia in critically ill patients. Blood 2009;114(22):1535 [abstract 3995].
39. Chan C, Woods C, Warkentin T, et al. Inter-rater variability of the 4Ts score and Chong score for heparin-induced thrombocytopenia. Crit Care Med 2010;38(12):[abstract 675].
40. Warkentin TE. Clinical picture of heparin-induced thrombocytopenia. In: Warkentin TE, Greinacher A, editors. Heparin-induced thrombocytopenia. 4th edition. New York: Informa Healthcare USA; 2007. p. 21–66.
41. Warkentin TE, Kelton JG. A 14-year study of heparin-induced thrombocytopenia. Am J Med 1996;101(5):502–7.
42. Vella A, Nippoldt TB, Morris JC III. Adrenal hemorrhage: a 25-year experience at the Mayo Clinic. Mayo Clin Proc 2001;76(5):161–8.
43. Kovacs KA, Lam YM, Pater JL. Bilateral massive adrenal hemorrhage. Assessment of putative risk factors by the case-control method. Medicine (Balt) 2001;80(1):45–53.

44. Ling E, Warkentin TE. Intraoperative heparin flushes and subsequent acute heparin-induced thrombocytopenia. Anesthesiology 1998;89(6):1567–9.
45. Warkentin TE, Greinacher A. Heparin-induced anaphylactic and anaphylactoid reactions: two distinct but overlapping syndromes. Expert Opin Drug Saf 2009; 8(2):129–44.
46. Hillis C, Warkentin TE, Taha K, et al. Chills and limb pain following administration of low-molecular-weight heparin for treatment of acute venous thromboembolism. Am J Hematol 2011;86(7):603–6.
47. Smythe MA, Koerber JM, Mattson JC. The incidence of recognized heparin-induced thrombocytopenia in a large, tertiary care teaching hospital. Chest 2007;131(6):1644–9.
48. Lee DH, Warkentin TE. Frequency of heparin-induced thrombocytopenia. In: Warkentin TE, Greinacher A, editors. Heparin-induced thrombocytopenia. 4th edition. New York: Informa Healthcare USA; 2007. p. 67–116.
49. Warkentin TE, Sheppard JI, Sigouin CS, et al. Gender imbalance and risk factor interactions in heparin-induced thrombocytopenia. Blood 2006;108(9):2937–41.
50. Lubenow N, Hinz P, Thomaschewski S, et al. The severity of trauma determines the immune response to PF4/heparin and the frequency of heparin-induced thrombocytopenia. Blood 2010;115(9):1797–1803.
51. Verma AK, Levine M, Shalansky SJ, et al. Frequency of heparin-induced thrombocytopenia in critical care patients. Pharmacotherapy 2003;23(6):745–53.
52. Crowther MA, Cook DJ, Meade MO, et al. Thrombocytopenia in medical-surgical critically ill patients: prevalence, incidence, and risk factors. J Crit Care 2005;20(4):348–53.
53. PROTECT Investigators for the Canadian Critical Care Trials Group and the Australian and New Zealand Intensive Care Society Clinical Trials Group; Cook D, Meade M, Guyatt G, et al. Dalteparin versus unfractionated heparin in critically ill patients. N Engl J Med 2011;364(14):1305–14.
54. Pouplard C, May MA, Iochmann S, et al. Antibodies to platelet factor 4-heparin after cardiopulmonary bypass in patients anticoagulated with unfractionated heparin or a low-molecular-weight heparin. Clinical implications for heparin-induced thrombocytopenia. Circulation 1999;99(19):2530–6.
55. Pouplard C, May RA, Regina S, et al. Changes in platelet count after cardiac surgery can effectively predict the development of pathogenic heparin-dependent antibodies. Br J Haematol 2005;128(6):837–41.
56. Selleng S, Malowsky B, Strobel U, et al. Early-onset and persisting thrombocytopenia in post-cardiac surgery patients is rarely due to heparin-induced thrombocytopenia, even when antibody tests are positive. J Thromb Haemost 2010;8(1):30–6.
57. Selleng S, Selleng K, Wollert HG, et al. Heparin-induced thrombocytopenia in patients requiring prolonged intensive care unit treatment after cardiopulmonary bypass. J Thromb Haemost 2007;6(3):428–35.
58. Warkentin TE. Heparin-induced thrombocytopenia: diagnosis and management. Circulation 2004;110(18):e454–8.
59. Warkentin TE, Greinacher A, Koster A, et al. Treatment and prevention of heparin-induced thrombocytopenia. American College of Chest Physicians evidence-based clinical practice guidelines (8th edition). Chest 2008;133(6 Suppl):340S–80S.
60. Heparin Sodium Injection, USP. Available at: www.hospira.com/Files/heparin_sodium_injection.pdf. Accessed September 3, 2011.
61. Lubenow N, Eichler P, Lietz T, et al;HIT Investigators Group. Lepirudin in patients with heparin-induced thrombocytopenia – results of the third prospective study (HAT-3) and a combined analysis of HAT-1, HAT-2, and HAT-3. J Thromb Haemost 2005; 3(11):2428–36.

62. Tardy B, Lecompte T, Boelhen F, et al. Predictive factors for thrombosis and major bleeding in an observational study in 181 patients with heparin-induced thrombocytopenia treated with lepirudin. Blood 2006;108(5):1492–6.
63. Tschudi M, Lämmle B, Alberio L. Dosing lepirudin in patients with heparin-induced thrombocytopenia and normal or impaired renal function: a single-center experience with 68 patients. Blood 2009;113(11):2402–9.
64. Hoffman WD, Czyz Y, McCollum DA, et al. Reduced argatroban doses after coronary artery bypass graft surgery. Ann Pharmacother 2008;42(3):309–16.
65. Beiderlinden M, Treschan TA, Görlinger K, et al. Argatroban anticoagulation in critically ill patients. Ann Pharmacother 2007;41(5):749–54.
66. Kiser TH, Jung R, MacLaren R, et al. Evaluation of diagnostic tests and argatroban or lepirudin therapy in patients with suspected heparin-induced thrombocytopenia. Pharmacotherapy 2005;25(12):1736–45.
67. Linkins LA, Warkentin TE. Heparin-induced thrombocytopenia: real-world issues. Semin Thromb Hemost 2011;37(6):653–63.
68. Warkentin TE, Sheppard JI, Moore JC, et al. Studies of the immune response in heparin-induced thrombocytopenia. Blood 2009;113(20):4963–9.
69. Warkentin TE, Greinacher A, Koster A. Bivalirudin. Thromb Haemost 2008;99:830–9.
70. Kiser TH, Burch JC, Klem PM, et al. Safety, efficacy, and dosing requirements of bivalirudin in patients with heparin-induced thrombocytopenia. Pharmacotherapy 2008;28(9):1115–24.
71. Skrupky LP, Smith JR, Deal EN, et al. Comparison of bivalirudin and argatroban for the management of heparin-induced thrombocytopenia. Pharmacotherapy 2010;30(12): 1229–38.
72. Warkentin TE. Agents for the treatment of heparin-induced thrombocytopenia. Hematol/Oncol Clin N Am 2010;24(4):755–75.
73. Warkentin TE, Greinacher A. So, does low-molecular-weight heparin cause less heparin-induced thrombocytopenia than unfractionated heparin or not? Chest 2007; 132:1108–10.

Treatment of Pulmonary Embolism: Anticoagulation, Thrombolytic Therapy, and Complications of Therapy

Victor F. Tapson, MD[a,b]

KEYWORDS

- Venous thromboembolism • Anticoagulation
- Thrombolytic therapy • Low molecular weight heparin
- Unfractionated heparin • Catheter-directed thrombolysis

During the last two decades, considerable progress in technology and clinical research methods have led to advances in the approach to the diagnosis, prevention, and treatment of acute venous thromboembolism (VTE).[1–5] Despite this, however, the diagnosis is often delayed and preventive methods are often ignored. Thus, the morbidity and mortality associated with VTE remain high. The therapeutic approach to acute VTE is discussed, with a particular focus on the intensive care unit (ICU) setting.

The primary goal of treatment of deep vein thrombosis (DVT) is the prevention of thrombus extension and pulmonary embolism (PE). Anticoagulation is the standard of care in patients with acute VTE, but other options in the treatment of PE include thrombolytic therapy, IVC filter placement, and surgical embolectomy. Each approach has specific indications as well as advantages and disadvantages. This article focuses on pharmacologic therapy. **Table 1** lists evidence-based recommendations for VTE management as they apply to critical care. While recommendations include low molecular weight heparin (LMWH), these anticoagulants are less commonly used in the ICU because they are longer acting and less easily reversed, both of which are disadvantages in critically ill patients with acute VTE.

ANTICOAGULATION

The anticoagulation regimens for the treatment of DVT and uncomplicated PE are generally similar. Although anticoagulants do not directly dissolve preexisting clot, they prevent thrombus extension and indirectly decrease clot burden by allowing the

The author has nothing to disclose.

[a] Division of Pulmonary and Critical Care Medicine, Duke University Medical Center, Durham, NC, USA

[b] Center for Pulmonary Vascular Disease, Duke University Medical Center, Durham, NC, USA

E-mail address: Tapso001@mc.duke.edu

Crit Care Clin 27 (2011) 825–839
doi:10.1016/j.ccc.2011.08.002
0749-0704/11/$ – see front matter © 2011 Published by Elsevier Inc.

criticalcare.theclinics.com

Table 1

Initial management of venous thromboembolism

1. For patients with objectively confirmed PE, we recommend short-term treatment with SC LMWH (Grade 1A), IV UFH (Grade 1A), monitored SC UFH (Grade 1A), fixed-dose SC UFH (Grade 1A), or SC fondaparinux (Grade 1A).[a]
2. Patients with acute PE should also be routinely assessed for treatment with thrombolytic therapy.
3. For patients in whom there is a high clinical suspicion of PE, we recommend treatment with anticoagulants while awaiting the outcome of diagnostic tests (Grade 1C).
4. In patients with acute PE, we recommend initial treatment with LMWH, UFH or fondaparinux for at least 5 days and until the INR is ≥2.0 for at least 24 hours (Grade 1C).
5. In patients with DVT or PE, thrombolytic treatment (Grade 2B) and mechanical (Grade 2C) or surgical embolectomy (Grade 2C) should be reserved for selected, highly compromised patients on a case-by-case basis and not performed routinely.
6. In the absence of contraindications, systemic thrombolytic therapy may be appropriate in selected patients with massive or submassive PE (Grade 2B).

Data from Kearon C, Kahn SR, Agnelli G, et al. Antithrombotic therapy for venous thromboembolic disease. American College of Chest Physicians evidence-based clinical practice guidelines (8th Edition). Chest 2008;133:454S–54; with permission.

[a] In general, standard UFH is favored in critically ill patients with acute VTE, based upon its shorter half-life and complete reversibility with protamine.

natural fibrinolytic system to proceed unopposed. When there is a strong clinical suspicion of PE, anticoagulation should be instituted immediately and before diagnostic confirmation, unless the risk of bleeding is deemed excessive.

Unfractionated Heparin

Therapy with unfractionated heparin (UFH) reduces the extension and recurrence of symptomatic proximal DVT as well as mortality in acute PE.[1,2] UFH is usually delivered by continuous intravenous infusion and therapy is monitored by measurement of the activated partial thromboplastin time (aPTT).[3] "Traditional" or physician-directed dosing of heparin often leads to subtherapeutic aPTT results, and validated dosing nomograms are generally favored.[4,5] Nomogram dosing reduces the time to achieve therapeutic anticoagulation that may be important in reducing the risk of recurrent VTE.[6] UFH should be administered as an intravenous bolus of 5000 U followed by a continuous infusion maintenance dose of 30,000 to 40,000 U every 24 hours (the lower dose being used if the patient is considered at risk for bleeding).[7] Two alternative dosing regimens include a 5000-U bolus followed by 1280 U per hour, or a bolus of 80 U/kg followed by 18 U/kg per hour.[4,5] After initiation, the aPTT should be measured at 6-hour intervals until it is consistently in the therapeutic range of 1.5 to 2.0 times control values, which corresponds to a heparin level of 0.2 to 0.4 U/mL as measured by protamine sulfate titration.[3] Further adjustment of the UFH dose should be weight based. In patients deemed to have heparin resistance (requiring >35,000 U of UFH per day to achieve a therapeutic aPTT), antifactor Xa levels may be used to guide effective therapy.[8]

Upper extremity thrombosis is common in the critically ill patient and is most often related to a central venous catheter (CVC). These clots should generally be treated with anticoagulation, as with uncomplicated DVT, but with an additional emphasis on prompt catheter removal once the diagnosis is established. The risk of clot embolization that accompanies CVC extraction appears to be outweighed by the risk for chronic thrombotic complications and potential infection.

LMWH

Multiple clinical trials have demonstrated that LMWH is at least as safe and effective as UFH for the treatment of acute VTE.[9-11] LMWH preparations offer certain advantages over UFH, including greater bioavailability, longer half-life, lack of need for an intravenous infusion, and a more predictable anticoagulant response to weight-based dosing. LMWH can be administered subcutaneously once or twice per day and does not require monitoring of the aPTT. Monitoring antifactor Xa levels (typically 4 hours after injection) may be reasonable in certain settings such as morbid obesity, very small patients (<40 kg), pregnancy, renal insufficiency, or with unanticipated bleeding or recurrent VTE despite appropriate weight-based dosing.[11-13] LMWH is often suitable for the outpatient treatment of DVT. However, because the anticoagulant effect of UFH is short acting and can be rapidly reversed, it is generally preferred over LMWH in the ICU, where patients are at increased risk for bleeding and may be undergoing fibrinolysis or need frequent procedures.

Fondaparinux is a highly bioavailable synthetic polysaccharide derived from heparin that is effective in the initial treatment and prophylaxis for VTE.[14] Despite a more limited therapeutic niche, fondaparinux does have some advantages over LMWH. Fondaparinux does not appear to interact with platelet factor 4, so that heparin-induced thrombocytopenia (HIT), although possible, appears to be an exceedingly unlikely event. Its specificity for antifactor Xa allows for very predictable anticoagulant dosing. The anticoagulant effect of fondaparinux is not reversible. Again, in the ICU, UFH is more practical.

Warfarin

For the same reasons as LMWH and fondaparinux, warfarin therapy is less frequently used as therapeutic anticoagulation for ICU patients. Also, oral warfarin therapy must take into account many drug and food interactions, as well as genetic variations in drug metabolism. When warfarin is employed, administration should generally overlap with therapeutic heparin anticoagulation. In patients with thrombophilia (Protein C or S deficiency), warfarin may cause a transient hypercoagulable state due to the abrupt decline in vitamin K–dependent coagulation inhibitors. With warfarin therapy, it is recommended that a heparin preparation be employed for at least 5 days and maintained at a therapeutic level until two consecutive international normalized ratio (INR) values of 2.0 to 3.0 have been documented at least 24 hours apart.[15] Warfarin may ultimately be appropriate for stable ICU patients with VTE once they are on heparin or LMWH therapy.

New Oral Anticoagulants

Advances in the understanding of thrombosis have led to the development of new anticoagulant therapies.[16] Among these are dabigatran, a direct thrombin inhibitor, approved for use in the United States for prevention of stroke in atrial fibrillation, and rivaroxaban, a factor Xa inhibitor approved in the United States in mid-2011 for use in prevention of DVT in hip and knee replacement surgery.[17] A number of other similar agents are being studied and may ultimately gain approval; apixaban, another Xa inhibitor, is included among these. A disadvantage of these newer agents includes lack of reversibility. In the ICU, careful control of anticoagulation generally mandates parenteral therapy. However, clinicians will increasingly encounter patients admitted to the ICU treated with these agents.

COMPLICATIONS OF ANTICOAGULATION

Hemorrhage and HIT are the major complications of anticoagulation. A pooled analysis of 11 clinical trials involving approximately 15,000 patients treated with either UFH or LMWH reported the frequency of major bleeding at 1.9% and a fatal hemorrhage rate of 0.2%.[9] Protamine may rapidly neutralize the anticoagulant effect of UFH, although allergy, hypotension, and bradycardia are possible adverse reactions to its administration. The anticoagulant effect of LMWH is partly but not completely reversed by protamine.[3]

Although anticoagulants clearly increase the risk of bleeding, a number of factors in the ICU also increase the risk. Placement and replacement of arterial and venous catheters, and sepsis with coagulopathy and thrombocytopenia are frequent in the ICU.[18] Renal failure affects platelet function, and hepatic failure is associated with thrombocytopenia and clotting factor deficiency.[19] Intracranial hemorrhage may occur due to trauma, status after procedures, or spontaneously. Retroperitoneal hemorrhage may occur due to femoral line placement and may remain undiagnosed until there is a significant drop in hematocrit.

HIT is an antibody-mediated adverse drug reaction that may lead to venous and arterial thrombosis. The principal clinical feature of HIT syndrome is the development of an otherwise unexplained drop in platelet count (absolute thrombocytopenia or >50% decrease if the platelet nadir remains in the normal range) after exposure to heparin. HIT generally develops 5 to 10 days after the initiation of heparin, but may occur earlier in the setting of prior heparin exposure. The frequency of HIT among patients treated with heparin is variable, and depends both on the preparation (bovine UFH > porcine UFH > LMWH) and the patient population (after surgery > medical > pregnancy).[20] Although relatively infrequent, HIT is one of the most serious causes of thrombocytopenia in the ICU, and careful evaluation and consideration is warranted in this setting.[21] Lepirudin (recombinant hirudin) and argatroban are direct thrombin inhibitors that make them unique in their ability to inactivate fibrin clot–bound thrombin. They are Food and Drug Administration (FDA)-approved parenteral drugs used for the treatment of heparin-induced thrombocytopenia (HIT). This topic is addressed in a separate article.

THROMBOLYTIC THERAPY

Thrombolytic agents may accelerate thrombus resolution by activating plasminogen to form plasmin, resulting in fibrinolysis as well as fibrinogenolysis. Given the paucity of data from randomized controlled trials, there remains considerable controversy regarding the indications for thrombolytic therapy because defining the patients in whom the benefit of a rapid reduction in clot burden outweighs the increased hemorrhagic risk may be difficult.[22–25] The case for thrombolysis is the strongest in patients with massive PE complicated by shock, where the mortality rate may be more than 30%.[22] Without question, thrombolytic therapy has been shown to accelerate clot lysis in PE and lead to a more rapid resolution of abnormal right ventricular (RV) dysfunction.[26–29] Evidence of a survival benefit, however, has been generally lacking and would appear to depend on identifying a cohort of patients with a very risk of dying if lysis is not accelerated. Accepting the limitations of registry data, a recent analysis of the International Cooperative Pulmonary Embolism Registry (ICOPER) nonetheless showed that thrombolysis for massive PE did not reduce mortality or the rate of recurrent PE at 90 days.[30] Thrombolytic treatment in patients with acute submassive PE (echocardiographic evidence of RV dysfunction without hypotension) may offer no survival benefit but may prevent clinical deterioration and

Table 2	
FDA-approved thrombolytic therapy regimens for acute PE	
Drug	**Protocol**
Streptokinase	250,000 U IV (loading dose during 30 minutes); then 100,000 U/h for 24 hours
Urokinase[a]	2000 U/lb IV (loading dose during 10 minutes); then 2,000 U/lb/h for 12–24 hours
tPA[b]	100 mg IV during 2 hours

[a] Not currently available in United States (since October 2010).
[b] The American College of Chest Physicians recommends shorter infusion regimens.[40]

the need for escalation of care.[31] The decision for thrombolysis should be made on a case-by-case basis. Even in the setting of a relative contraindication, thrombolytic therapy may be reasonable when a patient is extremely unstable from life-threatening PE. It is likely that with submassive PE (ie, RV dysfunction without associated hypotension), more severe RV dysfunction, a positive troponin, severe hypoxemia, or more extensive residual DVT might be more important to study and to consider in predicting improved outcome with thrombolytics.

No clear data indicate that one thrombolytic agent is superior to another, and each of the FDA-approved thrombolytic agents is administered at a fixed dose, making measurements of coagulation unnecessary during infusion (**Table 2**). Tissue-type plasminogen activator (tPA) (2-hour infusion) is most commonly used. Shorter regimens and even bolus dosing may be favored in cases of unstable patients with massive PE. After infusion of thrombolytics, the aPTT should be measured and repeated at 4-hour intervals until the aPTT is less than twice the upper limit of normal, after which continuous intravenous UFH should be administered without a loading bolus dose. Some clinicians elect to simply continue heparin through the thrombolytic infusion. Although thrombolytics have been administered as local intrapulmonary arterial infusions, standard systemic intravenous therapy appears adequate in most cases.[30–34]

Thrombolytic therapy is contraindicated in patients at high risk for bleeding (**Table 3**). Intracranial hemorrhage is the most devastating (and often fatal) complication of

Table 3	
Contraindications to thrombolytic therapy in PE	
Absolute	**Relative**
Previous hemorrhagic stroke	Bleeding diathesis/thrombocytopenia
Intracranial surgery or pathology, including trauma	Recent major trauma, internal bleeding, or nonhemorrhagic stroke
Active internal bleeding	Uncontrolled severe hypertension
	Cardiopulmonary resuscitation
	Recent major surgery[a]
	Pregnancy

Contraindications must be individualized based upon the minimal clinical trial data examining use in these settings. Less data are available with regard to risk involved with lower doses of thrombolytics delivered by catheter-based methods.
[a] This time frame may depend on the type of surgery, associated bleeding risk, and the level of critical illness.

thrombolytic therapy and occurs in 1% to 3% of patients.[35,36] Invasive procedures should be minimized around the time of therapy to decrease the risk of bleeding. A vascular puncture above the inguinal ligament can lead to retroperitoneal hemorrhage that is often initially silent but may be life threatening. Recent data from a randomized trial by Wang and colleagues from China suggest that a lower dose of tPA (50 mg intravenously over 2 hours) is as effective but results in less bleeding.[37] Thus, this may be considered, particularly in smaller patients.

Although there is some rationale for systemic thrombolytic therapy in DVT, such use is controversial and current guidelines are generally not supportive.[36]

CATHETER-DIRECTED THERAPY FOR ACUTE PE
Background and Indications

Catheter-directed thrombolysis is increasingly common, and appears to be a safer alternative for the management of extensive, symptomatic DVT.[38] A multicenter, prospective, randomized trial is currently in progress examining the efficacy of catheter-directed thrombolysis for acute DVT.[39] The focus here is on catheter intervention for acute PE. As with systemic thrombolysis and surgical embolectomy, clinical trial data for percutaneous catheter intervention for acute PE are insufficient for formulating strong recommendations. The potential for an aggressive approach with perhaps a lower bleeding risk than with systemic thrombolysis, and the avoidance of cardiopulmonary bypass, makes these interventional approaches attractive to consider in patients who are compromised enough to meet criteria for thrombolysis or embolectomy. It was demonstrated more than two decades ago that simple infusion of a thrombolytic agent directly into the pulmonary artery offered no benefit over systemic delivery.[34] A number of investigators have, however, found that directed mechanical techniques such as suctioning or fragmentation of large proximal emboli[40] or the combined "pharmacomechanical" approach with *intraembolic* infusion of thrombolytics into such clots[40,41] might be more beneficial and potentially safer than simply infusing thrombolytics via a peripherally vein or dripping them in the pulmonary artery. The 2008 ACCP recommendations did not discuss the various techniques, but suggested the use of interventional catheterization techniques if appropriate expertise is available, in selected highly compromised patients, unable to receive thrombolytic therapy because of bleeding risk, or whose critical status does not allow sufficient time for systemic thrombolytic therapy to be effective (Grade 2C).[36] The European Society of Cardiology Task Force indicated that catheter embolectomy or fragmentation of proximal pulmonary arterial clots may be considered as an alternative to surgical treatment in high-risk PE patients when thrombolysis is absolutely contraindicated or has failed.[42]

The presence of a contraindication to systemic thrombolytics increases the practicality of a catheter-directed approach. Of 304 patients from the ICOPER who received PE systemic thrombolysis, 66 (22%) experienced major bleeding and 9 (3%) experienced intracranial bleeding.[30] No randomized controlled clinical trials have compared surgical embolectomy with catheter embolectomy.

The General Approach to Catheter-directed Embolectomy

Acute PE should be proven before the procedure; alternatively, pulmonary arteriography can be performed in the interventional radiology laboratory in a patient with a high clinical suspicion for PE who is compromised enough to prompt consideration of aggressive treatment. In patients with massive PE, the amount of contrast material should be reduced. Because most compromised patients have large proximal emboli, manual injection of 10 to 15 mL of contrast agent is generally sufficient to document

Table 4
Catheter-based embolectomy techniques that can be considered in acute PE

Technique	Examples	Manufacturer
Aspiration	Greenfield embolectomy device[a]	Boston Scientific, Watertown, MA,USA
Fragmentation	Rotatable pigtail catheter	Cook Europe, The Netherlands
Mechanical rheolysis	Amplatz device	Bard-Microvena, White Bear Lake, MN, USA
	Aspirex device[b]	Straub Medical, Wangs, Switzerland
	Hydrolyser[b]	Cordis, Warren, NJ, USA
	AngioJet[b]	Possis, Minneapolis, MN, USA
	Oasis device	Boston Scientific, Watertown, MA, USA
Local thrombolysis[a]	tPA (alteplase)	Genentech (Roche), Switzerland
	Urokinase (Abbokinase)	Abbott Laboratories, Abbott Park, IL, USA
Ultrasound	Ultrasound[b]	EKOS Corporation, Bothell, WA, USA
Angioplasty/stenting	Wallstent	Schneider Europe AG, Bülach, Switzerland;
	Gianturco Z stents	Cook Europe, Bjaerskov, Denmark

There are no large, randomized trials favoring one technique over another.
[a] More than 100 cases reported.
[b] More than 20 cases reported.

emboli. Power injection of larger volumes is generally not necessary and may be dangerous in the setting of RV failure.

Specific Catheter-directed Techniques

Regardless of which approach is utilized, expertise is required. In most hospitals, the interventional radiologist performs catheter-directed embolectomy, and the level of interest and clinical expertise is variable. The optimal embolectomy catheter should be easily maneuverable; effective at suctioning, fragmenting, or infusing a thrombolytic agent; and safe, so as to avoid pulmonary arterial/cardiac perforation and mechanical hemolysis. Catheter-based techniques that have been clinically reported are listed in **Table 4**.

Aspiration embolectomy with the Greenfield suction embolectomy catheter (Boston Scientific/Meditech; Watertown, MA, USA) was introduced in 1969[43] and it remains the only device with FDA approval specifically for acute PE. This 10 French steerable catheter has a 5 to 7 mm plastic suction cup at its tip. Major disadvantages are that it requires insertion by venotomy via the femoral or jugular vein without a guidewire and the device and embolus must be removed as a unit through the surgical venotomy. This device has been utilized effectively in extracting pulmonary emboli in up to 83% of patients, with significant improvement in hemodynamics and a 30-day mortality rate of 30%.[44] Other techniques have been studied including catheter-directed embolus fragmentation,[45–48] and catheter-based rheolysis[49–57] (each of which can be done with or without thrombolytic therapy), as well as simple catheter-directed thrombolysis.

The latter simply requires an infusion catheter and involves intrapulmonary administration of a relatively low dose of a thrombolytic agent without the addition of a mechanical device. This has been reported in a number of small studies and case reports.[58–62] As described, simply infusing thrombolytics directly into the pulmonary

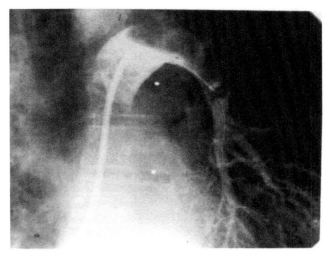

Fig. 1. Pulmonary arteriogram demonstrating large, central, pulmonary embolism (*black arrowhead*). Catheter-directed thrombolysis was performed. The guide catheter for contrast injection (*black arrow*) and infusion catheter (*white arrow*) are shown.

artery appears to offer no benefit over infusion via a peripheral vein.[34] The technique necessitates the positioning of an infusion catheter *within* the embolus, with injection of a bolus of thrombolytic drug followed by a continuous infusion.[41] The dose of intrapulmonary thrombolytic agents has generally been approximately 10% to 20% of the systemic dose. Short-acting, newer generation fibrinolytic drugs such as reteplase (2.5–5 U) or tenecteplase (5–10 mg) may be considered. A pulmonary arteriogram showing extensive proximal PE with a guide catheter and infusion catheter in place is shown in **Fig. 1**.

The mechanism for ultrasound-accelerated thrombolysis involves microstreaming and acoustic dispersion, which generates streams of high flow, consequently enhancing lytic drug infusion.[63,64]

There are no large, randomized controlled studies favoring one of these catheter-directed techniques over another.

Balloon Angioplasty and Stenting Procedures

Successful balloon angioplasty of obstructing acute emboli has been reported.[65] Too few data are available to speculate on efficacy and safety, and based on other available catheterization techniques, it is rarely undertaken. Pulmonary artery stents have been used successfully in the experimental animal model setting[66] as well as in isolated patient cases.[67] Self-expanding stents have been utilized in the setting of massive PE and failed thrombolysis or failed thrombus fragmentation.[67,68] It would appear that this approach, if used, should be reserved only in cases of acute PE in which other aggressive measures have failed.

Complications of Catheter-directed Embolectomy

Complications include those resulting from anticoagulation and contrast dye, including bleeding, contrast-induced nephropathy, and anaphylactic reactions to iodine contrast. Potential vascular access complications include bleeding, hematoma, arteriovenous fistula, and pseudoaneurysm. Major bleeding rates range from 0% to 17%.[40] Arrhythmias may occur when the catheter is advanced through the right heart. The most serious complication resulting from these catheter-directed procedures is perforation or dissection of a pulmonary artery, causing massive pulmonary hemorrhage and immediate death. The risk of perforation increases with smaller vessels.[40] Other serious complications include pericardial tamponade. To minimize the risk of perforation or dissection, embolectomy procedures should be performed only in the main and lobar pulmonary artery branches and not attempted in smaller vessels.

Device-related complications include hemorrhage and mechanical hemolysis. Acute pancreatitis due to mechanical hemolysis has been reported.[69]

Summary: Catheter-directed Embolectomy

There are no randomized, controlled data supporting catheter-based techniques but they have been used clinically with some success. Overall success rates range from 67% to 100%[40] but these rates suffer from significant potential reporting bias. Catheter-based embolectomy can be considered when systemic thrombolysis and surgical embolectomy cannot be performed. It is impossible to determine superiority of a particular catheter technique owing to the lack of comparative and randomized trial data. Many of the patients treated with fragmentation techniques have also received thrombolytic agents, making results and comparisons more difficult. At present, local expertise and familiarity with a particular device should guide the clinician when a catheter-based procedure appears indicated.

PULMONARY EMBOLECTOMY

Given the high morbidity and mortality associated with it, surgical embolectomy has traditionally been a treatment of last resort, often reserved for patients with documented central PE and refractory cardiogenic shock despite maximal therapy. Contemporary studies show improved outcomes and suggest that emergency surgical pulmonary embolectomy may be feasible in carefully selected patients and with an experienced surgical team.[70,71] Percutaneous embolectomy is a less well studied method of improving hemodynamics by reducing the burden of central pulmonary artery thromboembolism.

SPECIAL THERAPEUTIC CONSIDERATIONS: MASSIVE PE

In cases of massive PE, therapy should progress as directed by clinical likelihood and the diagnostic results. The mere suspicion of massive PE warrants immediate supportive therapy. Cautious infusion of intravenous saline may augment preload and improve impaired right ventricular function. Dopamine or norepinephrine are favored if hypotension remains, and combination therapy with dobutamine may boost right ventricular output, although it may exacerbate hypotension.[72] Supplemental oxygen and mechanical ventilation may be instituted as needed to support respiratory failure. Anticoagulation, thrombolytic therapy, and pulmonary embolectomy should be considered and employed as previously described.

VTE IN PREGNANCY

VTE is a leading cause of death in pregnant women, in whom the age-adjusted risk of VTE is at least five times higher compared to nonpregnant women.[73,74] DVT is more common during the antepartum period, and occurs with almost equal frequency in each of the three trimesters. In contrast, the incidence of PE is highest immediately post partum.

Therapy for VTE in pregnancy is generally similar to that in nonpregnant women, except that warfarin should be avoided because it is teratogenic and can cross the placental barrier. LMWH has been shown to be safe in pregnancy and is often preferred as long-term therapy; warfarin may be employed post partum.[75] Because of the risk of maternal hemorrhage and fetal demise, pregnancy is a relative contraindication for thrombolytic therapy. That being considered, controlled trials are lacking in this area, and thrombolysis may rarely be appropriate in cases of massive PE with hemodynamic instability.

NONTHROMBOTIC PULMONARY EMBOLI

While thrombotic PE is the most common and important syndrome in which embolic material reach the pulmonary circulation, nonthrombotic pulmonary emboli may rarely occur in several clinical settings. Fat embolism syndrome most commonly occurs after blunt trauma complicated by long-bone fractures. The characteristic findings of dyspnea, axillary and subconjunctival petechiae, and alterations in mental status generally occur between 12 and 48 hours after the primary event.[76] Cardiopulmonary derangement is likely due to venous obstruction by neutral fat and to a vasculitis and capillary leak syndrome caused by free fatty acids. The diagnosis of fat embolization syndrome is clinical; however, the identification of fat droplets within cells recovered by bronchoalveolar lavage may be helpful.[77] Therapy is generally prophylactic and supportive as more specific treatments have shown limited benefit. The syndrome is usually mild and the prognosis good.

Amniotic fluid embolism is uncommon but it represents one of the leading causes of maternal death in the United States.[78] The condition may occur during or shortly after either spontaneous or cesarean delivery and there exist no consistent identifiable risk factors. Clinical hallmarks include hypoxemia, cardiogenic shock, altered mental status, and disseminated intravascular coagulation. The diagnosis is clinical and the therapy is primarily supportive. Amniotic fluid embolism is frequently fatal and permanent neurologic deficits are found in 85% of survivors. Septic emboli generally present as multiple bilateral peripheral nodules that are often poorly marginated and may have cavitary changes. Right-sided endocarditis and septic thrombophlebitis are the most common sources of septic pulmonary emboli.[79] Fever, chills, and pleuritic chest pain may be more impressive in septic PE as compared with bland PE. Treatment centers on appropriate antibiotic therapy, but anticoagulation and surgical management may be appropriate in certain circumstances. Intensive care is generally not necessary unless there is significant associated cardiopulmonary dysfunction.

Air embolism requires communication between the air and the venous circulation when venous blood pressure is below atmospheric pressure. Predisposing settings include invasive procedures, barotrauma, and the use of indwelling catheters. Air may gain entry into the arterial system by incomplete filtering of a large air embolus by the pulmonary capillaries or via paradoxical embolization through a patent foramen ovale.[80] The clinical picture is critical in raising the suspicion of disease because the signs and symptoms are generally nonspecific. Immediate Trendelenburg and left lateral decubitus positioning may open an obstructed RV outflow tract, and air aspiration should be attempted if there is a central venous catheter in the right atrium. Administration of 100% oxygen aids in bubble reabsorption via nitrogen washout, and hyperbaric oxygen therapy may also be beneficial.

Other miscellaneous nonthrombotic causes of pulmonary vascular obstruction include cancer cells, schistosomal disease, and inorganic injected material such as talc crystals or various fibers.

REFERENCES

1. Hull RD, Raskob GE, Hirsh J, et al. Continuous intravenous heparin compared with intermittent subcutaneous heparin in the initial treatment of proximal-vein thrombosis. N Engl J Med 1986;315:1109–14.
2. Barritt DW, Jordan SC. Anticoagulant drugs in the treatment of pulmonary embolism. A controlled trial. Lancet 1960;1:1309–12.
3. Hirsh J, Warkentin TE, Shaughnessy SG, et al. Heparin and low-molecular-weight heparin: mechanisms of action, pharmacokinetics, dosing, monitoring, efficacy, and safety. Chest 2001;119(1 Suppl):64S–94S.
4. Cruickshank MK, Levine MN, Hirsh J, et al. A standard heparin nomogram for the management of heparin therapy. Arch Intern Med 1991;151:333–7.
5. Raschke RA, Reilly BM, Guidry JR, et al. The weight-based heparin dosing nomogram compared with a "standard care" nomogram. A randomized controlled trial. Ann Intern Med 1993;119:874–81.
6. Hull RD, Raskob GE, Brant RF, et al. Relation between the time to achieve the lower limit of the APTT therapeutic range and recurrent venous thromboembolism during heparin treatment for deep vein thrombosis. Arch Intern Med 1997;157:2562–8.
7. Hull RD, Raskob GE, Rosenbloom D, et al. Optimal therapeutic level of heparin therapy in patients with venous thrombosis. Arch Intern Med 1992;152:1589–95.
8. Levine MN, Hirsh J, Gent M, et al. A randomized trial comparing activated thromboplastin time with heparin assay in patients with acute venous thromboembolism requiring large daily doses of heparin. Arch Intern Med 1994;154:49.
9. Gould MK, Dembitzer AD, Doyle RL, et al. Low-molecular-weight heparins compared with unfractionated heparin for treatment of acute deep venous thrombosis. A meta-analysis of randomized, controlled trials. Ann Intern Med 1999;130:800–9.
10. Dolovich LR, Ginsberg JS, Douketis JD, et al. A meta-analysis comparing low-molecular-weight heparins with unfractionated heparin in the treatment of venous thromboembolism: examining some unanswered questions regarding location of treatment, product type, and dosing frequency. Arch Intern Med 2000;160:181–8.
11. Weitz JI. Low-molecular-weight heparins. N Engl J Med 1997;337:688–98.
12. Wilson SJ, Wilbur K, Burton E, et al. Effect of patient weight on the anticoagulant response to adjusted therapeutic dosage of low-molecular-weight heparin for the treatment of venous thromboembolism. Haemostasis 2001;31:42–8.
13. Nagge J, Crowther M, Hirsh J. Is impaired renal function a contraindication to the use of low-molecular-weight heparin? Arch Intern Med 2002;162:2605–9.
14. Buller HR, Davidson BL, Decousus H, et al. Fondaparinux or enoxaparin for the initial treatment of symptomatic deep venous thrombosis: a randomized trial. Ann Intern Med 2004;140:867–73.
15. Ansell J, Hirsh J, Poller L, et al. The pharmacology and management of the vitamin K antagonists: the Seventh ACCP Conference on Antithrombotic and Thrombolytic Therapy. Chest 2004;126(3 Suppl):204S–33S.
16. Weitz JI, Bates SM. New anticoagulants. J Thromb Haemost 2005;3:1843–53.
17. Rybak I, Ehle M, Buckley L, et al. Efficacy and safety of novel anticoagulant compared with established agents. Therapeutic Advances in Hematology doi: 10.1177/2040620711408489.
18. Crowther MA, Cook DJ, Meade MO, et al. Thrombocytopenia in medical-surgical critically ill patients: prevalence, incidence, and risk factors. J Crit Care 2005;20:348–53.
19. Redei I, Rubin RN. Techniques for evaluating the cause of bleeding in the ICU. Diagnostic clues and keys to interpreting hemostatic tests. J Crit Illn 1995;10:133–7.

20. Warkentin TE, Greinacher A. Heparin-induced thrombocytopenia: recognition, treatment, and prevention: the Seventh ACCP Conference on Antithrombotic and Thrombolytic Therapy. Chest 2004;126(3 Suppl):311S–37S.

21. Warkentin TE, Cook DJ. Heparin, low molecular weight heparin, and heparin-induced thrombocytopenia in the ICU. Crit Care Clin 2005;21:513–29.

22. Dalen JE, Alpert JS, Hirsh J. Thrombolytic therapy for pulmonary embolism: is it effective? Is it safe? When is it indicated? Arch Intern Med 1997;157:2550–6.

23. Agnelli G, Becattini C, Kirschstein T. Thrombolysis vs heparin in the treatment of pulmonary embolism: a clinical outcome-based meta-analysis. Arch Intern Med 2002;162:2537–41.

24. Dalen JE. The uncertain role of thrombolytic therapy in the treatment of pulmonary embolism. Arch Intern Med 2002;162:2521–3.

25. Wan S, Quinlan DJ, Agnelli G, et al. Thrombolysis compared with heparin for the initial treatment of pulmonary embolism: a meta-analysis of the randomized controlled trials. Circulation 2004;110:744–9.

26. Levine M, Hirsh J, Weitz J, et al. A randomized trial of a single bolus dosage regimen of recombinant tissue plasminogen activator in patients with acute pulmonary embolism. Chest 1990;98:1473–9.

27. Tissue plasminogen activator for the treatment of acute pulmonary embolism. A collaborative study by the PIOPED Investigators. Chest 1990;97:528.

28. Dalla-Volta S, Palla A, Santolicandro A, et al. PAIMS 2: alteplase combined with heparin versus heparin in the treatment of acute pulmonary embolism. Plasminogen activator Italian multicenter study 2. J Am Coll Cardiol 1992;20:520–6.

29. Goldhaber SZ, Haire WD, Feldstein ML, et al. Alteplase versus heparin in acute pulmonary embolism: randomised trial assessing right-ventricular function and pulmonary perfusion. Lancet 1993;341:507–11.

30. Goldhaber SZ, Visni L, De Rosa M. Acute pulmonary embolism: clinical outcomes in the International Cooperative Pulmonary Embolism Registry (ICOPER). Lancet 1999; 353,1386–9.

31. Konstantinides S, Geibel A, Heusel G, et al. Heparin plus alteplase compared with heparin alone in patients with submassive pulmonary embolism. N Engl J Med 2002;347:1143–50.

32. The UKEP Study Research Group. The UKEP study: multicentre clinical trial on two local regimens of urokinase in massive pulmonary embolism. Eur Heart J 1987;8:2.

33. Leeper KV Jr, Popovich J Jr, Lesser BA, et al. Treatment of massive acute pulmonary embolism. The use of low doses of intrapulmonary arterial streptokinase combined with full doses of systemic heparin. Chest 1988;93:234–40.

34. Verstraete M, Miller GA, Bounameaux H, et al. Intravenous and intrapulmonary recombinant tissue-type plasminogen activator in the treatment of acute massive pulmonary embolism. Circulation 1988;77:353–60.

35. Kanter DS, Mikkola KM, Patel SR, et al. Thrombolytic therapy for pulmonary embolism. Frequency of intracranial hemorrhage and associated risk factors. Chest 1997; 111:1241–5.

36. Kearon C, Kahn SR, Agnelli G, et al. Antithrombotic therapy for venous thromboembolic disease. American College of Chest Physicians evidence-based clinical practice guidelines. 8th edition. Chest 2008;133:454S–545S.

37. Wang C, Zhai Z, Yang Y, et al. Efficacy and safety of low dose recombinant tissue-type plasminogen activator for the treatment of acute pulmonary thromboembolism: a randomized, multicenter, controlled trial. Chest 2010;137:254–62.

38. Mewissen MW, Seabrook GR, Meissner MH, et al. Catheter-directed thrombolysis for lower extremity deep venous thrombosis: report of a national multicenter registry. Radiology 1999;211:39–49.
39. Acute venous thrombosis: thrombus removal with adjunctive catheter-directed thrombolysis (ATTRACT). Available at: http://clinicaltrials.gov/ct2/show/NCT00790335. Accessed April 10, 2011.
40. Kucher N. Catheter embolectomy for acute pulmonary embolism. Chest 2007;132: 657–63.
41. Tapson VF, Gurbel PA, Stack RS. Pharmacomechanical thrombolysis of experimental pulmonary emboli: rapid low-dose intraembolic therapy. Chest 1994;106:1558–62.
42. Torbicki A, Perrier A, Konstantinides S, et al. Guidelines on the diagnosis and management of acute pulmonary embolism. The Task Force for the Diagnosis and Management of Acute Pulmonary Embolism of the European Society of Cardiology (ESC). Eur Heart J 2008;29:2276–315.
43. Greenfield LJ, Greenfield LJ, Kimmell GO, et al. Transvenous removal of pulmonary emboli by vacuum-cup catheter technique. J Surg Res 1969;9:347–52.
44. Greenfield LJ, Proctor MC, Williams DM, et al. Long-term experience with transvenous catheter pulmonary embolectomy. J Vasc Surg 1993;18:450–7.
45. Brady AJ, Crake T, Oakley CM. Percutaneous catheter fragmentation and distal dispersion of proximal pulmonary embolus. Lancet 1991;338:1186–9.
46. Brady AJ, Crake T, Oakley CM. Percutaneous catheter fragmentation and distal dispersion of proximal pulmonary embolus. Lancet 1991;338:1186–9.
47. Kucher N, Windecker S, Banz Y, et al. Percutaneous catheter thrombectomy device for acute pulmonary embolism: in vitro and in vivo testing. Radiology 2005;236: 852–8.
48. Schmitz-Rode T, Janssens U, Schild HH, et al. Fragmentation of massive pulmonary embolism using a pigtail rotation catheter. Chest 1998;114:1427–36.
49. Schmitz-Rode T, Janssen U, Duda SH, et al. Massive pulmonary embolism: percutaneous emergency treatment by pigtail rotation catheter. J Am Coll Cardiol 2000;36: 375–80.
50. Müller-Hülsbeck S, Brossmann J, Jahnke T, et al. Mechanical thrombectomy of major and massive pulmonary embolism with use of the Amplatz thrombectomy device. Invest Radiol 2001;36:317–22.
51. Erne P, Yamshidi P. Percutaneous aspiration of inverior vena cava thrombus. J Invasive Cardiol 2006;18:E149–51.
52. Fava M, Loyola S, Huete I. Massive pulmonary embolism: treatment with the hydrolyser thrombectomy catheter. J Vasc Interv Radiol 2000;11:1159–64.
53. Reekers JA, Baarslag HJ, Koolen MG, et al. Mechanical thrombectomy for early treatment of massive pulmonary embolism. Cardiovasc Intervent Radiol 2003;26: 246–50.
54. Michalis LK, Tsetis DK, Rees MR. Case report: percutaneous removal of pulmonary artery thrombus in a patient with massive pulmonary embolism using the hydrolyser catheter; the first human experience. Clin Radiol 1997;52:158–61.
55. Siablis D, Karnabatidis D, Katsanos K, et al. AngioJet rheolytic thrombectomy versus local intrapulmonary thrombolysis in massive pulmonary embolism: a retrospective data analysis. J Endovasc Ther 2005;12:206–14.
56. Margheri M, Vittori G, Vecchio S, et al. Early and long-term clinical results of AngioJet rheolytic thrombectomy in patients with acute pulmonary embolism. Am J Cardiol 2008;101(2):252–8.

57. Angiojet rheolytic thrombectomy in case of massive pulmonary embolism. An ongoing clinical trial. Available at: http://clinicaltrials.gov/ct2/show/NCT00780767. Accessed April 12, 2011.
58. Fava M, Loyola S, Bertoni H, et al. Massive pulmonary embolism: percutaneous mechanical thrombectomy during cardiopulmonary resuscitation. J Vasc Interven Radiol 2005;16:119–23.
59. Eid-Lidt G, Gaspar J, Sandoval J, et al. Combined clot fragmentation and aspiration in patients with acute pulmonary embolism. Chest 2008;134:54–60.
60. Vujic I, Young JWR, Gobien RP, et al. Massive pulmonary embolism treatment with full heparinization and topical low-dose streptokinase. Radiology 1983;148:671–5.
61. Gonzales-Juanatey JR, Valdes L, Amaro A, et al. Treatment of massive pulmonary thromboembolism with low intrapulmonary dosages of urokinase: short term angiographic and hemodynamic evolution. Chest 1992;102:341–6.
62. Molina HE, Hunter DW, Yedlick JW, et al. Thrombolytic therapy for post operative pulmonary embolism. Am J Surg 1992;163,375–81.
63. Kelly P, Carroll N, Grant C, et al. Successful treatment of massive pulmonary embolism with prolonged catheter-directed thrombolysis. Heart and Vessels 2006; 21:124–6.
64. Lin P, Annambhotla S, Bechara CF, et al. Comparison of percutaneous ultrasound-accelerated thrombolysis versus catheter-directed thrombolysis in patients with acute massive pulmonary embolism. Vascular 2009;17(Suppl 3):S137–47.
65. Stambo GW, Montague B. Bilateral EKOS EndoWave™ catheter thrombolysis of acute bilateral pulmonary embolism in a hemodynamically unstable patient. South Med J 2010;3(5):455–7.
66. Handa K, Sasaki Y, Kiyonaga A, et al. Acute pulmonary thromboembolism treated successfully by balloon angioplasty: a case report. Angiology 1988;8:775–8.
67. Schmitz-Rode T, Verma R, Pfeffer JG, et al. Temporary pulmonary stent placement as emergency treatment of pulmonary embolism: first experimental evaluation. J Am Coll Cardiol 2006;48:812–6.
68. Haskal ZJ, Soulen MC, Huetti EA, et al. Life-threatening pulmonary emboli and cor pulmonale: treatment with percutaneous pulmonary artery stent placement. Radiology 1994;191:473–5.
69. Koizumi J, Kusano S, Akima T, et al. Emergent Z stent placement for treatment of cor pulmonale due to pulmonary emboli after failed lytic treatment: technical considerations. Cardiovasc Intervent Radiol 1998;21:254–5.
70. Danetz JS, McLafferty RB, Ayerdi J, et al. Pancreatitis caused by rheolytic thrombolysis: an unexpected complication. J Vasc Interv Radiol 2004;15:857–60.
71. Aklog L, Williams CS, Byrne JG, et al. Acute pulmonary embolectomy: a contemporary approach. Circulation 2002;105:1416–9.
72. Yalamanchili K, Fleisher AG, Lehrman SG, et al. Open pulmonary embolectomy for treatment of major pulmonary embolism. Ann Thorac Surg 2004;77:819–23.
73. Tapson VF, Witty LA. Massive pulmonary embolism. Diagnostic and therapeutic strategies. Clin Chest Med 1995;16:329–40.
74. Douketis JD, Kearon C, Bates S, et al. Risk of fatal pulmonary embolism in patients with treated venous thromboembolism. JAMA 1998;279:458–62.
75. Toglia MR, Weg JG. Venous thromboembolism during pregnancy. N Engl J Med 1996;335:108–14.
76. Fabian TC, Unravelling the fat embolism syndrome. N Engl J Med 1993;329: 961–3.

77. Chastre J, Fagon JY, Soler P, et al. Bronchoalveolar lavage for rapid diagnosis of the fat embolism syndrome in trauma patients. Ann Intern Med 1990;113:583–8.

78. Clark SL, Hankins GD, Dudley DA, et al. Amniotic fluid embolism: analysis of the national registry. Am J Obstet Gynecol 1995;172(4 Pt 1):1158–67.

79. Fred HL, Harle TS. Septic pulmonary embolism. Dis Chest 1969;55:483–6.

80. O'Quin RJ, Lakshminarayan S. Venous air embolism. Arch Intern Med 1982;142:2173–6.

Diagnostic Approach to Deep Venous Thrombosis and Pulmonary Embolism in the Critical Care Setting

Marisa Magaña, MD*, Robert Bercovitch, MD, Peter Fedullo, MD

KEYWORDS

- Pulmonary embolism • Venous thrombosis • Critical care
- Computed tomography • Ventilation–perfusion scanning
- Clinical prediction rules

Estimates of the incidence and case-fatality rates of venous thromboembolism in the United States vary widely owing to limitations in the accuracy of clinical diagnosis and the dearth of autopsy data. Even the most conservative estimate, however, would suggest an incidence of 200,000 episodes of venous thromboembolism annually in the United States, resulting in approximately 30,000 to 50,000 deaths.[1,2]

Considerable progress has been made during the last 30 years in the prevention, diagnosis, and therapy of the disease. Its epidemiology has been investigated and both clinical and genetic risk factors have been identified, defining patient groups at risk.[3,4] Effective methods of venous thrombosis prophylaxis have been evaluated in a wide range of patient populations, and recommendations for their application have been widely disseminated.[5] Noninvasive diagnostic techniques for venous thrombosis and pulmonary embolism (PE) have been developed and carefully validated against the traditional diagnostic "gold standards," contrast venography and pulmonary angiography.[6–8] Objective clinical prediction rules, capable of defining the pretest probability of disease and guiding subsequent diagnostic and therapeutic decisions, have been derived and validated.[9,10] Therapeutic guidelines for acute thromboembolic disease as well as for postthrombotic prophylaxis have been developed and new therapeutic agents have been introduced into clinical practice.[11]

Although embolism-related mortality appears to have been favorably influenced by these advances, venous thromboembolism remains a major and often unexpected cause of death in hospitalized patients.[12,13] The prevention, diagnosis, and management of venous thromboembolism in critically ill patients pose unique challenges. In this population, the utilization of pharmacologic thromboprophylaxis can be problematic because

Division of Pulmonary and Critical Care Medicine, Department of Medicine, University of California, San Diego, 200 West Arbor Drive, San Diego, CA 92103, USA
* Corresponding author.
E-mail address: mmmagana@ucsd.edu

Crit Care Clin 27 (2011) 841–867
doi:10.1016/j.ccc.2011.08.003
0749-0704/11/$ – see front matter

of active bleeding or perceived bleeding risk. Clinical prediction rules, diagnostic algorithms, and exclusionary studies such as D-dimer testing applicable to ambulatory or noncritically ill patients are poorly transferable to those who are critically ill. The usual presenting symptoms and signs of venous thromboembolism in intensive care unit (ICU) patients are commonly present or masked by elements of the underlying disease. Safety concerns regarding the administration of contrast agents in patients with compromised cardiac or renal function and the complexities of safe transportation can become determining factors in the diagnostic approach. As a result, management decisions in critically ill patients with suspected embolism are often empiric, based on incomplete clinical data and the assumed risk of anticoagulant therapy in the individual patient.

The overwhelming majority of deaths from PE are the result of diagnostic oversight associated with the often subtle, nonspecific presentation of the disease, especially in hospitalized patients, and not a failure of existing therapeutic options.[14,15] Therefore, any discussion of diagnostic approach must include a review of basic concepts related to venous thromboembolism.

EPIDEMIOLOGY

Surprisingly little data are available regarding the incidence of venous thromboembolism and its impact on outcome in critically ill patients. Incidence estimates vary widely and range from 5% to 25%.[16–19] This wide estimate range reflects the different populations studied, the rate and type of thromboprophylaxis provided, and the diagnostic criteria used to confirm the presence of the disease.

Most critically ill patients have one or more recognizable risk factors for venous thromboembolism. The risk imposed by a major surgical procedure is well recognized. Without prophylaxis, venous thrombosis occurs after approximately 20% of all major surgical procedures with associated embolism after 1% to 2% of such procedures.[20] The incidence of thromboembolism without prophylaxis is even higher in orthopedic patients, with more than 50% of major orthopedic procedures complicated by venous thrombosis.[21] In the absence of prophylaxis, the frequency of fatal postoperative PE ranges from 0.1% to 0.4% in patients undergoing elective general surgery and from 1% to 5% in patients undergoing elective hip or knee surgery, emergency hip surgery, major trauma, or spinal cord injury.

Recent data have demonstrated that the risk of venous thromboembolism in medical patients in the absence of prophylaxis approximates 15%, comparable to that in moderate risk surgical patients.[22] In the nonsurgical population, a number of risk factors common to an ICU population have been identified as increasing thrombotic risk and include advancing age, cancer, prolonged immobilization, prior venous thromboembolism, ischemic stroke, myocardial infarction, congestive heart failure, chronic obstructive pulmonary disease, chronic inflammatory disease, and acute infectious disease.[23] A recent meta-analysis suggested that 25% of patients with chronic obstructive pulmonary disease who require hospitalization for an acute exacerbation of their lung disease may have PE.[24]

The use of thromboprophylaxis is capable of substantially reducing the risk of venous thrombosis, proximal vein thrombosis, and fatal PE in both medical and surgical populations.[5] It is important to recognize, however, that it does not eliminate the possibility. Although only limited data are available in critically ill patients, pharmacologic prophylaxis with unfractionated heparin (UFH) or a low molecular weight heparin (LMWH) in general surgical and medical patients appears to result in a 60% to 70% risk reduction for venous thrombosis and fatal PE. A large international trial comparing the efficacy of UFH with dalteparin in a critically ill population demonstrated an overall thrombosis rate of 5.5%. Dalteparin was not superior to UFH in decreasing the incidence of proximal deep venous thrombosis (DVT).[25] Initiation of the diagnostic sequence, therefore, should not be dissuaded by the concurrent use of prophylaxis.

PATHOPHYSIOLOGY

The effect of PE on oxygenation and hemodynamics depends on the extent of obstruction of the pulmonary vascular bed and the severity of underlying cardiopulmonary disease. Hypoxemia develops in the preponderance of patients with PE and has been attributed to various mechanisms including intrapulmonary or intracardiac right-to-left shunting, elevated alveolar dead space, regional perfusion redistribution with associated ventilation–perfusion (V/Q) inequality, and decreases in the mixed venous O_2 level, which magnifies the effect of the normal venous admixture.[26-31] The two latter mechanisms are proposed to account for the majority of hypoxemia and hypocarbia associated with acute embolism. Shunt can occur due to atelectasis related to loss of surfactant, alveolar hemorrhage, or from bronchoconstriction related to regional areas of hypocarbia. Hypoxemia leads to an increase in sympathetic tone, with systemic vasoconstriction, and may actually increase venous return with augmentation of stroke volume, at least initially, if there is no significant underlying cardiac or pulmonary pathology already present.

The creation of alveolar dead space and depression of cardiac output associated with embolism may also result in a reduction in end-tidal carbon dioxide ($etco_2$) and an increase in the arterial-$etco_2$ gradient.[32]

The hemodynamic effects of embolism are related to the degree of reduction of the cross-sectional area of the pulmonary vascular bed, the preexisting status of the cardiopulmonary system, and the physiologic consequences of both hypoxic and neurohumorally mediated vasoconstriction.[33-37] Obstruction of the pulmonary vascular bed by embolism acutely increases the workload on the right ventricle (RV), a chamber ill equipped to deal with high pressure load. In patients without preexisting cardiopulmonary disease, obstruction of less than 20% of the pulmonary vascular bed results in a number of compensatory events that minimize adverse hemodynamic consequences. Recruitment and distension of pulmonary vessels occur, resulting in a normal or near-normal pulmonary artery pressure and pulmonary vascular resistance; cardiac output is maintained by increases in the RV stroke volume and increases in the heart rate. As the degree of pulmonary vascular obstruction exceeds 30% to 40%, increases in pulmonary artery pressure and modest increases in right atrial pressure occur. The Frank–Starling mechanism maintains RV stroke work and cardiac output. When the degree of pulmonary artery obstruction exceeds 50% to 60%, compensatory mechanisms are overcome, cardiac output begins to fall, and right atrial pressure increases dramatically. With acute obstruction beyond this amount, the right heart dilates, RV wall tension increases, RV ischemia may develop, the cardiac output falls, and systemic hypotension develops. In patients without prior cardiopulmonary disease, the maximal *mean* pulmonary artery pressure capable of being generated by the RV appears to be 40 mm Hg. The correlation between the extent of pulmonary vascular obstruction and the pulmonary vascular resistance is hyperbolic, reflecting at its lower end the expansible nature of the pulmonary vascular bed and at its upper the precipitous decline in cardiac output that may occur as the RV fails.

The hemodynamic response to acute PE in patients with preexisting cardiopulmonary disease, a population common in the critical care setting, is considerably different.[35] Patients with cardiopulmonary disease demonstrate degrees of pulmonary hypertension that are disproportionate to the degree of pulmonary vascular obstruction. As a result, severe pulmonary hypertension and subsequent RV failure may develop in response to a relatively small reduction in pulmonary artery cross-sectional area. In critically ill patients with limited cardiopulmonary reserve even a small embolic event might have severe or fatal hemodynamic consequences.

CLINICAL PRESENTATION

The acceptance of venous thrombosis and PE as manifestations of a common disease process represented a major conceptual advance in our understanding of the natural history of venous thromboembolism. The often silent nature of lower extremity venous thrombosis along with the often dramatic presentation of PE tended to obscure the unitary nature of the disease and to focus attention on the complication, rather than the origin, of the underlying process. Although the overwhelming majority of pulmonary emboli arise from thrombi in the deep veins of the lower extremity, emboli may arise from other sites. Thrombi can develop in the pelvic and periprostatic veins, the renal veins, and the right cardiac chamber. The increasing use of central venous catheters and transvenous pacing devices has resulted in an increased incidence of venous thrombosis involving the veins of the upper extremities.

Physical examination findings in symptomatic venous thrombosis depend on the extent of vascular obstruction as well as the degree of inflammation and include pain, erythema, warmth, and swelling of the involved extremity. Individual clinical features, used in isolation, have limited diagnostic value.[10] In as many as 50% to 85% of patients with clinical signs and symptoms suggestive of venous thrombosis the diagnosis will not be confirmed by objective testing.[38,39] Alternatively, screening studies in high-risk populations have demonstrated that a substantial number of lower extremity venous thrombi will not be apparent clinically.[40] Crowther and colleagues, in a study of 261 critically ill patients, found that 25 developed proximal venous thrombosis confirmed by ultrasonography during their ICU stay. Only 3 of these 25 (12%) were suspected based on signs or symptoms before ultrasonographic confirmation.[18,41]

The clinical presentation of PE varies widely, ranging from limited symptoms to cardiogenic shock. The presenting syndromes of PE were characterized in the Prospective Investigation of Pulmonary Embolism Diagnosis (PIOPED) and PIOPED II trials and included: (1) the pulmonary infarction syndrome with hemoptysis or pleuritic pain or both, which occurred in 65% of patients in PIOPED and 44% in PIOPED II; (2) the isolated dyspnea syndrome, which occurred in 22% of patients in PIOPED and in 36% of patients in PIOPED II; and (3) the circulatory collapse syndrome with shock or syncope or both, which occurred in 8% of patients in both PIOPED and PIOPED II.[42,43] Although such a classification has merit, it likely understates the incidence of uncomplicated PE events. The clinical presentation of PE may often be atypical and embolic episodes may occur with minimal clinical effect. At least one third of patients with proximal venous thrombosis have PE in the absence of pulmonary symptoms.[44]

Among patients without preexisting cardiac or pulmonary disease in PIOPED II, dyspnea either at rest or with exertion occurred in 73% of patients. Other prominent symptoms included pleuritic chest pain (44%), nonpleuritic chest pain (19%), cough (34%), and edema (41%). Tachypnea, defined as a respiratory rate of 20 breaths/min, was present in 54% of patients without preexisting cardiopulmonary disease. Other physical findings included tachycardia (24%), an abnormal cardiac examination (21%), rales (18%), and decreased breath sounds (17%). Fewer than half of the patients had clinical evidence of venous thrombosis (edema, erythema, tenderness, or a palpable cord). Fever, defined as a temperature greater than 37.8°C (100 °F), has been reported in 14% of patients with embolism.[45]

The clinical diagnosis of venous thromboembolism is especially problematic in critically ill patients in whom the usual presenting symptoms, signs, and laboratory/imaging findings may be obscured by elements of a patient's underlying disease or attributed to any of the myriad cardiopulmonary derangements that accompany an ICU stay. Berlot and colleagues published an autopsy series of 600 patients who died in an ICU that highlights the scope of the problem.[16] In this series, the overall incidence of embolism confirmed at autopsy was 14.3%. In 33 patients with the antemortem clinical diagnosis of embolism, only 39% had autopsy confirmation of that diagnosis. Of the 86 patients with autopsy-confirmed embolism, the diagnosis was considered clinically in 13 patients (15%) and discovered only at autopsy in the remainder. Of the 73 patients in whom the diagnosis was not clinically considered, embolism was considered the cause of death in 45%.

These precautionary statements regarding clinical diagnosis are meant as a reminder that the clinical presentation of PE, rather than being a dramatic event as commonly perceived, may be atypical or subtle and should serve to generate a suspicion of that diagnosis. A reliance on presenting symptoms and signs that are considered to be "classic" before making the decision to proceed to objective testing will ultimately lead to underdiagnosis and avoidable mortality.

DIAGNOSTIC OPTIONS: DVT
Clinical Prediction Rules

The most widely used clinical prediction rule for DVT is the Wells score, which uses a combination of clinical features to assess the pretest probability of DVT (**Table 1**). The Wells score was initially proposed in 1995, then revised and incorporated into a diagnostic algorithm in 1997.[46] The original score utilized nine clinical criteria to stratify patients into low, moderate, or high likelihood of having DVT. The score was modified further in 2003 by adding an item for a prior history of documented DVT and

Table 1 Revised Wells score for DVT	
Variable	**Points**
Active cancer (treatment ongoing or within the previous 6 months or palliative)	+ 1
Paralysis, paresis, or recent plaster immobilization of the lower extremities	+ 1
Recently bedridden for >3 days or major surgery within 4 weeks	+ 1
Localized tenderness along the distribution of the deep venous system	+ 1
Entire leg swollen	+ 1
Calf swelling by >3 cm when compared to the asymptomatic leg (measured below tibial tuberosity)	+ 1
Pitting edema (greater in the symptomatic leg)	+ 1
Collateral superficial veins (nonvaricose)	+ 1
Previously document DVT	+ 1
Alternate diagnosis as likely or greater than DVT	− 2
Low risk: ≤0 points	
Intermediate risk: 1 or 2 points	
High risk: ≥3 points	

Data from Engelberger RP, Aujesky D, Calanca L, et al. Comparison of the diagnostic performance of the original and modified Wells score in inpatients and outpatients with suspected deep vein thrombosis. Thromb Res 2011;127:535–9.

stratifying the patients into two categories: DVT-likely and DVT-unlikely.[47] The Wells score provides a simplified diagnostic approach to reliably diagnose or exclude DVT. A DVT-unlikely score coupled with a negative D-dimer is capable of safely excluding the diagnosis; a DVT-likely score requires ultrasound confirmation. One criticism of the Wells score is that it relies, in part, on the clinician's subjective assessment of whether an alternative diagnosis to DVT is more likely. The Wells score was originally validated in symptomatic outpatients suspected of having DVT. It has since been validated in the emergency department in combination with D-dimer testing.[48] The utility of the Wells score in critically ill patients is unclear. In a recent publication, neither the original nor modified score appeared to be useful in hospitalized patients.[47]

Other scoring systems include the six-component St. Andre hospital score, the four-component Kahn score, the six-component ambulatory score, and the seven-component Hamilton score. As is the case with the Wells score, none has been derived or validated in a critically ill population.[49–52]

D-dimer

The use of D-dimer testing, which detects the degradation product of cross-linked fibrin, has gained widespread acceptance in the diagnostic evaluation of suspected DVT. The addition of D-dimer testing to the Wells score improves the negative predictive value of the prediction rule, effectively excluding DVT in outpatients with a negative D-dimer and low pretest probability.[39] However, although the test is highly sensitive, a negative D-dimer test alone does not reliably exclude DVT.[53] The clinical utility of the test is limited by poor specificity, as an elevated plasma D-dimer can be found in numerous conditions common to hospitalized patients.

The clinical utility of D-dimer testing is also complicated by the different performances of available assays. There is substantial heterogeneity in the types of D-dimer assays used in clinical studies, including qualitative whole blood assays (such as SimpliRED), plasma enzyme-linked immunosorbent assays (ELISA), and immunoturbidometric assays, which provide quantitative levels. Comparisons of commercially available tests show significant variability in sensitivity, specificity, and optimal cutoff values.[54,55]

Contrast Venography

Contrast venography is considered the "gold standard" test for DVT.[56,57] Contrast is injected into a superficial vein on the dorsum of the foot and a series of images obtained extending from the calf to the pelvis. The technique has changed little since its introduction nearly four decades ago. The presence of a filling defect or abrupt termination of the opaque column is used as a criterion for DVT. Other than being used for the detection of asymptomatic DVT in clinical trials of anticoagulant agents, it is rarely performed because of the availability of accurate noninvasive diagnostic techniques. The use of contrast venography in critically ill patients is also limited by the need for patient transport, lack of venous access, the risk of post-venographic phlebitis, and the presence of acute renal failure or chronic kidney disease, which are relative contraindications to the procedure.

Duplex Ultrasonography

Duplex ultrasonography has become the diagnostic procedure of choice for the diagnosis of symptomatic lower extremity DVT. The advantages of the test include noninvasiveness, portability, and high sensitivity and specificity. Among the sonographic features for diagnosis, noncompressibility of the common femoral

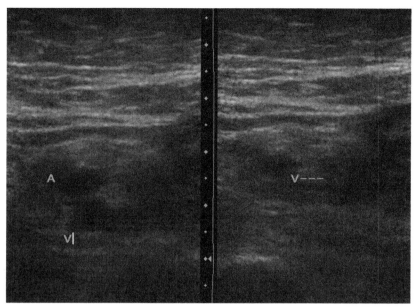

Fig. 1. Lower extremity DUS demonstrating normal compression of the femoral vein. The A denotes the femoral artery. The V denotes the femoral vein. The image on the left is without compression and the image on the right is with compression.

and popliteal veins is highly sensitive and specific for DVT (**Figs. 1** and **2**).[58] The addition of duplex or color Doppler flow has increased the accuracy of ultrasound, and has replaced limited B-mode compression ultrasonography as the preferred technique.

Although duplex ultrasonography (DUS) is highly sensitive and specific in the diagnosis of DVT in symptomatic patients, its accuracy in the diagnosis of asymptomatic DVT is less clear. A meta-analysis of studies comparing ultrasound to contrast venography in asymptomatic patients found that ultrasound was accurate for the detection of asymptomatic proximal DVT, but the data were limited almost entirely to postoperative orthopedics patients.[59] The practice of screening asymptomatic high-risk patients for DVT with ultrasound is controversial. The sensitivity of ultrasound for screening depends on the prevalence of asymptomatic DVT in the target population. Although most screening for DVT is performed in high-risk postoperative orthopedic or critically ill trauma patients, a high prevalence of asymptomatic DVT has also been reported in the medical ICU, post-coronary artery bypass graft surgery, and in advanced malignancy, raising the question of the role of screening in other high-risk populations.[60–62]

Ultrasound has a lower sensitivity and specificity for the detection of calf vein thrombosis than it does for proximal DVT.[63] The clinical significance of isolated calf vein thrombosis is uncertain. Although isolated calf vein thrombosis has a low risk of PE, it is estimated that 20% of symptomatic calf vein thrombosis may extend to the proximal veins.[64] Little is known about the risk of proximal extension in asymptomatic isolated calf vein thrombosis. Due to the risk of proximal extension, it is generally recommended that serial ultrasounds examinations be performed when an isolated calf vein thrombosis is found. The practice of serial ultrasound in symptomatic

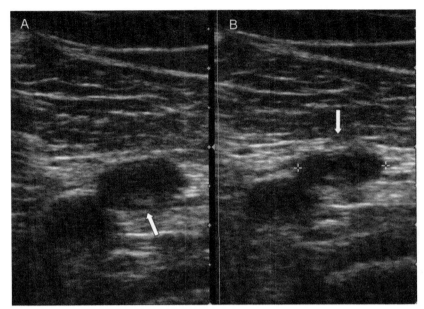

Fig. 2. Lower extremity DUS demonstrating incomplete compression of the popliteal vein with the presence of intraluminal thrombus. The image on the left is without compression. The arrow denotes the popliteal vein with intramural thrombus. The image on the right is with compression and the arrow demonstrates incomplete compression of the popliteal vein.

patients after an initial negative ultrasound is more controversial. Although a very low incidence of venous thromboembolic events is found after an initial negative ultrasound study because of the low sensitivity of ultrasound for calf vein thrombosis, it is recommended that serial ultrasound be performed when symptoms of DVT are present but initial ultrasound is negative.[65,66]

After an initial episode of DVT, there is a high rate of recurrence, with more than 20% of patients experiencing recurrent DVT within 5 years.[67] In addition, approximately 50% of patients will have residual vascular obstruction after an initial episode of acute venous thrombosis. Whereas certain sonographic features, including echogenicity, compressibility, vein diameter, and thrombus length may help differentiate acute on chronic DVT from chronic disease, the differentiation of acute from chronic disease can represent a diagnostic challenge.[68,69]

Upper extremity DVT represents approximately 5% of total cases of DVT.[70,71] This is more commonly seen in the ICU owing to use of central venous catheters, a major risk factor for the development of upper extremity DVT. There is an estimated 10% to 15% risk of PE with upper extremity DVT.[25,71,72] The accuracy of ultrasonography for diagnosis of upper extremity DVT remains unclear. Two systematic reviews found a paucity of quality evidence on the topic.[73,74]

Computed Tomographic Venography

Because many patients undergoing evaluation of DVT will also be evaluated for PE, there has been growing interest in combining computed tomography (CT) angiography (CTA) for the diagnosis of PE with CT venography (CTV) of the lower extremities for diagnosis of DVT. The obvious advantage of this technique is that evaluation for

DVT and PE can be accomplished with a single test. In addition, CTV has the theoretical advantage of imaging pelvic clots, which are not easily visualized by ultrasonography.[75] In reality, isolated pelvic thrombosis is rare. The PIOPED II study showed similar performance of CTV and ultrasonography in diagnosing or excluding DVT.[76] The accuracy of CTV for detection of calf thrombosis is unknown, and the calf may not be routinely included in the examination. The disadvantages of CTV include need for patient transport, risks associated with contrast agent, and radiation exposure.

Magnetic Resonance Imaging

Magnetic resonance imaging (MRI) has also been used for diagnosis of DVT although it has not been nearly as well studied as ultrasonography or CTV. Like CT imaging, MRI can be performed as a combined procedure to evaluate for DVT and PE simultaneously.[77] MRI techniques for detection of DVT include gadolinium-enhanced venography, phase contrast–enhanced venography and magnetic resonance direct thrombus imaging that does not require the use of gadolinium.[77,78] A recent meta-analysis showed a pooled estimate sensitivity of 91.5% and specificity of 94.8% for DVT diagnosis. The disadvantages of MRI include cost, time of examination, and need for patient transport.[79]

DIAGNOSTIC OPTIONS: PE
Clinical Prediction Rules

In a recent review, nine different clinical prediction rules for the evaluation of PE pretest probability were evaluated. All of these rules have been prospectively validated in multiple studies and have similar accuracy.[9] The most extensively validated rules are the three-level and two-level Wells scores (**Table 2**), the Geneva score, the Revised Geneva score (**Table 3**), and the Charlotte rule.[80–84] Only the Wells rule and the Geneva score have been applied to inpatients, and only in a minority of patients.

Applying these scores to patients in the ICU would result in most patients being placed into the intermediate or high-risk categories in which the pretest probability of

Table 2	
Wells dichotomous clinical decision rule for PE	
Variable	**Points**
Clinical signs and symptoms of DVT (minimum of leg swelling and pain with palpation of the deep veins)	3.0
Alternative diagnosis less likely than PE	3.0
Heart rate > 100 beats/min	1.5
Immobilization (>3 days) or surgery in the previous 4 weeks	1.5
Previous PE or DVT	1.5
Hemoptysis	1.0
Malignancy (receiving treatment, treat in the last 6 months, or palliative)	1.0
Clinical probability of PE unlikely: ≤4 points	
Clinical probability of PE likely: >4 points	

Data from Wells PS, Anderson DR, Rodger M, et al. Derivation of a simple clinical model to categorize patients probability of pulmonary embolism: increasing the models utility with the SimpliRED D-dimer. Thromb Haemost 2000;83:416–20.

Table 3	
Revised Geneva score for PE	
Variable	**Points**
Risk factors:	
Age >65 years	1
Previous DVT or PE	3
Surgery (under general anesthesia) or fracture (of the lower limbs) within 1 month	2
Active malignant condition (solid or hematologic malignant condition, currently active or considered cured <1 year)	2
Symptoms:	
Unilateral lower limb pain	3
Hemoptysis	2
Clinical signs:	
Heart rate	
75–94 beats/min	3
95 beats/min	5
Pain on lower-limb deep venous palpation and unilateral edema	4
Clinical probability low: 0–3 total	
Clinical probability intermediate: 4–10 total	
Clinical probability high: ≥11 total	

Data from Le Gal G, Righini M, Roy PM, et al. Prediction of pulmonary embolism in the emergency department: the revised Geneva score. Ann Intern Med 2006;144:165–71.

PE would range from 25% to 75%. For example, a heart rate greater than or equal to 95 beats/min alone would place a patient in the moderate clinical probability group based on the revised Geneva score. A heart rate greater than 100 beats/min in the setting of immobilization or surgery within the prior 4 weeks would do the same using the Wells rule. For these reasons, the clinical prediction rules described have limited if any utility in the diagnosis of PE in the ICU.

Electrocardiogram

Electrocardiographic abnormalities have been reported in as many as 70% of patients with PE.[42] A variety of findings have been reported ranging from no abnormalities to disturbances of rate, rhythm, repolarization, and conduction and include sinus tachycardia, nonspecific ST abnormalities, T-wave inversion in the precordial leads, right bundle branch block, and an $S_1Q_3T_3$ pattern (**Fig. 3**). Although certain electrocardiographic findings may have prognostic value, the findings are nonspecific and have little diagnostic value.[85,86]

Chest Radiograph

The majority of patients with PE have an abnormal chest radiograph. The abnormalities encountered are nonspecific and commonly include atelectasis, parenchymal abnormalities, an elevated hemidiaphragm, cardiomegaly, and small pleural effusions.[42,87] In embolic suspects, however, these findings are encountered just as often in patients without PE, thereby severely limiting the discriminatory value of the study. Findings previously thought to be characteristic of PE such as the Westermark sign (focal area of avascularity or oligemia), the Fleischner sign (prominent central

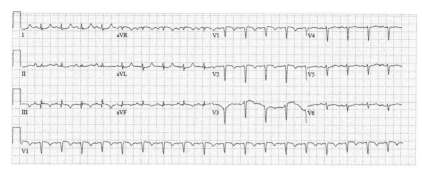

Fig. 3. Electrocardiogram in patient with massive PE demonstrating a $S_1Q_3T_3$ pattern along with inverted T waves in anterior precordial leads.

pulmonary artery), and the Hampton hump (pleural-based wedge shaped opacity) do not have sufficient diagnostic accuracy to be useful in confirming or excluding PE.[87] In critically ill patients, especially those being mechanically ventilated, the chest radiograph is very unlikely to be normal. Therefore, it is most useful in eliminating other potential diagnoses that may have a similar clinical presentation to that of PE and in raising the clinical suspicion of the disease in symptomatic patients in the instances when it is normal.

Arterial Blood Gases

Arterial hypoxemia may be present, and the more massive the obstruction, the more severe the hypoxemia is likely to be. However, many other conditions also cause hypoxemia, and embolism does not necessarily cause hypoxemia or even a widening of the $(A-a)O_2$ gradient.[88,89] In the PIOPED trial, no combinations of blood gases were identified that reliably excluded PE.[89] Although most patients with embolism have a low PaO_2, low $PaCO_2$, or high $P(A-a)O_2$ gradient, the absence of such abnormal values, alone or in combination, did not exclude PE. Although hypocapnia usually is present with embolism, hypercapnia may occur in patients with marked antecedent ventilatory limitation or when such limitation has been imposed because the patient is on controlled mechanical ventilation when embolism occurs.

etCO$_2$

Obstruction of the pulmonary vascular bed can be expected to cause an increased dead space ventilation (V_d/V_t). Kline and coworkers demonstrated that patients with proven PE had a statistically significant increase in V_d/V_t ratio.[32] Methods for measuring V_d/V_t, are cumbersome and investigators have attempted to use bedside capnography as a surrogate measure of dead space ventilation. Preliminary studies suggest that this may be a useful adjunct in excluding embolism in low-risk patients.[90,91] In a study that evaluated 298 patients suspected of PE, a statistically significant difference in the $etCO_2$ was found in patients with PE compared to those in whom PE had been excluded (30.5 ± 5.5 mm Hg vs 35.5 ± 6.8 mm Hg). Using a cutoff value of 36 mm Hg, the negative predictive value was 96.8%. This study specifically excluded patients with hypercapneic respiratory failure, mechanical ventilation, neuromuscular disease, or who required more than 5 L/min of supplemental oxygen, making it difficult to predict its utility in a critically ill patient population.[90] Kline and coworkers evaluated the $etCO_2/O_2$ ratio in conjunction with D-dimer testing as a screening strategy for segmental or larger embolism. In moderate-risk patients with a positive D-dimer, an $etco_2/o_2$ ratio less than 0.28 significantly increased the probability of segmental or larger PE and the $etco_2/o_2$ greater than 0.45 predicted the absence of segmental or larger PE on multidetector computerized tomographic pulmonary angiography.[91]

D-dimer

The D-dimer test has emerged as a useful test in the diagnostic algorithm of suspected PE. Algorithms exist that combine clinical prediction rules and the D-dimer assay to determine the need for further invasive diagnostic workup in patients suspected of having PE. Wells and coworkers validated their revised dichotomous score in combination with a D-dimer test to categorize patients' probability of embolism. In a mixed inpatient and outpatient group, 46% of patients were designated "PE unlikely" and had a negative D-dimer test. Only 2.2% of patients had PE in the derivation set and 1.7% in the validation set. The Christopher study enrolled 3306 patients in whom PE was suspected and confirmed these results. Patients underwent assessment with the dichotomous Wells as well as D-dimer testing. In patients who were unlikely to have PE by the Wells criteria and had a normal D-dimer assay, PE was safely excluded without any further testing, with only a 0.5% event rate at the 3-month follow-up.[92] These algorithms have become very useful in the evaluation of outpatients presenting with signs and symptoms concerning for PE and allow risk stratification and the judicious use of more invasive testing only in patients in whom PE cannot be safely excluded based on the prediction rule and D-dimer alone.

The same issues that limit the diagnostic utility of D-dimer testing for venous thrombosis in critically ill patients are associated with its use in suspected PE. In a recent study that evaluated the use of the Wells prediction rule in conjunction with a latex-agglutination or rapid ELISA D-dimer assay in hospitalized patients, only 10% of more than 600 patients tested fell into the low-probability category.[93] It is probable that comorbidities responsible for D-dimer elevation would be even more prevalent in critically ill patients, making the D-dimer assay even less useful in this setting.

CTA

CT pulmonary angiography (CT-PA) has supplanted ventilation–perfusion scanning as the imaging modality of choice when PE is suspected (**Fig. 4**).

The PIOPED II trial represents the largest trial evaluating the diagnostic accuracy of CT-PA in the diagnosis of suspected embolism.[7,94] Although the trial included inpatients, the majority of those enrolled (89%) were outpatients. Exclusion criteria included critical illness, ventilatory support, shock, recent myocardial infarction, abnormal serum creatinine, allergy to contrast material, pregnancy, treatment with long-term anticoagulants, inferior vena cava filter, and upper extremity DVT. To establish a diagnosis of PE, one of the following criteria had to be met: a high-probability V/Q scan, an abnormal digital subtraction pulmonary angiogram (DSA), or an abnormal compression venous ultrasound and a nondiagnostic V/Q scan. To exclude the diagnosis of PE, one of the following criteria had to be met: a normal DSA, a normal V/Q scan, or a low or very low probability V/Q scan in the setting of a Wells score of less than 2 and a normal compression venous ultrasound.

Of the 824 patients who were enrolled, embolism was diagnosed in 192 for a prevalence of 23%. The specificity for CT-PA alone was 96%; sensitivity for CT-PA alone was 83%, which increased to 90% when CTV was added. The positive predictive value of CT-PA alone depended significantly on the location of the embolism: 97% for involvement of the main and lobar arteries, 68% for segmental

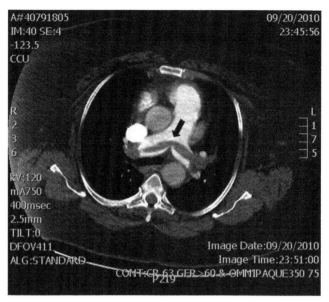

Fig. 4. CTA demonstrating "saddle" embolus (*black arrow*) straddling bifurcation of right and left main pulmonary arteries.

disease, and 25% for subsegmental disease. When the Wells clinical prediction rule was applied, the positive predictive and negative predictive values improved significantly. In patients with an intermediate or high probability of PE and a positive CT-PA, the positive predictive value was 92%; in patients with a low probability of PE and a negative CT-PA the negative predictive value was 96%. As noted previously, however, formalized clinical prediction rules are rarely applicable to critically ill patients and empiric assessment is often inaccurate. The relatively high false-negative rate (17%) of CT-PA alone in the PIOPED II study suggests that additional information must be added to it to safely exclude PE if the clinical prediction rule cannot be appropriately applied.

Considerable controversy accompanies the question of whether indirect CTV or DUS should be utilized as an adjunct to CTA as part of the diagnostic pathway for PE. In ambulatory patients, lower extremity imaging adds little to the overall diagnostic yield and 3-month follow-up demonstrates the same recurrence rates as for those with negative CTA-only examinations.[76,95] In critically ill patients, however, the incremental benefit, albeit small, may prove valuable given that the CTA may be suboptimal due to motion artifact or may represent a false-negative examination. Given the substantial pelvic radiation exposure associated with CTV, DUS would appear to be the procedure of choice.

Ventilation–Perfusion Scanning

Despite limitations, ventilation–perfusion (V/Q) lung scanning is valuable if interpreted appropriately. A negative study rules out the diagnosis of PE with the same degree of certainty as a negative pulmonary angiogram and with a higher degree of certainty than is achieved by a negative CT pulmonary angiogram (**Fig. 5**). In the PIOPED trial, a high-probability study (one characterized by multiple, segmental-sized, mismatched

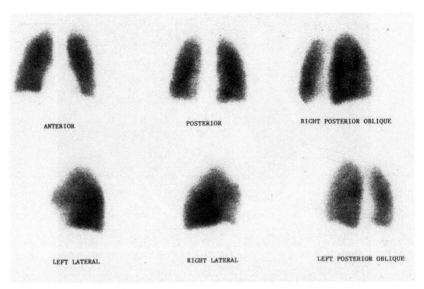

ANTERIOR   POSTERIOR   RIGHT POSTERIOR OBLIQUE

LEFT LATERAL   RIGHT LATERAL   LEFT POSTERIOR OBLIQUE

Fig. 5. Normal six-view perfusions scan.

defects) was associated with embolism in approximately 87% of patients; when coupled with a high clinical probability of embolism, the positive predictive value increased to 96% (**Fig. 6**). However, the PIOPED data also highlighted the limitations of the technique: (1) the overwhelming majority of patients with suspected embolism did not have scan findings that fell into a high probability or normal category, the only categories that can be considered definitive; (2) the majority of patients with embolism

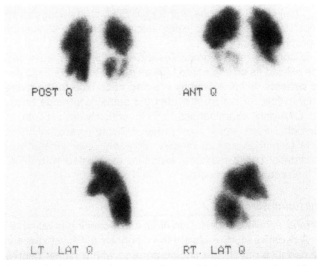

POST Q   ANT Q

LT. LAT Q   RT. LAT Q

Fig. 6. Four-view perfusions scan demonstrating multiple segmental and larger perfusion defects.

did not have a high-probability scan finding; (3) the overwhelming majority of patients without embolism did not have a normal scan; and (4) a substantial and clinically significant percentage of patients with scan findings interpreted as intermediate probability (33%) and low probability (16%) were subsequently demonstrated to have angiographic evidence of embolism.

In a prospective cohort study, the reliability of ventilation–perfusion lung scanning was compared in 223 critically ill patients, 46 of whom were receiving mechanical ventilatory support, and 627 noncritically ill patients. The sensitivity, specificity, and positive predictive value of a high-probability lung scan were not statistically different than values in noncritically ill patients. However, the study was diagnostic (high probability or normal/near normal scan interpretation) in only 18% of the critically ill patients and only 11% of those receiving mechanical ventilatory support.[96]

To improve perfusion scan specificity, traditional interpretive criteria, including the PIOPED criteria, rely on the number and size of the perfusion defects as well as on the results of a concurrent ventilation image. The intended basis for doing so is to differentiate pulmonary vascular obstruction ("mismatched" defects) from primary parenchymal disorders that result in compensatory pulmonary vasoconstriction ("matched" defects). The PISA-PED (Prospective Investigative Study of Acute Pulmonary Embolism Diagnosis) investigators utilized a fundamentally different, dichotomous interpretive scheme that relied on the shape of the perfusion defects regardless of their number or size or their association with ventilation findings.[97,98] Although not specifically applied to an ICU population, the majority of patients enrolled in PISA-PED were inpatients in whom the majority of chest radiographs were interpreted as abnormal. Perfusion scans were graded as being consistent with embolism (PE+) if they demonstrated single or multiple wedge-shaped defects; scans not consistent with embolism (PE–) demonstrated defects that were other than wedge shaped. Most patients with angiographically proven PE had PE+ scans (sensitivity: 92%). Conversely, most patients without emboli on angiography had PE– scans (specificity: 87%). A positive scan associated with a very likely or possible clinical presentation of PE had positive predictive values of 99% and 92%, respectively. A negative scan paired with an unlikely clinical presentation had a negative predictive value of 97%.

Stein and coworkers subsequently evaluated a sample of the PIOPED data and compared perfusion scans alone with ventilation–perfusion scans using modified PIOPED interpretive criteria. There was no difference in the positive predictive value of a high-probability perfusion scan (93%) when compared with the positive predictive value of a high-probability V/Q scan (94%). However, a higher number of perfusion scans were interpreted as intermediate-probability compared with V/Q scans.

Although not specifically applied to an ICU population in whom the likelihood of indeterminate results would be expected to be higher, these results suggest that perfusion scanning may have a role in the diagnostic pathway in selected patients.

There are certain situations in which V/Q scanning may be preferred over CT-PA. IV contrast is not required for V/Q scanning, making it a more desirable option in patients with renal dysfunction or iodinated contrast allergy. In addition, with a portable gamma scintillation camera the perfusion portion of the study can be performed at the bedside, which may be a major advantage in a critically ill patient in whom transportation to the CT scanner may be deemed too high risk.

Echocardiography

Echocardiography, although not a primary diagnostic technique, may play a valuable adjunctive role in critically ill patients, especially those with acute, unexplained hemodynamic deterioration.[99] A number of echocardiographic findings have been described associated with acute embolism including McConnell's sign (RV hypokinesis with sparing of apical motion) and the "60/60" sign (pulmonary acceleration time <60 ms in the presence of an echocardiographically derived pulmonary artery pressure ≤60 mm Hg). Both signs are associated with a specificity exceeding 90% but a substantially lower sensitivity in the range of 15% to 25%. Kurzyna and coworkers evaluated various echocardiographic findings in 100 consecutive patients with suspected PE, 62 of whom were in a critical care unit.[100] They reported a positive predictive value of 100% and 90% for McConnell's sign and the "60/60" sign, respectively, and a negative predictive value of 37% and 38% for McConnell's sign and the "60/60" sign, respectively. The prevalence of PE in this study was unusually high (67%), so these predictive values may not be generally applicable to all patients in a critical care setting.

RV dysfunction independent of embolism is not uncommon in critically ill patients, especially those with acute lung injury on mechanical ventilatory support.[101] In the setting of a patient with acute hemodynamic deterioration, however, a negative study (ie, absence of RV dilation, RV strain, or pulmonary hypertension) would strongly suggest a nonembolic basis (such as pneumothorax, sepsis, pericardial tamponade) for the patient's deterioration and might avoid the delay in management and risk of transportation for pulmonary vascular imaging.

Transesophageal echocardiography (TEE) is capable of directly imaging the right-sided cardiac structures, the main pulmonary artery, a significant portion of the right pulmonary artery, and the proximal portion of the left pulmonary artery. Pruszcyk and coworkers prospectively compared the value of TEE and spiral CT in 49 consecutive patients with clinical suspicion of PE and RV overload noted on transthoracic echocardiography. PE was diagnosed in 40 patients by means of reference diagnostic methods (ventilation–perfusion scan in 27, pulmonary angiography in 13). Sensitivity for central embolism was noted to be 90% for spiral CT and 80% for TEE, with 100% specificity for both methods.[102] The role of TEE in the diagnosis of peripheral pulmonary emboli is limited because of its inability to image the more distal pulmonary vessels.

Magnetic Resonance Angiography

The PIOPED III trial was the largest, multicenter study designed to assess magnetic resonance angiography (MRA) for the diagnosis of PE.[8] Three hundred and seventy-one patients were enrolled in whom PE was confirmed or excluded by CT-PA or V/Q. Approximately 25% of studies were technically inadequate and could not be interpreted. However, this seemed to vary by site (11%–52%), suggesting that some sites may have more experience and may be able to limit their number of inadequate scans. The sensitivity and specificity of MRA among patients with technically adequate scans was 78% and 99% respectively. These figures fell considerably when the technically inadequate scans were included in the calculations. Sensitivity for emboli involving the main or lobar pulmonary arteries was only 79%.

There are patients in whom CT-PA may not be possible because of IV contrast allergy or in whom avoidance of radiation is preferred (eg, pregnancy). In these patients, MRA may be a reasonable alternative. However, in the critically ill patient population this is a cumbersome and impractical modality in most circumstances.

Most MRI scanners are physically located outside of hospitals, requiring significant cost and risk associated with transportation; monitoring within the MRI requires special equipment and may not always be readily accessible. In addition, the study is contraindicated in patients with pacemakers or other implantable devices and the administration of gadolinium is relatively contraindicated in patients with kidney disease owing to the risk of nephrogenic systemic fibrosis.

Conventional Pulmonary Angiography

Pulmonary angiography has long been considered the gold standard for diagnosing PE. As is the case with contrast venography, however, pulmonary angiography has a number of limitations as a gold standard. First, the procedure in invasive and not without risk, especially in patients with acute RV failure. Recent experience, however, has demonstrated that the perception of risk associated with angiography outweighs the actual risk. Pulmonary angiography can be performed quite safely if certain safeguards are observed and experienced personnel are involved. In the 1111 angiograms performed in the original PIOPED trial, pulmonary angiography was nondiagnostic in 3% of patients and associated with a major complication rate of 1% and death rate of 0.5%.[103] Major complications occurred more frequently among patients sent for angiography from the medical ICU than in patients from elsewhere (4% vs 1%). The procedure has other limitations. One is accessibility and the need for transportation. The other limitation is interpretation. Interpretation of pulmonary angiograms is heavily influenced by three factors: the location of the thromboembolic obstruction, the quality of the images, and the experience of the interpreters. Only two angiographic findings are diagnostic of acute embolism: the filling defect and abrupt cutoff of a vessel (**Fig. 7**). Technical adequacy of the angiogram is critical to accurate identification of both. Flow artifacts can falsely suggest a filling defect. It is essential that good vessel opacification be obtained and that the filling defects be identified as real on a sequence of films.

Angiography should be considered in patients in whom the diagnosis has not been confirmed or excluded using noninvasive techniques and when it is considered unsafe to withhold anticoagulation and when the results of noninvasive diagnostic testing are at such odds with the clinical impression to warrant the risk of the procedure. As noted by Dr Kenneth Moser more than two decades ago, it is an odd commentary that few would advise against performance of a coronary angiogram in a patient with suspected coronary ischemia because of risk, yet the question of risk often deters pulmonary angiography in patients with suspected embolism.

Pulmonary angiography may be contraindicated in patients with severe renal dysfunction, coagulopathy, and severe hemodynamic instability. In addition, because of its decreasing utilization it may not be available at all centers and some centers may have insufficient interpretive experience for it to be a useful test in the critical care setting.

DIAGNOSTIC APPROACH

The initiating point for the diagnostic pathway begins with clinical suspicion. In ambulatory or hospitalized noncritically ill patients, clinical suspicion is most commonly generated by a patient's symptomatic complaints and is supported by clinical signs. In the ICU setting, in which patients may have limited communication ability and the clinical manifestations of venous thromboembolism, with the exception of unilateral edema, are often present or are masked by elements of the primary disease, clinical suspicion is commonly generated by physiologic criteria such as unexplained

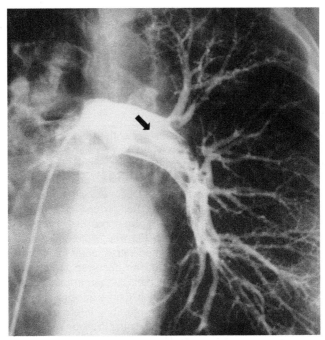

Fig. 7. Conventional pulmonary angiogram demonstrating filling defects (*black arrow*) within left main, left upper lobe, and left lower lobe pulmonary arteries consistent with acute embolism.

tachycardia, hypoxemia, hypotension, an increase in minute ventilation, or reduction in $etCO_2$.

In ambulatory or hospitalized, noncritically ill patients an empirical or explicit assessment of the clinical probability of embolism would be calculated that would define a pretest likelihood of disease. This pretest likelihood would subsequently define the weight of objective clinical evidence necessary to accurately confirm the diagnosis of venous thromboembolism or safely exclude it with a predefined degree of certainty.

An explicit rule has not been derived for critically ill patients. Extrapolation from studies in noncritically ill populations, though inviting, is problematic. D-dimer testing, the central exclusionary study in ambulatory patients with a low or moderate probability of disease, is not applicable to a critically ill population. Critically ill patients have multiple comorbid conditions such as advanced age, systemic inflammation, surgical trauma, or advanced liver or kidney disease capable of causing an elevated D-dimer level in the absence of venous thromboembolism. D-dimer levels are routinely elevated in the postoperative period and remain so for several weeks postoperatively.[104] In a prospective cohort study of 197 critically ill medical–surgical patients, the overwhelming majority of patients had markedly elevated D-dimer results throughout their ICU stay. In this study, a total of 804 bedside D-dimer tests were also performed. Of these, only 29 tests (3.6%) in 5 patients were normal.[105]

Until further data are available applicable to a critically ill population, an empirical assessment based on available clinical and physiologic criteria will continue to be utilized, with subsequent diagnostic studies based on individual patient factors including the pretest likelihood of disease, the ease and safety of transportation, renal function, and hemodynamic status. As is the case with ambulatory or noncritically ill patients, once the diagnosis has been considered, objective testing is required to either confirm or exclude the diagnosis.

Venous Thrombosis

Lower extremity DUS represents the procedure of choice for symptomatic venous thrombosis. In this setting, the sensitivity of the test for proximal vein thrombosis approaches 100%. The sensitivity is substantially less for asymptomatic patients and those with isolated calf-limited disease.

The sensitivity and specificity of the study when used as a surveillance tool in critically ill patients are unknown and remain controversial. Adams and coworkers, in a study of 2939 trauma patients, 772 considered to be at high thromboembolic risk, noted an overall 3.2% incidence of thromboembolism. Incidence in the high-risk group was 10.1%, the overwhelming majority of which were asymptomatic and detected only on routine screening.[106] Similar rates of asymptomatic thrombosis were noted by Cook and Crowther.[41] Conversely, Borer and coworkers found no significant difference in the rate of PE in 972 patients with fractures of the pelvis or acetabulum when comparing those who were screened versus those who were not.[107]

Isolated pelvic vein thrombosis is rare and when present often extends into the thigh, where it can be detected by ultrasonography. However, in patients with pelvic fracture or other pelvic pathology with suspected thrombosis, CTV or MR venography is sensitive in detecting the disease.

PE

CTA would appear to represent the imaging procedure of choice in patients who are capable of being transported and who can safely tolerate a contrast load. In the PIOPED II trial, the sensitivity of CTA was 83% and the specificity 95% in those patients whose study was sufficient for a conclusive interpretation. The positive predictive value of CTA, however, was dependent on the proximal location of the thrombus. Positive predictive values for CTA in PIOPED II were 97% for emboli in the main or lobar arteries, 68% for segmental vessels, and 25% for subsegmental involvement. It is important to recognize, therefore, that if discordance exists between the pretest likelihood of disease and the CTA findings, additional diagnostic tests may be necessary. In PIOPED II, if results of CTA were negative in a patient with a high-probability clinical assessment, embolism was actually present in 40%. Alternatively, if CTA was positive in a patient with a low-probability clinical assessment, PE was present in only 58%.[94]

MRA appears to provide diagnostic yield that is inferior to CTA. Further, the study suffers from the same limitations in terms of transportation and utilization in those with renal dysfunction. Given the longer examination time required, high likelihood of an inadequate exam, limited access, its contraindication in patients with pacemakers or other implanted devices, and, unlike CTA, its inability to diagnose an alternative basis for the patient's symptomatic complaints or physiologic abnormality, its role in critically ill patients would appear limited until additional data have been accrued.

For patients who cannot be safely transported or are at risk of a contrast load, a somewhat less direct diagnostic pathway should be considered. Risk factors for contrast-induced kidney injury include preexisting chronic renal disease (creatinine clearance >60 mL/min), diabetes mellitus, volume depletion, concurrent use of nephrotoxic drugs including nonsteroidal anti-inflammatory agents, and hemodynamic instability. The short-term and long-term consequences of contrast-induced acute kidney injury cannot be understated. In a retrospective analysis of 7586 patients exposed to iodinated contrast during a percutaneous coronary intervention, 3.3% developed contrast-induced kidney injury. The amount of contrast administered, however, was substantially more than that administered with CTA. The in-hospital death rate was 22% in those who did develop acute kidney injury compared with 1.4% in patients who did not. The mortality rates at 1 and 5 years after development of contrast-induced kidney injury were 12.1% and 44.6%, respectively, compared to 3.7% and 14.5% in patients who were free of renal injury. If contrast must be used, interventions designed to avoid nephrotoxicity (volume expansion, withdrawal of nephrotoxic drugs, and perhaps N-acetylcysteine) should be utilized.

Lower extremity DUS appears to provide a diagnostic yield equivalent to that of indirect CTV. The prevalence of detectable DVT in patients with symptomatic PE has not been widely investigated and varies greatly among studies. Girard and coworkers, in a study of 281 patients with CTA-documented embolism, demonstrated that DUS-detectable venous thrombosis was present in 60% of patients, 75% which were in the proximal veins.[108] Similar results were obtained in the PIOPED study. Given the low prevalence of embolism in those suspected of the disease, DUS would be diagnostic in only 10% to 15% of patients. Compression ultrasonography, however, does have a number of advantages over other imaging techniques. It provides direct rather than indirect diagnostic information and can be performed rapidly and at the bedside. The finding of proximal vein thrombosis, although not confirming that embolism has occurred, would have the same therapeutic implications. A negative study obviously would be insufficient to exclude the disease and additional testing would be required.

In patients who are hemodynamically stable and with a less than high probability of embolism, a strategy of preventive surveillance might be considered. Although not applied to a critically ill population, such a strategy has proven effective in ambulatory and hospitalized patients. Wells and coworkers demonstrated a negative predictive value of normal serial lower extremity ultrasound studies (days 3, 7, and 14) of 99.5% in 679 embolic suspects with a low or moderate pretest clinical probability and a non–high-probability lung scan.[109]

Ventilation–perfusion also may provide valuable diagnostic information. Further, with the use of a portable gamma scintillation camera, the study can be performed at the bedside. A normal study would exclude embolism with a higher degree of certainty than a negative CTA.

Transthoracic or transesophageal echocardiography, although not primary diagnostic techniques, may also play a valuable role in critically ill patients, especially those with acute, unexplained hemodynamic deterioration. Direct visualization of main or lobar thrombi by transesophageal echocardiography would serve to confirm the diagnosis. The finding of normal right ventricular size and function would strongly suggest that the basis for the hemodynamic deterioration was not thromboembolic in nature.

SUMMARY

The one certainty surrounding the issue of thromboembolism diagnosis in critically ill patients is that considerable uncertainty remains. Until further randomized studies are performed, physicians caring for a critically ill population will have to live with the limitations imposed by this uncertainty, maintaining a high level of suspicion for the disease and remaining cognizant of the strengths and limitations of the diagnostic tools available to them. Any discussion of venous thromboembolism diagnosis as an entity implies a certain homogeneity among patients and among diagnostic options.

In actuality, critically ill patients at risk for thromboembolism cover a wide spectrum in terms of the context in which the disease arises, the individual risk, the coexistence of other disorders, and the variability of individual response.

Until further data are accumulated, there is usually no one answer to guide the diagnostic sequence for critically ill patients with suspected venous thromboembolism. Optimal evaluation of a patient with suspected venous thromboembolism requires an acceptance that there is no ideal study, an understanding of the capabilities and limitations of existing diagnostic techniques, and an acceptance that a systematic and sequential diagnostic approach may be necessary. In certain patients in a critical care setting, attempts to confirm or exclude the diagnosis may be so fraught with risk that the only clinically feasible options, based on existing data and an informed estimate of risk/benefit, are to institute empirical therapy or to pursue a strategy of surveillance intended to prevent recurrent episodes. The central goal of the process is to avoid, on the one hand, the morbid and potentially mortal complications of unnecessary anticoagulant therapy and, on the other, to minimize the potentially fatal consequences of overlooking the diagnosis.

Existing data would suggest that thromboembolism is underdiagnosed in critically ill patients, a population in whom the adverse hemodynamic effects of embolism may be enhanced as a result of the patients' existing compromise in cardiopulmonary reserve. Although the overall number of hospital beds in the United States has declined, critical care medicine beds increased by 36% between 1985 and 2005.[110,111] Given the future expansion in critical care demand that will occur as a result of an aging population with multiple comorbidities and the development of new therapeutic modalities for previously untreatable diseases, there would appear to be a pressing need for additional thromboembolism research endeavors in this population similar to those achieved so comprehensively in the ambulatory population. The recently published PROTECT trial (PROphylaxis for ThromboEmbolism in Critical Care Trial) represented a valuable first step in this process.[25] Ongoing efforts are now required in the areas of epidemiology, clinical presentation, diagnosis, and management to provide intensivists an evidence-based approach to venous thromboembolism in this growing and susceptible population.

REFERENCES

1. Anderson FA Jr, Wheeler HB, Goldberg RJ, et al. A population-based perspective of the hospital incidence and case-fatality rates of deep vein thrombosis and pulmonary embolism. The Worcester DVT Study. Arch Intern Med 1991;151:933–8.
2. Gillum RF. Pulmonary embolism and thrombophlebitis in the United States, 1970–1985. Am Heart J 1987;114:1262–4.
3. Stein PD, Matta F. Epidemiology and incidence: the scope of the problem and risk factors for development of venous thromboembolism. Clin Chest Med 2010;31:611–28.
4. Anderson JA, Weitz JI. Hypercoagulable states. Clin Chest Med 2010;31:659–73.
5. Geerts WH, Bergqvist D, Pineo GF, et al. Prevention of venous thromboembolism: American College of Chest Physicians evidence-based clinical practice guidelines. 8th edition. Chest 2008;133:381S–453S.
6. The PIOPED Investigators. Value of the ventilation/perfusion scan in acute pulmonary embolism. Results of the prospective investigation of pulmonary embolism diagnosis (PIOPED). JAMA 1990;263:2753–9.
7. Stein PD, Fowler SE, Goodman LR, et al. Multidetector computed tomography for acute pulmonary embolism. N Engl J Med 2006;354:2317–27.

8. Stein PD, Chenevert TL, Fowler SE, et al. Gadolinium-enhanced magnetic resonance angiography for pulmonary embolism: a multicenter prospective study (PIOPED III). Ann Intern Med 2010;152:434–43.

9. Ceriani E, Combescure C, Le Gal G, et al. Clinical prediction rules for pulmonary embolism: a systematic review and meta-analysis. J Thromb Haemost 2010; 8:957–70.

10. Goodacre S, Sutton AJ, Sampson FC. Meta-analysis: the value of clinical assessment in the diagnosis of deep venous thrombosis. Ann Intern Med 2005;143:129–39.

11. Kearon C, Kahn SR, Agnelli G, et al. Antithrombotic therapy for venous thromboembolic disease: American College of Chest Physicians evidence-based clinical practice guidelines. 8th Edition. Chest 2008;133:454S–545S.

12. Stein PD, Kayali F, Olson RE. Estimated case fatality rate of pulmonary embolism, 1979 to 1998. Am J Cardiol 2004;93:1197–9.

13. Hoffmann B, Gross CR, Jockel KH, et al. Trends in mortality of pulmonary embolism—an international comparison. Thromb Res 2010;125:303–8.

14. Carson JL, Kelley MA, Duff A, et al. The clinical course of pulmonary embolism. N Engl J Med 1992;326:1240–5.

15. Kearon C. Natural history of venous thromboembolism. Circulation 2003;107: I22–30.

16. Berlot G, Calderan C, Vergolini A, et al. Pulmonary embolism in critically ill patients receiving antithrombotic prophylaxis: a clinical-pathologic study. J Crit Care 2011; 26:28–33.

17. Cook DJ, Crowther MA, Meade MO, et al. Prevalence, incidence, and risk factors for venous thromboembolism in medical-surgical intensive care unit patients. J Crit Care 2005;20:309–13.

18. Cook D, Crowther M, Meade M, et al. Deep venous thrombosis in medical-surgical critically ill patients: prevalence, incidence, and risk factors. Crit Care Med 2005;33: 1565–71.

19. Ibrahim EH, Iregui M, Prentice D, et al. Deep vein thrombosis during prolonged mechanical ventilation despite prophylaxis. Crit Care Med 2002;30:771–4.

20. Prevention of fatal postoperative pulmonary embolism by low doses of heparin. An international multicentre trial. Lancet 1975;2:45–51.

21. Freedman KB, Brookenthal KR, Fitzgerald RH Jr, et al. A meta-analysis of thromboembolic prophylaxis following elective total hip arthroplasty. J Bone Joint Surg Am 2000;82-A:929–38.

22. Samama MM, Cohen AT, Darmon JY, et al; Prophylaxis in Medical Patients with Enoxaparin Study Group. A comparison of enoxaparin with placebo for the prevention of venous thromboembolism in acutely ill medical patients. N Engl J Med 1999;341:793–800.

23. Cook DJ, Crowther MA. Thromboprophylaxis in the intensive care unit: focus on medical-surgical patients. Crit Care Med 2010;38:S76–82.

24. Rizkallah J, Man SF, Sin DD. Prevalence of pulmonary embolism in acute exacerbations of COPD: a systematic review and metaanalysis. Chest 2009;135:786–93.

25. The PROTECT Investigators for the Canadian Critical Care Trials Group and the Australian and New Zealand Intensive Care Society Clinical Trials Group. Dalteparin versus unfractionated heparin in critically ill patients. N Engl J Med 2011; 364:1305–14.

26. Huet Y, Lemaire F, Brun-Buisson C, et al. Hypoxemia in acute pulmonary embolism. Chest 1985;88:829–36.

27. D'Angelo E. Lung mechanics and gas exchange in pulmonary embolism. Haematologica 1997;82:371–4.
28. Prediletto R, Paoletti P, Fornai E, et al. Natural course of treated pulmonary embolism. Evaluation by perfusion lung scintigraphy, gas exchange, and chest roentgenogram. Chest 1990;97:554–61.
29. Severinghaus JW, Swenson EW, Finley TN, et al. Unilateral hypoventilation produced in dogs by occluding one pulmonary artery. J Appl Physiol 1961;16:53–60.
30. Manier G, Castaing Y, Guenard H. Determinants of hypoxemia during the acute phase of pulmonary embolism in humans. Am Rev Respir Dis 1985;132:332–8.
31. D'Alonzo GE, Bower JS, DeHart P, et al. The mechanisms of abnormal gas exchange in acute massive pulmonary embolism. Am Rev Respir Dis 1983;128:170–2.
32. Kline JA, Meek S, Boudrow D, et al. Use of the alveolar dead space fraction (Vd/Vt) and plasma D-dimers to exclude acute pulmonary embolism in ambulatory patients. Acad Emerg Med 1997;4:856–63.
33. Wood KE. Major pulmonary embolism: review of a pathophysiologic approach to the golden hour of hemodynamically significant pulmonary embolism. Chest 2002;121:877–905.
34. Elliott CG. Pulmonary physiology during pulmonary embolism. Chest 1992;101:163S–71S.
35. McIntyre KM, Sasahara AA. The hemodynamic response to pulmonary embolism in patients without prior cardiopulmonary disease. Am J Cardiol 1971;28:288–94.
36. McIntyre KM, Sasahara AA. Hemodynamic alterations related to extent of lung scan perfusion defect in pulmonary embolism. J Nucl Med 1971;12:166–70.
37. McIntyre KM, Sasahara AA. Hemodynamic and ventricular responses to pulmonary embolism. Prog Cardiovasc Dis 1974;17:175–90.
38. Haeger K. Problems of acute deep venous thrombosis. I. The interpretation of signs and symptoms. Angiology 1969;20:219–23.
39. Wells PS, Anderson DR, Rodger M, et al. Evaluation of D-dimer in the diagnosis of suspected deep-vein thrombosis. N Engl J Med 2003;349:1227–35.
40. Mismetti P, Laporte S, Darmon JY, et al. Meta-analysis of low molecular weight heparin in the prevention of venous thromboembolism in general surgery. Br J Surg 2001;88:913–30.
41. Crowther MA, Cook DJ, Griffith LE, et al. Deep venous thrombosis: clinically silent in the intensive care unit. J Crit Care 2005;20:334–40.
42. Stein PD, Terrin ML, Hales CA, et al. Clinical, laboratory, roentgenographic, and electrocardiographic findings in patients with acute pulmonary embolism and no pre-existing cardiac or pulmonary disease. Chest 1991;100:598–603.
43. Stein PD, Beemath A, Matta F, et al. Clinical characteristics of patients with acute pulmonary embolism: data from PIOPED II. Am J Med 2007;120:871–9.
44. Stein PD, Matta F, Musani MH, et al. Silent pulmonary embolism in patients with deep venous thrombosis: a systematic review. Am J Med 2010;123:426–31.
45. Stein PD, Afzal A, Henry JW, et al. Fever in acute pulmonary embolism. Chest 2000;117:39–42.
46. Wells PS, Anderson DR, Bormanis J, et al. Value of assessment of pretest probability of deep-vein thrombosis in clinical management. Lancet 1997;350:1795–8.
47. Engelberger RP, Aujesky D, Calanca L, et al. Comparison of the diagnostic performance of the original and modified Wells score in inpatients and outpatients with suspected deep vein thrombosis. Thromb Res 2011;127:535–9.

48. Anderson DR, Wells PS, Stiell I, et al. Management of patients with suspected deep vein thrombosis in the emergency department: combining use of a clinical diagnosis model with D-dimer testing. J Emerg Med 2000;19:225–30.

49. Constans J, Nelzy ML, Salmi LR, et al. Clinical prediction of lower limb deep vein thrombosis in symptomatic hospitalized patients. Thromb Haemost 2001;86: 985–90.

50. Kahn SR, Joseph L, Abenhaim L, et al. Clinical prediction of deep vein thrombosis in patients with leg symptoms. Thromb Haemost 1999;81:353–7.

51. Constans J, Boutinet C, Salmi LR, et al. Comparison of four clinical prediction scores for the diagnosis of lower limb deep venous thrombosis in outpatients. Am J Med 2003;115:436–40.

52. Subramaniam RM, Chou T, Heath R, et al. Importance of pretest probability score and D-dimer assay before sonography for lower limb deep venous thrombosis. AJR Am J Roentgenol 2006;186:206–12.

53. Farrell S, Hayes T, Shaw M. A negative SimpliRED D-dimer assay result does not exclude the diagnosis of deep vein thrombosis or pulmonary embolus in emergency department patients. Ann Emerg Med 2000;35:121–5.

54. Gosselin RC, Owings JT, Kehoe J, et al. Comparison of six D-dimer methods in patients suspected of deep vein thrombosis. Blood Coagul Fibrinolysis 2003;14: 545–50.

55. Gardiner C, Pennaneac'h C, Walford C, et al. An evaluation of rapid D-dimer assays for the exclusion of deep vein thrombosis. Br J Haematol 2005;128:842–8.

56. Rabinov K, Paulin S. Roentgen diagnosis of venous thrombosis in the leg. Arch Surg 1972;104:134–44.

57. Sidhu PS, Alikhan R, Ammar T, et al. Lower limb contrast venography: a modified technique for use in thromboprophylaxis clinical trials for the accurate evaluation of deep vein thrombosis. Br J Radiol 2007;80:859–65.

58. Lensing AW, Prandoni P, Brandjes D, et al. Detection of deep-vein thrombosis by real-time B-mode ultrasonography. N Engl J Med 1989;320:342–5.

59. Kassai B, Boissel JP, Cucherat M, et al. A systematic review of the accuracy of ultrasound in the diagnosis of deep venous thrombosis in asymptomatic patients. Thromb Haemost 2004;91:655–66.

60. Hirsch DR, Ingenito EP, Goldhaber SZ. Prevalence of deep venous thrombosis among patients in medical intensive care. JAMA 1995;274:335–7.

61. Reis SE, Polak JF, Hirsch DR, et al. Frequency of deep venous thrombosis in asymptomatic patients with coronary artery bypass grafts. Am Heart J 1991;122: 478–82.

62. Beck-Razi N, Kuzmin A, Koren D, et al. Asymptomatic deep vein thrombosis in advanced cancer patients: the value of venous sonography. J Clin Ultrasound 2010;38:232–7.

63. Tomkowski WZ, Davidson BL, Wisniewska J, et al. Accuracy of compression ultrasound in screening for deep venous thrombosis in acutely ill medical patients. Thromb Haemost 2007;97:191–4.

64. Philbrick JT, Becker DM. Calf deep venous thrombosis. A wolf in sheep's clothing? Arch Intern Med 1988;148:2131–8.

65. Elias A, Mallard L, Elias M, et al. A single complete ultrasound investigation of the venous network for the diagnostic management of patients with a clinically suspected first episode of deep venous thrombosis of the lower limbs. Thromb Haemost 2003;89:221–7.

66. Tapson VF, Carroll BA, Davidson BL, et al. The diagnostic approach to acute venous thromboembolism. Clinical practice guideline. American Thoracic Society. Am J Respir Crit Care Med 1999;160:1043–66.
67. Hansson PO, Sorbo J, Eriksson H. Recurrent venous thromboembolism after deep vein thrombosis: incidence and risk factors. Arch Intern Med 2000;160:769–74.
68. Gaitini D. Current approaches and controversial issues in the diagnosis of deep vein thrombosis via duplex Doppler ultrasound. J Clin Ultrasound 2006;34:289–97.
69. Linkins LA, Pasquale P, Paterson S, et al. Change in thrombus length on venous ultrasound and recurrent deep vein thrombosis. Arch Intern Med 2004;164:1793–6.
70. Isma N, Svensson PJ, Gottsater A, et al. Upper extremity deep venous thrombosis in the population-based Malmo thrombophilia study (MATS). Epidemiology, risk factors, recurrence risk, and mortality. Thromb Res 2010;125:e335–8.
71. Munoz FJ, Mismetti P, Poggio R, et al. Clinical outcome of patients with upper-extremity deep vein thrombosis: results from the RIETE Registry. Chest 2008;133: 143–8.
72. Monreal M, Raventos A, Lerma R, et al. Pulmonary embolism in patients with upper extremity DVT associated to venous central lines—a prospective study. Thromb Haemost 1994;72:548–50.
73. Mustafa BO, Rathbun SW, Whitsett TL, et al. Sensitivity and specificity of ultrasonography in the diagnosis of upper extremity deep vein thrombosis: a systematic review. Arch Intern Med 2002;162:401–4.
74. Di Nisio M, Van Sluis GL, Bossuyt PM, et al. Accuracy of diagnostic tests for clinically suspected upper extremity deep vein thrombosis: a systematic review. J Thromb Haemost 2010;8:684–92.
75. Kalva SP, Jagannathan JP, Hahn PF, et al. Venous thromboembolism: indirect CT venography during CT pulmonary angiography—should the pelvis be imaged? Radiology 2008;246:605–11.
76. Goodman LR, Stein PD, Matta F, et al. CT venography and compression sonography are diagnostically equivalent: data from PIOPED II. AJR Am J Roentgenol 2007;189:1071–6.
77. Kluge A, Mueller C, Strunk J, et al. Experience in 207 combined MRI examinations for acute pulmonary embolism and deep vein thrombosis. AJR Am J Roentgenol 2006;186:1686–96.
78. Fraser DG, Moody AR, Morgan PS, et al. Diagnosis of lower-limb deep venous thrombosis: a prospective blinded study of magnetic resonance direct thrombus imaging. Ann Intern Med 2002;136:89–98.
79. Sampson FC, Goodacre SW, Thomas SM, et al. The accuracy of MRI in diagnosis of suspected deep vein thrombosis: systematic review and meta-analysis. Eur Radiol 2007;17:175–81.
80. Wells PS, Anderson DR, Rodger M, et al. Derivation of a simple clinical model to categorize patients probability of pulmonary embolism: increasing the models utility with the SimpliRED D-dimer. Thromb Haemost 2000;83:416–20.
81. Wolf SJ, McCubbin TR, Feldhaus KM, et al. Prospective validation of Wells Criteria in the evaluation of patients with suspected pulmonary embolism. Ann Emerg Med 2004;44:503–10.
82. Wicki J, Perneger TV, Junod AF, et al. Assessing clinical probability of pulmonary embolism in the emergency ward: a simple score. Arch Intern Med 2001;161:92–7.
83. Le Gal G, Righini M, Roy PM, et al. Prediction of pulmonary embolism in the emergency department: the revised Geneva score. Ann Intern Med 2006;144: 165–71.

84. Kline JA, Nelson RD, Jackson RE, et al. Criteria for the safe use of D-dimer testing in emergency department patients with suspected pulmonary embolism: a multicenter US study. Ann Emerg Med 2002;39:144–52.

85. Daniel KR, Courtney DM, Kline JA. Assessment of cardiac stress from massive pulmonary embolism with 12-lead ECG. Chest 2001;120:474–81.

86. Ferrari E, Imbert A, Chevalier T, et al. The ECG in pulmonary embolism. Predictive value of negative T waves in precordial leads— 80 case reports. Chest 1997;111: 537–43.

87. Worsley DF, Alavi A, Aronchick JM, et al. Chest radiographic findings in patients with acute pulmonary embolism: observations from the PIOPED Study. Radiology 1993; 189:133–6.

88. Rodger MA, Carrier M, Jones GN, et al. Diagnostic value of arterial blood gas measurement in suspected pulmonary embolism. Am J Respir Crit Care Med 2000;162:2105–8.

89. Stein PD, Goldhaber SZ, Henry JW, et al. Arterial blood gas analysis in the assessment of suspected acute pulmonary embolism. Chest 1996;109:78–81.

90. Hemnes AR, Newman AL, Rosenbaum B, et al. Bedside end-tidal CO_2 tension as a screening tool to exclude pulmonary embolism. Eur Respir J 2010;35:735–41.

91. Kline JA, Hogg MM, Courtney DM, et al. D-dimer and exhaled CO_2/O_2 to detect segmental pulmonary embolism in moderate-risk patients. Am J Respir Crit Care Med 2010;182:669–75.

92. van Belle A, Buller HR, Huisman MV, et al. Effectiveness of managing suspected pulmonary embolism using an algorithm combining clinical probability, D-dimer testing, and computed tomography. JAMA 2006;295:172–9.

93. Kruip MJ, Sohne M, Nijkeuter M, et al. A simple diagnostic strategy in hospitalized patients with clinically suspected pulmonary embolism. J Intern Med 2006; 260:459–66.

94. Stein PD, Woodard PK, Weg JG, et al. Diagnostic pathways in acute pulmonary embolism: recommendations of the PIOPED II investigators. Am J Med 2006;119: 1048–55.

95. Anderson DR, Kahn SR, Rodger MA, et al. Computed tomographic pulmonary angiography vs ventilation-perfusion lung scanning in patients with suspected pulmonary embolism: a randomized controlled trial. JAMA 2007;298:2743–53.

96. Henry JW, Stein PD, Gottschalk A, et al. Scintigraphic lung scans and clinical assessment in critically ill patients with suspected acute pulmonary embolism. Chest 1996;109:462–6.

97. Miniati M, Pistolesi M, Marini C, et al. Value of perfusion lung scan in the diagnosis of pulmonary embolism: results of the Prospective Investigative Study of Acute Pulmonary Embolism Diagnosis (PISA-PED). Am J Respir Crit Care Med 1996; 154:1387–93.

98. Invasive and noninvasive diagnosis of pulmonary embolism. Preliminary results of the Prospective Investigative Study of Acute Pulmonary Embolism Diagnosis (PISA-PED). Chest 1995;107:33S–8S.

99. Stawicki SP, Seamon MJ, Meredith DM, et al. Transthoracic echocardiography for suspected pulmonary embolism in the intensive care unit: unjustly underused or rightfully ignored? J Clin Ultrasound 2008;36:291–302.

100. Kurzyna M, Torbicki A, Pruszczyk P, et al. Disturbed right ventricular ejection pattern as a new Doppler echocardiographic sign of acute pulmonary embolism. Am J Cardiol 2002;90:507–11.

101. Bouferrache K, Vieillard-Baron A. Acute respiratory distress syndrome, mechanical ventilation, and right ventricular function. Curr Opin Crit Care 2011;17:30–5.

102. Pruszczyk P, Torbicki A, Pacho R, et al. Noninvasive diagnosis of suspected severe pulmonary embolism: transesophageal echocardiography vs spiral CT. Chest 1997; 112:722–8.
103. Stein PD, Athanasoulis C, Alavi A, et al. Complications and validity of pulmonary angiography in acute pulmonary embolism. Circulation 1992;85:462–8.
104. Dindo D, Breitenstein S, Hahnloser D, et al. Kinetics of D-dimer after general surgery. Blood Coagul Fibrinolysis 2009;20:347–52.
105. Crowther MA, Cook DJ, Griffith LE, et al. Neither baseline tests of molecular hypercoagulability nor D-dimer levels predict deep venous thrombosis in critically ill medical-surgical patients. Intensive Care Med 2005;31:48–55.
106. Adams RC, Hamrick M, Berenguer C, et al. Four years of an aggressive prophylaxis and screening protocol for venous thromboembolism in a large trauma population. J Trauma 2008;65:300–6 [discussion: 306–8].
107. Borer DS, Starr AJ, Reinert CM, et al. The effect of screening for deep vein thrombosis on the prevalence of pulmonary embolism in patients with fractures of the pelvis or acetabulum: a review of 973 patients. J Orthop Trauma 2005;19:92–5.
108. Girard P, Sanchez O, Leroyer C, et al. Deep venous thrombosis in patients with acute pulmonary embolism: prevalence, risk factors, and clinical significance. Chest 2005;128:1593–600.
109. Wells PS, Ginsberg JS, Anderson DR, et al. Use of a clinical model for safe management of patients with suspected pulmonary embolism. Ann Intern Med 1998;129:997–1005.
110. Halpern NA, Pastores SM. Critical care medicine in the United States 2000–2005: An analysis of bed numbers, occupancy rates, payer mix, and costs. Crit Care Med 2010;38:65–71.
111. Halpern NA, Pastores SM, Thaler HT, et al. Changes in critical care beds and occupancy in the United States 1985–2000: differences attributable to hospital size. Crit Care Med 2006; 34:2105–12.

Natural History of Venous Thromboembolism

Timothy A. Morris, MD

KEYWORDS

- Venous thromboembolism • Deep venous thrombosis
- Chronic thrombotic venous disease • Pulmonary embolism
- Chronic thromboembolic pulmonary hypertension

Venous thromboembolism (VTE), originates in systemic venous thrombosis, and has different etiological mechanisms and natural history from arterial thrombosis. VTE typically originates as deep venous thrombosis (DVT) in a lower extremity, where it may give rise to acute symptoms "upstream" from the obstructed vein, result in pulmonary embolism (PE) and/or cause chronic venous obstruction. PE may result in acute respiratory symptoms, cardiovascular collapse and, uncommonly, may also cause chronic disease.

ETIOLOGICAL FACTORS

Conditions that favor venous thromboembolism (VTE) may fall into 3 categories, as observed by Virchow more than a century ago: venous stasis, injury to the venous intima, and alterations in the coagulation-fibrinolytic system.[1] The relative importance of the 3 factors varies among clinical situations. Venous stasis is associated with deep vein thrombosis (DVT) in the lower extremities during medically indicated bed rest and with right (and left) atrial thrombosis during atrial fibrillation.[2] Intermittent compression stockings that restore venous flow reduce the risk for DVT.[3–5] It may be, however, that the risk of stasis in the absence of medical illness or injury, as may occur during air flight, is more modest.[6] Injury to the venous wall is the most likely mechanism of the large number of lower extremity DVTs observed in proximity to sites of trauma and major orthopedic surgery.[7–9] Coagulation abnormalities that occur alone or in concert with other conditions can promote clinical venous thrombosis. For example, there is an increased risk for VTE associated with mutations in factor V (factor V Leiden)[10] and in the untranslated region of the gene-encoding prothrombin (although the procoagulant mechanism of the latter mutation is still under investigation).[11] Other less prevalent, but probably more potent, "thrombophilias" include deficiencies of

This work was supported by grant number HL095089 from the National Institutes of Health. The author has nothing to disclose.

Division of Pulmonary and Critical Care Medicine, Department of Medicine, University of California, San Diego School of Medicine, 200 West Arbor Drive, San Diego, CA 92103-8378, USA
E-mail address: t1morris@ucsd.edu

Crit Care Clin 27 (2011) 869–884
doi:10.1016/j.ccc.2011.09.001
0749-0704/11/$ – see front matter © 2011 Published by Elsevier Inc.

criticalcare.theclinics.com

antithrombin III, protein C, and protein S; aberrations in the thrombolytic system; and the presence of antibodies responsible for the antiphospholipid syndrome ("lupus anticoagulant"). Clinical conditions that involve combinations of these fundamental risk factors are associated with higher risks of thrombosis.

DEEP VENOUS THROMBOSIS

The events initiating DVT are not fully understood. The initial event is typically the development of a small nidus of thrombosis in 1 or more valves of the lower extremity veins, especially in the calves where eddy currents arise, or at the site of intimal injury.[12] A positive feedback cascade leads to the elaboration of clot-potentiating materials that trigger prolongation of the thrombus with red blood cells (RBCs), fibrin and, to a lesser degree, platelets. Once formed, the thrombus grows by accumulating additional RBC, fibrin, and platelet "layers," seen pathologically as the lines of Zahn.

Even as thrombosis is occurring, the process of resolution is beginning. The thrombi resolve by 1 or both of 2 mechanisms: fibrinolysis and organization. Fibrinolysis refers to actual dissolution of the thrombus by plasma enzymes. It is a relatively rapid process, proceeding over a period of hours to several days. As thrombus extension occurs, local fibrinolytic activity is enhanced. Thus, thrombus behavior becomes a dynamic process that may result in complete dissolution, partial resolution resulting in a variable degree of intimal narrowing and valvular damage, progressive proximal extension, or embolization.

If fibrinolysis is not totally successful, organization may either complete the job of resolution or form permanent intravascular scars. Reparative cells infiltrate the residual thrombus and replace the "thrombotic components" with connective tissue. The fibrotic residuum is then incorporated into the venous wall and re-endothelialized. Organization usually thickens the venous wall, which may provide loci for further thrombus formation. The thickening may also incorporate 1 or more venous valves, rendering them incompetent. Whatever the fate of a given thrombus, the organizational phase of resolution is typically underway within 7 to 10 days. By that time, the initial thrombus is gone or has been incorporated into the venous wall. In more than half of patients, some degree of permanent venous wall scarring occurs, which is visible on ultrasound.[13] If the venous wall scarring causes severe obstruction, collateral veins develop. At that point, the pathology is more accurately termed a venous scar than an old clot.

The duration of venous obstruction after DVT appears to be much longer than can be accounted for by the presence of "pure" thrombi.[14,15] Acute thrombi themselves are impermanent structures. Histologically, they are composed of layers of platelets, fibrin, and erythrocytes.[16] Fibrin-entrapped erythrocytes constitute most of the volume in acute thromboemboli. The life expectancy of new erythrocytes within the circulation is between 2 and 4 months,[17,18] and it seems reasonable to expect that erythrocytes entrapped within thrombi would disintegrate within this period. The duration of time that fibrin persists within thromboemboli may be inferred by plasma levels of fibrin D-dimer, a principal fragment resulting from fibrinolytic digestion. When patients are treated with anticoagulants to prevent the deposition of new fibrin, elevated blood D-dimer levels can be found in about two-fifths of patients at the end of 1 month.[19] However, by 3 months only about one-tenth of patients remain positive and about half of those are positive because of recurrence. The long-term outlook is influenced principally by the extent of residual venous obstruction and valvular damage. If significant obstruction or valvular damage persists, downstream stasis will be present, leading to a risk of recurrent deep venous thrombosis and development of the post-phlebitic syndrome.[14,20]

CHRONIC THROMBOTIC VENOUS DISEASE

If, after DVT, the thrombotic material in the vasculature does not resolve by fibrinolysis, it is remodeled into organized scars that may be termed "chronic thrombotic venous disease" (CTVD). The extent to which remodeling occurs, and the severity of the resulting vascular obstruction, vary among patients. In some patients with DVT the venous lumen is rapidly restored,[21] although the resolution in the first month is typically incomplete. Recovery continues at a slower pace for the next 3 to 6 months, during which clot remodeling may be occurring.[20] Residual defects persist commonly beyond this period, suggesting that the clots have been remodeled into permanent vascular scars.[20] These findings suggest that incomplete clot resolution occurs in a significant proportion of patients with acute DVT.

Incomplete clot lysis after thromboembolism may predispose patients toward developing CTVD, and may be a useful marker of this risk.[22] However, delayed fibrinolysis could be implicated in the development of symptomatic disease only if the acute thromboembolism was large enough to create a substantial local nidus for remodeling and intravascular scar formation. It is in the presence of large focal thromboemboli that cellular reparative and organizational mechanisms would have the greatest clinical importance. The resulting persistent large vessel obstruction, combined with various degrees of vascular reaction, lead to progressively worsening symptoms.[23]

In the case of CTVD, damage to the integrity of adjacent venous valves by the intravascular scarring is particularly problematic.[24,25] Permanent valvular reflux may result in postthrombotic syndrome (PTS), manifested by chronic pain and swelling in the affected limb.[26,27] Although the involvement of any particular venous valve may be subject to random chance, it stands to reason that the probability of venous valve damage would be increased if the vascular scarring process is extensive.

The reason that a fraction of patients with DVT go on to have fulminant CTVD is unclear. Most patients who present with these disorders were previously diagnosed with DVT, but their presentations (clot burden, clinical stability, etc) are not entirely distinct from patients who resolve their acute clots.[26,28] Some insights may be gained by the clinical conditions associated with PTS, although the definition of this syndrome does not require anatomical evidence of CTVD. PTS is associated with DVT after a previous venous thrombosis episode,[26] an idiopathic etiology of the venous thrombosis episode,[26] the presence of venous reflux[25] in the lower extremity veins,[24] advancing age,[29] female sex,[29] hormone therapy,[26,29] varicose veins,[29] DVT postabdominal surgery,[29] and an increased body mass index.[29,30] These findings raise the possibility that an acquired or inherited predisposition toward incomplete clot resolution is present in at least some patients with CTVD.

PULMONARY EMBOLISM

Of course, DVT is the principal cause of acute pulmonary embolism (APE). The risk of embolism is highest early in thrombus development before significant fibrinolysis or organization occurs. Approximately 90% of pulmonary emboli that elicit clinical attention arise from venous thrombosis in the deep veins of the lower extremities.[31] Uncommonly, venous thrombi capable of embolization arise from other sites. Primary iliac or proximal femoral thrombi may develop in patients undergoing surgery involving the hip, and pelvic vein thrombosis can occur in patients undergoing pelvic or prostatic surgery. Axillosubclavian vein thrombosis may be spontaneous, resulting from congenital abnormalities of the thoracic outlet, or may be related to indwelling central venous catheters, pulmonary artery catheters, or transvenous pacing wires.[32]

Thrombi may also form dilated right heart chambers and embolize into the pulmonary artery.

The location of the DVT has a profound influence on the likelihood of embolism. Upper extremity proximal DVT appears to pose at least as high a risk of clinically significant PE as lower extremity proximal DVT.[32,33] Although the majority of lower extremity thrombi originate in the veins of the calf, thrombi that remain limited to the calf veins rarely result in PE.[34] If left untreated, however, one-fourth of symptomatic, isolated calf thrombi will extend to involve the proximal veins (popliteal, superficial femoral and common femoral veins, or even more proximally).[35] Proximal extension poses a risk of embolization that approaches 50%.[36,37]

It is becoming apparent that the composition of the thrombi themselves may also influence the likelihood of PE. Patients in whom VTE is manifested by PE tend to recur with PE rather than with DVT alone.[38] A provocative finding in some of the patients with PE is the presence of a fibrinogen mutation,[39-41] which gives rise to highly cross-linked, and therefore tightly compressed, thrombi.[42] DVT arising in patients with the mutation may be predisposed to embolization. Whether other genetic or acquired fibrinogen variants may also influence the risk of embolization is not yet known.

Because PE is typically a complication of DVT, rather than a de novo disorder, the natural history of DVT has several important clinical implications. Because the vast majority of emboli arise from thrombi in the proximal veins in the lower extremity, diagnostic approaches to deep venous thrombosis can be focused on techniques that detect lower extremity DVT. Techniques that detect above-knee thrombi are of particular value regardless of whether they can detect calf-limited thrombi. However, although calf-limited thrombi rarely embolize, it would be incorrect to assume that symptomatic, calf-limited deep venous thrombosis represents a clinically irrelevant condition. Proximal extension of calf vein thrombi may occur, at which point PE is a significant risk. In addition, symptomatic calf vein thrombosis appears to be subject to recurrence, albeit at a lower risk than proximal vein thrombosis.[43]

Acute Effects of Acute Pulmonary Emboli

When emboli arise and lodge in 1 or more pulmonary arteries, hemodynamic and respiratory consequences occur. The hemodynamic consequences stem from a decrease in the available cross-sectional area of the pulmonary arterial system through both mechanical obstruction and release of vasoconstrictive thrombus metabolites directly into the vascular bed. The pulmonary vascular resistance rises, causing an increased pulmonary arterial pressure, and therefore an increased right ventricular workload. If these consequences are severe, the right ventricle may not tolerate the workload and the cardiac output will fall. The respiratory effects are due to alterations in the patterns of pulmonary perfusion and ventilation that result from the mechanical obstruction itself, passive redistribution of blood flow and active compensatory mechanisms.

Hemodynamic Effects

The cardiac and hemodynamic effects of embolism are related to the degree of reduction of the cross-sectional area of the pulmonary vascular bed, the preexisting status of the cardiopulmonary system, and the physiologic consequences of hypoxic and neurohumorally mediated vasoconstriction.[44-49] Mechanical obstruction of the pulmonary vascular bed by embolism is accompanied by release of vasoconstrictive substances such as thromboxane-A(2) and serotonin.[50] The combination acutely increases the workload on the right ventricle, a chamber ill equipped to deal with high pressure load. In patients without preexisting cardiopulmonary disease, obstruction of less than 20% of the pulmonary vascular bed results in a number of compensatory events that minimize adverse hemodynamic consequences. Recruitment and distention of pulmonary vessels occur, resulting in a normal or near-normal pulmonary artery pressure and pulmonary vascular resistance; cardiac output is maintained by increases in the right ventricular stroke volume and increases in the heart rate. As the degree of pulmonary vascular obstruction exceeds 30% to 40%, increases in pulmonary artery pressure and modest increases in right atrial pressure occur. The Frank-Starling mechanism maintains right ventricular stroke work and cardiac output. When the degree of pulmonary artery obstruction exceeds 50% to 60%, compensatory mechanisms are overcome, cardiac output begins to fall, and right atrial pressure increases dramatically. With acute obstruction beyond this amount, the right heart dilates, right ventricular wall tension increases, right ventricular ischemia may develop, the cardiac output falls, and systemic hypotension develops. The myocardium of the right ventricle is at particular risk of ischemia, because its coronary artery perfusion pressure drops as a result of the decrease in mean arterial pressure and the increase in right ventricular pressure.

In patients without prior cardiopulmonary disease, the maximal mean pulmonary artery pressure capable of being generated by the right ventricle appears to be 40 mm Hg (representing a pulmonary artery systolic pressure of approximately 70 mm Hg). The correlation between the extent of pulmonary vascular obstruction and the pulmonary vascular resistance appears to be hyperbolic, reflecting at its lower end the expansible nature of the pulmonary vascular bed and at its upper the precipitous decline in cardiac output that may occur as the right ventricle fails.[51]

The hemodynamic response to APE in patients with preexisting cardiopulmonary disease may be considerably different.[49] Unlike patients without prior cardiopulmonary disease, in whom there is a general relationship between the degree of pulmonary vascular obstruction and the level of the pulmonary artery pressure, patients with prior cardiopulmonary disease demonstrate degrees of pulmonary hypertension that are disproportionate to the degree of pulmonary vascular obstruction. As a result, severe pulmonary hypertension may develop in response to a relatively small reduction in pulmonary artery cross-sectional area. Thus, evidence of right ventricular hypertrophy (rather than right ventricular dilation) associated with a mean pulmonary artery pressure in excess of 40 mm Hg (pulmonary artery systolic pressure in excess of approximately 70 mm Hg) in a patient suspected of embolism should suggest an element of chronic pulmonary hypertension resulting from a potentially diverse group of etiologic possibilities (chronic thromboembolic pulmonary hypertension, left ventricular failure, valvular disease, right-to-left cardiac shunts, etc).

Respiratory Effects

Respiratory consequences of PE include altered ventilation-perfusion relationships, which, combined with a fall in cardiac output and resulting lowered venous oxygen concentration, may lead to arterial hypoxemia, development of 1 or more zones of alveolar dead space (zones that are ventilated but not perfused), transient pneumoconstriction of these same zones, and hyperventilation (the reasons for which are debated).

At least some degree of hypoxemia is common in patients with acute PE, primarily because of the regional obstruction to pulmonary blood flow, diversion of the flow to unobstructed portions of the lung, and alterations in the ventilation/perfusion balance in both the obstructed and the unobstructed regions.[52,53] According to Mason in

Murray and Nadel's Textbook of Respiratory Medicine, "If regional pulmonary vascular obstruction is total, alveolar dead space is created."[54] If a region's blood flow is severely obstructed, bronchoconstriction may occur in the lung distal to the area of obstruction as the result of alveolar hypocapnia.[55] This is probably uncommon in patients because they are free to inhale carbon dioxide–rich dead space air into the associated lung regions, and because obstruction is rarely total. Hyperventilation almost always occurs, the mechanism for which remains uncertain. Arterial hypoxemia may be worsened when acute increases in right ventricular afterload lower the cardiac output enough to widen the arteriovenous oxygen difference and decrease the saturation of mixed venous gas.[56] This lowering of the mixed venous oxygen content magnifies the effects of the normal venous admixture, thereby lowering the arterial pO_2. Another potential mechanism for hypoxemia in patients with massive pulmonary embolism is right-to-left shunt, either on an intrapulmonary or an intracardiac basis.[57] With embolic occlusion sufficient to increase pulmonary artery pressure, hypoxic vasoconstrictive mechanisms can be overcome, and perfusion to poorly ventilated or nonventilated lung regions may occur. On occasion, embolic events massive enough to increase right atrial pressure may result in intracardiac right-to-left shunting through a patent foramen ovale.

Surfactant loss may occur if severe pulmonary artery occlusion occurs for a sufficient duration to deplete the nutrient supply necessary to produce alveolar surfactant[58]: typically at least 24 hours. Once this occurs, surfactant becomes depleted in the obstructed alveolar zones. The 2 major consequences of surfactant depletion are atelectasis and an increase in permeability of the alveolocapillary membrane, causing further problems with gas exchange. If partial thrombus resolution and reperfusion to this atelectatic region develop, hypoxemia can result.

Pulmonary infarction is a rare consequence of embolism; fewer than 10% of emboli lead to infarction. Infarction is uncommon because the pulmonary parenchyma has 3 potential sources of oxygen: the pulmonary arteries, the bronchial arteries, and the airways.[59] In patients with no coexisting cardiopulmonary disease, large infarctions (such as those visible by chest radiography) are rare.[60,61] However, autopsy series suggest that infarctions of smaller pulmonary arteries are more common.[62,63] Infarction occurs in approximately 20% to 33% of patients with significant cardiac or pulmonary disease that compromises either bronchial arterial flow or airway patency. In patients with left ventricular failure, increased pulmonary venous pressure may decrease bronchial flow and infarction may result.[64]

EFFECT OF PLASMINOGEN ACTIVATION ON SHORT-TERM OUTCOME AFTER ACUTE PULMONARY EMBOLISM

The effect of plasminogen-activating drugs on the resolution of acute PE, and on its subsequent outcome, is unclear and based at least partly on indirect information rather than by comparative clinical trials in the appropriate patient population. The Urokinase in Pulmonary Embolism Trial[65] (UPET), the largest trial to randomize patients into thrombolytic or standard heparin therapy, was performed on patients who were hemodynamically stable. There was a very short-term hemodynamic benefit: cardiac outputs and pulmonary pressures were improved on the day after thrombolytics. No positive effects on morbidity or mortality were demonstrated, nor was the ultimate degree of embolic resolution any greater. By 1 week, the treatment groups were identical (except for an increase in bleeding in the thrombolytic group). Multiple studies have confirmed that these agents promote rapid embolic resolution.[66] However, there does not appear to be a long-term benefit to more rapid (but not necessarily more complete) clot resolution.[67]

Patients with massive PE have much higher mortality rates than the patients evaluated in the UPET trial. The mortality for patients with high right ventricular pressures and high pulmonary artery pressures is about double the mortality for more stable patients with PE. The mortality increases exponentially as patients progress to hypotension, shock, and then the need for CPR.[68] It is likely that the acute hemodynamic benefits of thrombolytics will have a much higher impact on these patients than on the stable patients in the UPET trial. The outcome benefit of thrombolytics in unstable patients has been studied in uncontrolled, retrospective studies. One study reported a lower mortality rate in patients treated with thrombo-lytics,[68] whereas the other reported a higher mortality rate (because of bleeding).[69]

A study of "submassive" pulmonary embolism (ie, with evidence of right ventricular strain)[70] randomized patients to either thrombolytics plus heparin or heparin plus placebo. The groups were compared on the basis of a "combined" primary endpoint including death and escalation of treatment (including subsequent thrombolytic therapy). Although the group receiving thrombolytics had a lower incidence of the combined endpoint, the only actual "outcome" difference between the groups was that those treated with heparin-placebo received more thrombolytic therapy during the follow-up period. No other outcome, such as death and the need for mechanical ventilation or vasopressors, was different between the groups, begging the question of whether "rescue" thrombolytic therapy was necessary. Unfortunately, the results did not answer the question of whether thrombolytic therapy is beneficial initially or even during follow-up for patients with evidence of right heart strain.

Thrombolytics carry significant risks. A review of clinical trials disclosed a 2.1% intracranial hemorrhage rate and 1.6% fatal intracranial hemorrhage rate when thrombolytics were used for thromboembolic disease.[71] For this reason, the potential short-term benefits of thrombolytics on the hemodynamic and respiratory effects of PE must be weighed against the risk of catastrophic bleeding.

An important clinical question concerns the hemodynamic deterioration observed in some patients with PE in the first few days after embolization. Although PE can be immediately fatal, a large number of patients who eventually succumb do so 1 or more days after presentation.[72] It stands to reason that these "late fatalities" are caused by either progressively deteriorating myocardial fatigue (right ventricular infarction or other myocyte injury) or increase in workload because of recurrent emboli, or are caused by factors such as embolus propagation, or further release of vasoactive mediators from the embolus. The hypothesis that acute recurrent emboli (even clinically undetected emboli) are the source of the risk is supported by the findings in 2 case series that adjunctive inferior vena cava filter placement was associated with substantial reductions in mortality rates during treatment of hemodynamically signif-icant pulmonary embolism.[73,74]

The phenomenon of embolic fragments entrapped in the right atrium and ventricle has been recognized in experimental embolism for some time; as cardiac echocardiography is more extensively utilized, this phenomenon has become more widely recognized in human disease as well. The clinical significance of these sessile cardiac thrombi has not been studied in a controlled fashion. However, it is likely that these thrombi may embolize; therefore, larger cardiac thrombi may warrant emergent surgical removal, especially in the presence of preexisting hemodynamic compromise.[75]

LONG-TERM EFFECTS OF ACUTE PULMONARY EMBOLISM

Beyond these acute events, most PE, like most DVT, tends to resolve if prevented from propagating by anticoagulants. The behavior of PE parallels that previously described DVT: they undergo resolution by fibrinolysis, by organization and recanalization, or both. Although there is a great deal of interpatient variability, resolution of pulmonary emboli typically is substantial during the first week, somewhat more gradual for the next 4 to 8 weeks, and then very slow thereafter.[54,76–81]

Despite the heterogeneity of the clinical data, several generalizations can be made with respect to the time course of perfusion recovery after acute PE. The percentage of patients experiencing complete scintigraphic resolution during the first week is very low. By 1 month, roughly one-fifth to one-third of patients on average will go on to complete recovery. Between 1 and 3 months, an additional small percentage of patients may recover. After 3 months, additional patients will recover, although the data vary so widely that it is difficult to draw conclusions regarding the proportion of who will eventually recover perfusion completely.

Some of the hemodynamic manifestations of pulmonary emboli may also persist beyond the acute episode. Serial echocardiography of patients with PE suggests a rapid, but often incomplete phase of recovery in the systolic pulmonary artery pressure (as estimated from the tricuspid regurgitation jet velocities) during the first month, followed by a much more gradual rate of recovery in the subsequent year.[82,83] High pulmonary artery pressures during the initial phase were associated with increased risk of persistent pulmonary hypertension, further supporting the etiological role of incomplete thrombus resolution in the development of chronic disease.

LUNG PERFUSION RECOVERY AFTER ACUTE PULMONARY EMBOLISM

Persistent perfusion defects may have other consequences besides the risk of pulmonary hypertension. Pulmonary arterial obstruction can lead to ventilation/perfusion mismatching sufficient to affect gas exchange.[84–87] Up to 15% of acute patients with PE remain symptomatically compromised 2 years after treatment[88] and may have abnormal alveolar-arterial O_2 gradients and increased dead space ratios and decreased DL_{CO} values.[54]

The likelihood of recovery is influenced by the size of the initial defect as well as the existence of other cardiopulmonary diseases. Larger initial perfusion defects lower the incidence of complete recovery at all time points after PE. Short-term recovery of perfusion occurred in one-third of patients with small initial perfusion defects (<15%), but only in about one-fifth of those with larger defects.[89] Likewise, the frequency of complete resolution 4 months after PE varied from 67% in patients with minimal initial perfusion defects (≤15%) to 20% in patients with severe defects (31%–50%).[90] Another study reported complete recovery in 49% of patients whose initial defects were less than 30% compared with only 14% among those with initial defects of 30% or greater, a statistically significant difference.[80]

Preexisting cardiac or pulmonary disease at the time of PE has been associated with a lower likelihood of complete resolution of perfusion defects. One series reported complete recovery by 3 months in 32% (16 of 51) of patients without heart disease compared with only 5% (1 of 19) with heart disease.[89] A longer follow-up of 48 patients surviving acute massive PE reported complete scintigraphic normalization in 46% of patients without concomitant cardiopulmonary disease versus 22% of patients with concomitant cardiopulmonary disease.[91] These observations may reflect slower rates of PE resolution in these patients or may be explained by the effect of the concomitant diseases themselves on lung perfusion.

Incomplete recovery after PE occurs with about the same pattern as it does after DVT.[22,90–97] The proportions of patients completely resolving their intravascular defects after acute DVT and acute PE are quite comparable. Similar to DVT, residual defects after acute PE commonly persist beyond the expected survival of erythrocytes and fibrin.[81]

The average degree of resolution by 6 months is about half of the initial vascular defect in patients with DVT[20,21] and in patients with acute PE.[54,65,76–80,94] The similarity in resolution rates raises the possibility that similar phenomena may interfere with thrombus resolution in both patients with DVT and patients with PE. It follows from these observations that long-term residual defects within the pulmonary arteries would be attributed to processes beyond the initial thrombotic episode.

The resolution or persistence of thrombotic material in the pulmonary arteries depends on the balance between fibrinolysis and the cellular remodeling processes that produce scars within the pulmonary arterial lumen. Early after pulmonary thromboembolism, inflammation and associated intimal hyperplasia occur within the pulmonary arteries,[98] similar to what is observed with chronic thromboembolic pulmonary hypertension.[99,100] The extent to which this histological process occurs in actual patients must be inferred from clinical outcome studies.

Relative perfusion recovery is influenced by the presence of underlying cardiopulmonary disease. One may expect that, in patients with acute PE and preexisting cardiopulmonary disorders, the degree of perfusion recovery will be about one-third less than the degree of recovery in other patients with acute PE.[79,81,89,90] It is likely that underlying cardiopulmonary conditions themselves are responsible for some of the perfusion abnormalities observed during PE, but it is also possible that underlying cardiopulmonary disease predisposes to persistent or recurrent thromboembolism. The contribution of each of these factors is difficult to sort through, because the persistence of a perfusion defect in the same position from one scan to another may reflect the failure of an initial thrombus to resolve, the recurrence of thrombus in the same location, or simply decreased perfusion from parenchymal or cardiac disease.

CHRONIC THROMBOEMBOLIC PULMONARY HYPERTENSION

In a small proportion of patients with PE, pulmonary artery scarring develops residual obstruction sufficient to cause chronic thromboembolic pulmonary hypertension (CTEPH).[22] The persistent large vessel obstruction, combined with various degrees of an incompletely understood small vessel reaction, lead to progressively worsening pulmonary hypertension.[23] The reason that a fraction of patients with PE go on to have CTEPH is unclear. Most patients who present with CTEPH who were previously diagnosed with acute pulmonary emboli had initial presentations (clot burden, clinical stability, etc) that were indistinguishable from patients who went on to resolve their acute clots.[101] A prospective study of patients presenting with PE disclosed that, in addition to the size of the initial PE, factors such as recurrent PE, idiopathic PE, and PE at a young age were associated with a higher risk for CTEPH.[22] These findings raise the possibility that an inherited or acquired predisposition toward incomplete clot resolution is present in at least some patients who develop CTEPH.

Although the specific etiologies leading to CTEPH after PE are not fully understood, there is evidence to suggest the fibrin clots themselves are relatively resistant to lysis in some patients with CTEPH.[102] Persistent fibrin after thrombosis may be important to pulmonary artery remodeling. Fibrin activates pulmonary artery endothelial cells[103] via the fibrin receptor vascular endothelial cadherin.[104] Fibrin induces expression of interleukin-8 and facilitates the migration of repair cells along endothelial cells by interactions with the intracellular adhesion molecule-1[105] and the leukocyte adhesion receptor Mac-1.[106] Incomplete thrombus resolution would result in pulmonary vascular scarring after an acute PE only if there was a persistence of ligands within the residual thrombotic material that would stimulate inflammation and remodeling by connective tissue cells. Interestingly, there is a clinical association between chronic inflammatory conditions and the development of CTEPH after acute PE.[107]

In some cases, fibrinogen variants might be involved with CTEPH development. For example, 5 heterozygous fibrinogen gene mutations (fibrinogens$_{San\ Diego\ 1-5}$) with abnormalities in fibrin polymer structure and susceptibility to lysis were discovered in a series of 33 patients with CTEPH.[108] Another variant, fibrinogen$_{Bellingham}$, includes a γ275 Arg→Cys substitution that confers a relative resistance to tissue type plasminogen activator-mediated fibrinolysis.[109] The mechanism of resistance was presumably related to steric interference with the normal polymerization/crosslinking structure due to the cysteine residue or a structure bound to it.

Interestingly, family studies demonstrate that fibrinogen mutations alone are not sufficient to cause CTEPH. Rather, CTEPH requires the combination of acute PE (eg, to knee replacement surgery as well as an additive thrombogenic genetic risk factor[108]) along with the resistance to fibrinolysis. For this reason, the absence of disease in family members of patients with CTEPH does not rule out the presence of fibrinogen abnormalities.

POTENTIAL MEDIATORS OF CTEPH, CTVD, AND OTHER CHRONIC CONDITIONS AFTER VTE

Several inflammatory mediators may be stimulated by thrombosis, and may be implicated in the connection between acute pulmonary thromboemboli and vascular scaring.[110] For example, E-selectin and P-selectin may play a role in the balance between thrombus resolution and vascular remodeling after acute VTE.[111–118] In fact, heparin-type medications, in addition to their anticoagulant properties, may block selectin[119] and attenuate the inflammation and remodeling that can lead to poor resolution of the thromboemboli within the pulmonary arteries.[120,121] Despite these insights, it still remains unclear why some patients with acute VTE have poor thrombus resolution and why a few go on to develop CTVD or CTEPH. There are many factors that perturb the complex balance between coagulation and fibrinolysis and the normal processes of pulmonary vascular remodeling and inflammation. Although it is widely believed that there is a thromboembolic basis in the development of CTEPH, the detailed genetic, molecular, and cellular mechanism underlying its pathogenesis has yet to be fully explained.

SUMMARY

A great deal is known about the natural history of VTE, from its typical origin as lower extremity DVT to its gravest dangers as acute and chronic pulmonary emboli. Some questions still remain, however. The identification of patients at the greatest risk is for VTE still imprecise, and further work in this area can improve prophylactic strategies. The pathophysiological mechanisms underlying pulmonary embolism have been well investigated, although it remains a challenge to identify and predict how they affect any particular patient. Finally, we are only at the beginning of our understanding of why some patients resolve their thromboemboli rapidly, while in others, the clots organize into intravascular scars that can cause considerable morbidity and can even be life-threatening.

REFERENCES

1. Bagot CN, Arya R. Virchow and his triad: a question of attribution. Br J Haematol 2008;143:180–90.
2. Lowe GD. Virchow's triad revisited: abnormal flow. Pathophysiol Haemost Thromb 2003;33:455–7.

3. Christen Y, Wutschert R, Weimer D, et al. Effects of intermittent pneumatic compression on venous haemodynamics and fibrinolytic activity. Blood Coagul Fibrinolysis 1997;8:185–90.

4. Hull RD, Raskob GE, Gent M, et al. Effectiveness of intermittent pneumatic leg compression for preventing deep vein thrombosis after total hip replacement [see comments]. JAMA 1990;263:2313–7.

5. Woolson ST, Watt JM. Intermittent pneumatic compression to prevent proximal deep venous thrombosis during and after total hip replacement. A prospective, randomized study of compression alone, compression and aspirin, and compression and low-dose warfarin. J Bone Joint Surg [Am] 1991;73:507–12.

6. Belcaro G, Geroulakos G, Nicolaides AN, et al. Venous thromboembolism from air travel: the LONFLIT study. Angiology 2001;52:369–74.

7. Wolf LD, Hozack WJ, Rothman RH. Pulmonary embolism in total joint arthroplasty. Clin Orthop Relat Res 1993;288:219–33.

8. Planaes A, Vochelle N, Fafola M. Venous thromboembolic prophylaxis in orthopedic surgery: knee surgery. Semin Thromb Hemost 1999;25(Suppl 3):73–7.

9. Geerts WH, Bergqvist D, Pineo GF, et al. Prevention of venous thromboembolism: American College of Chest Physicians Evidence-based Clinical Practice Guidelines (8th edition). Chest 2008;133:381S–453S.

10. Koster T, Rosendaal FR, de Ronde H, et al. Venous thrombosis due to poor anticoagulant response to activated protein C: leiden thrombophilia study. Lancet 1993;342:1503–6.

11. Poort SR, Rosendaal FR, Reitsma PH, et al. A common genetic variation in the 3'-untranslated region of the prothrombin gene is associated with elevated plasma prothrombin levels and an increase in venous thrombosis. Blood 1996;88:3698–703.

12. Kearon C. Natural history of venous thromboembolism. Circulation 2003;107:I22–30.

13. Prandoni P, Cogo A, Bernardi E, et al. A simple ultrasound approach for detection of recurrent proximal-vein thrombosis. Circulation 1993;88:1730–5.

14. Prandoni P, Lensing AW, Cogo A, et al. The long-term clinical course of acute deep venous thrombosis. Ann Intern Med 1996;125:1–7.

15. Prandoni P, Villalta S, Bagatella P, et al. The clinical course of deep-vein thrombosis. Prospective long-term follow-up of 528 symptomatic patients. Haematologica 1997;82:423–8.

16. Wagenvoort CA. Pathology of pulmonary thromboembolism. Chest 1995;107:10S–7S.

17. Landaw SA. Homeostasis, survival, and red cell kinetics: measurement and imaging of red cell production. In: Hoffman R, Benz EJ, Shattil SJ, et al, editors. Hematology: basic principles and practice. New York: Churchill Livingston; 1995. p. 274–90.

18. Franco RS. The measurement and importance of red cell survival. Am J Hematol 2008;84:109–14.

19. Kuruvilla J, Wells PS, Morrow B, et al. Prospective assessment of the natural history of positive d-dimer results in persons with acute venous thromboembolism (DVT or PE). Thromb Haemost 2003;89:284–7.

20. Prandoni P, Lensing AW, Prins MH, et al. Residual venous thrombosis as a predictive factor of recurrent venous thromboembolism. Ann Intern Med 2002;137:955–60.

21. van Ramshorst B, van Bemmelen PS, Hoeneveld H, et al. Thrombus regression in deep venous thrombosis. Quantification of spontaneous thrombolysis with duplex scanning. Circulation 1992;86:414–9.

22. Pengo V, Lensing AW, Prins MH, et al. Incidence of chronic thromboembolic pulmonary hypertension after pulmonary embolism. N Engl J Med 2004;350: 2257–64.
23. Skoro-Sajer N, Becherer A, Klepetko W, et al. Longitudinal analysis of perfusion lung scintigrams of patients with unoperated chronic thromboembolic pulmonary hypertension. Thromb Haemost 2004;92:201–7.
24. Labropoulos N, Patel PJ, Tiongson JE, et al. Patterns of venous reflux and obstruction in patients with skin damage due to chronic venous disease. Vasc Endovasc Surg 2007;41:33–40.
25. Labropoulos N, Tiongson J, Pryor L, et al. Definition of venous reflux in lower-extremity veins. J Vasc Surg 2003;38:793–8.
26. Kahn SR, Ginsberg JS. Relationship between deep venous thrombosis and the postthrombotic syndrome. Arch Intern Med 2004;164:17–26.
27. Kahn SR, Shrier I, Julian JA, et al. Determinants and time course of the postthrombotic syndrome after acute deep venous thrombosis. Ann Intern Med 2008;149: 698–707.
28. Fedullo PF, Auger WR, Kerr KM, et al. Chronic thromboembolic pulmonary hypertension. N Engl J Med 2001;345:1465–72.
29. Wille-Jorgensen P, Jorgensen T, Andersen M, et al. Postphlebitic syndrome and general surgery: an epidemiologic investigation. Angiology 1991;42:397–403.
30. Biguzzi E, Mozzi E, Alatri A, et al. The post-thrombotic syndrome in young women: retrospective evaluation of prognostic factors. Thromb Haemost 1998;80:575–7.
31. Sevitt S, Gallagher N. Venous thrombosis and pulmonary embolism. A clinico-pathological study in injured and burned patients. Br J Surg 1961;48:475–89.
32. Prandoni P, Bernardi E. Upper extremity deep vein thrombosis. Curr Opin Pulm Med 1999;5:222–6.
33. Hingorani A, Ascher E, Hanson J, et al. Upper extremity versus lower extremity deep venous thrombosis. Am J Surg 1997;174:214–7.
34. Moser KM, LeMoine JR. Is embolic risk conditioned by location of deep venous thrombosis? Ann Intern Med 1981;94:439–44.
35. Huisman MV, Buller HR, ten Cate JW. Utility of impedance plethysmography in the diagnosis of recurrent deep-vein thrombosis. Arch Intern Med 1988;148:681–3.
36. Moser KM, Fedullo PF, LitteJohn JK, et al. Frequent asymptomatic pulmonary embolism in patients with deep venous thrombosis [published erratum appears in JAMA 1994;271(24):1908] [see comments]. JAMA 1994;271:223–5.
37. Huisman MV, Buller HR, ten Cate JW, et al. Unexpected high prevalence of silent pulmonary embolism in patients with deep venous thrombosis. Chest 1989;95:498–502.
38. Eichinger S, Weltermann A, Minar E, et al. Symptomatic pulmonary embolism and the risk of recurrent venous thromboembolism. Arch Intern Med 2004;164:92–6.
39. Carter AM, Catto AJ, Kohler HP, et al. Alpha-fibrinogen thr312ala polymorphism and venous thromboembolism. Blood 2000;96:1177–9.
40. Le Gal G, Delahousse B, Lacut K, et al. Fibrinogen Aalpha-Thr312Ala and factor XIII-A Val34Leu polymorphisms in idiopathic venous thromboembolism. Thromb Res 2007;121:333–8.
41. Suntharalingam J, Goldsmith K, van Marion V, et al. Fibrinogen Aalpha Thr312Ala polymorphism is associated with chronic thromboembolic pulmonary hypertension. Eur Respir J 2008;31:736–41.
42. Standeven KF, Grant PJ, Carter AM, et al. Functional analysis of the fibrinogen aalpha thr312ala polymorphism: effects on fibrin structure and function. Circulation 2003;107:2326–30.

43. Schulman S, Rhedin AS, Lindmarker P, et al. A comparison of six weeks with six months of oral anticoagulant therapy after a first episode of venous thromboembolism. Duration of anticoagulation trial study group [see comments]. N Engl J Med 1995;332:1661–5.

44. Wood KE. Major pulmonary embolism: review of a pathophysiologic approach to the golden hour of hemodynamically significant pulmonary embolism. Chest 2002;121: 877–905.

45. Elliott CG. Pulmonary physiology during pulmonary embolism. Chest 1992;101: 163S–71S.

46. McIntyre KM, Sasahara AA. The hemodynamic response to pulmonary embolism in patients without prior cardiopulmonary disease. Am J Cardiol 1971;28:288–94.

47. McIntyre KM, Sasahara AA. Hemodynamic alterations related to extent of lung scan perfusion defect in pulmonary embolism. J Nucl Med 1971;12:166–70.

48. McIntyre KM, Sasahara AA. Correlation of pulmonary photoscan and angiogram as measures of the severity of pulmonary embolic involvement. J Nucl Med 1971;12: 732–8.

49. McIntyre KM, Sasahara AA. Hemodynamic and ventricular responses to pulmonary embolism. Prog Cardiovasc Dis 1974;17:175–90.

50. Smulders YM. Pathophysiology and treatment of haemodynamic instability in acute pulmonary embolism: the pivotal role of pulmonary vasoconstriction. Cardiovasc Res 2000;48:23–33.

51. Azarian R, Wartski M, Collignon MA, et al. Lung perfusion scans and hemodynamics in acute and chronic pulmonary embolism. J Nucl Med 1997;38:980–3.

52. Huet Y, Lemaire F, Brun-Buisson C, et al. Hypoxemia in acute pulmonary embolism. Chest 1985;88:829–36.

53. D'Angelo E. Lung mechanics and gas exchange in pulmonary embolism. Haematologica 1997;82:371–4.

54. Prediletto R, Paoletti P, Fornai E, et al. Natural course of treated pulmonary embolism. Evaluation by perfusion lung scintigraphy, gas exchange, and chest roentgenogram. Chest 1990;97:554–61.

55. Severinghaus JW, Swenson EW, Finley TN, et al. Unilateral hypoventilation produced in dogs by occluding one pulmonary artery. J Appl Physiol 1961;16:53–60.

56. Manier G, Castaing Y, Guenard H. Determinants of hypoxemia during the acute phase of pulmonary embolism in humans. Am Rev Respir Dis 1985;132:332–8.

57. D'Alonzo GE, Bower JS, DeHart P, et al. The mechanisms of abnormal gas exchange in acute massive pulmonary embolism. Am Rev Respir Dis 1983;128: 170–2.

58. Chernick V, Hodson WA, Greenfield LJ. Effect of chronic pulmonary artery ligation on pulmonary mechanics and surfactant. J Appl Physiol 1966;21:1315–20.

59. Bjork L, McNeil BJ. Blood flow in pulmonary and bronchial arteries in acute experimental pneumonia and pulmonary embolism. Acta Radiol 1977;18:393–9.

60. Dalen JE, Haffajee CI, Alpert JS 3rd, et al. Pulmonary embolism, pulmonary hemorrhage and pulmonary infarction. N Engl J Med 1977;296:1431–5.

61. Ellis FH Jr, Grindlay JH, Edwards JE. The bronchial arteries. II. Their role in pulmonary embolism and infarction. Surgery 1952;31:167–79.

62. Schraufnagel DE, Tsao MS, Yao YT, et al. Factors associated with pulmonary infarction. A discriminant analysis study. Am J Clin Pathol 1985;84:15–8.

63. Tsao MS, Schraufnagel D, Wang NS. Pathogenesis of pulmonary infarction. Am J Med 1982;72:599–606.

64. Jandik J, Endrys J, Rehulova E, et al. Bronchial arteries in experimental pulmonary infarction: angiographic and morphometric study. Cardiovasc Res 1993;27: 1076–83.
65. The urokinase pulmonary embolism trial. A national cooperative study. Circulation 1973;47:II1–108.
66. Meneveau N, Schiele F, Vuillemenot A, et al. Streptokinase vs alteplase in massive pulmonary embolism. A randomized trial assessing right heart haemodynamics and pulmonary vascular obstruction [see comments]. Eur Heart J 1997;18:1141–8.
67. Meneveau N, Schiele F, Metz D, et al. Comparative efficacy of a two-hour regimen of streptokinase versus alteplase in acute massive pulmonary embolism: immediate clinical and hemodynamic outcome and one-year follow-up. J Am Coll Cardiol 1998;31:1057–63.
68. Kasper W, Konstantinides S, Geibel A, et al. Management strategies and determinants of outcome in acute major pulmonary embolism: results of a multicenter registry [see comments]. J Am Coll Cardiol 1997;30:1165–71.
69. Hamel E, Pacouret G, Vincentelli D, et al. Thrombolysis or heparin therapy in massive pulmonary embolism with right ventricular dilation: results from a 128-patient monocenter registry. Chest 2001;120:120–5.
70. Konstantinides S, Geibel A, Heusel G, et al. Heparin plus alteplase compared with heparin alone in patients with submassive pulmonary embolism. N Engl J Med 2002;347:1143–50.
71. Dalen JE, Alpert JS, Hirsh J. Thrombolytic therapy for pulmonary embolism: is it effective? Is it safe? When is it indicated? Arch Intern Med 1997;157:2550–6.
72. Morgenthaler TI, Ryu JH. Clinical characteristics of fatal pulmonary embolism in a referral hospital. Mayo Clin Proc 1995;70:417–24.
73. Kucher N, Rossi E, De Rosa M, et al. Massive pulmonary embolism. Circulation 2006;113:577–82.
74. Jha VM, Lee-Llacer J, Williams J, et al. Adjunctive inferior vena cava filter placement for acute pulmonary embolism. Cardiovasc Intervent Radiol 2010;33:739–43.
75. Rose PS, Punjabi NM, Pearse DB. Treatment of right heart thromboemboli. Chest 2002;121:806–14.
76. Donnamaria V, Palla A, Petruzzelli S, et al. Early and late follow-up of pulmonary embolism. Respiration 1993;60:15–20.
77. Menendez R, Nauffal D, Cremades MJ. Prognostic factors in restoration of pulmonary flow after submassive pulmonary embolism: a multiple regression analysis. Eur Respir J 1998;11:560–4.
78. Murphy ML, Bulloch RT. Factors influencing the restoration of blood flow following pulmonary embolization as determined by angiography and scanning. Circulation 1968;38:1116–26.
79. Palla A, Donnamaria V, Petruzzelli S, et al. Follow-up of pulmonary perfusion recovery after embolism. J Nucl Med Allied Sci 1986;30:23–8.
80. Walker RH, Goodwin J, Jackson JA. Resolution of pulmonary embolism. Br Med J 1970;4:135–9.
81. Wartski M, Collignon MA. Incomplete recovery of lung perfusion after 3 months in patients with acute pulmonary embolism treated with antithrombotic agents. THESEE study group. Tinzaparin ou Heparin Standard: Evaluation dans l'Embolie Pulmonaire Study. J Nucl Med 2000;41:1043–8.
82. Ribeiro A, Lindmarker P, Johnsson H, et al. Pulmonary embolism: one-year follow-up with echocardiography doppler and five-year survival analysis. Circulation 1999;99:1325–30.

83. Miller RL, Das S, Anandarangam T, et al. Association between right ventricular function and perfusion abnormalities in hemodynamically stable patients with acute pulmonary embolism. Chest 1998;113:665–70.

84. Dantzker DR, Wagner PD, Tornabene VW, et al. Gas exchange after pulmonary thromboemoblization in dogs. Circ Res 1978;42:92–103.

85. Wagner PD, Laravuso RB, Goldzimmer E, et al. Distribution of ventilation-perfusion ratios in dogs with normal and abnormal lungs. J Appl Physiol 1975;38:1099–109.

86. Wagner PD, Laravuso RB, Uhl RR, et al. Distributions of ventilation-perfusion ratios in acute respiratory failure. Chest 1974;65(Suppl):35S.

87. Tsang JY, Lamm WJ, Starr IR, et al. Spatial pattern of ventilation-perfusion mismatch following acute pulmonary thromboembolism in pigs. J Appl Physiol 2005;98: 1862–8.

88. Phear D. Pulmonary embolism. A study of late prognosis. Lancet 1960;2:832–5.

89. Winebright JW, Gerdes AJ, Nelp WB. Restoration of blood flow after pulmonary embolism. Arch Intern Med 1970;125:241–7.

90. Tow DE, Wagner HN Jr. Recovery of pulmonary arterial blood flow in patients with pulmonary embolism. N Engl J Med 1967;276:1053–9.

91. Hall RJ, Sutton GC, Kerr IH. Long-term prognosis of treated acute massive pulmonary embolism. Br Heart J 1977;39:1128–34.

92. James WS 3rd, Menn SJ, Moser KM. Rapid resolution of a pulmonary embolus in man. West J Med 1978;128:60–4.

93. Dalen JE, Banas JS, Brooks HL, et al. Resolution rate of acute pulmonary embolism in man. N Engl J Med 1969;280(22):1194–9.

94. Wartski M, Collignon MA. Incomplete recovery of lung perfusion after 3 months in patients with acute pulmonary embolism treated with antithrombotic agents. Thesee study group. Tinzaparin ou heparin standard: Evaluation dans l'embolie pulmonaire study. J Nucl Med 2000;41:1043–8.

95. Paraskos JA, Adelstein SJ, Smith RE, et al. Late prognosis of acute pulmonary embolism. N Engl J Med 1973;289:55–8.

96. Sutton GC, Hall RJ, Kerr IH. Clinical course and late prognosis of treated subacute massive, acute minor, and chronic pulmonary thromboembolism. Br Heart J 1977; 39:1135–42.

97. De Soyza ND, Murphy ML. Persistent post-embolic pulmonary hypertension. Chest 1972;62:665–8.

98. Eagleton MJ, Henke PK, Luke CE, et al. Southern Association for Vascular Surgery William J. von Leibig Award. Inflammation and intimal hyperplasia associated with experimental pulmonary embolism. J Vasc Surg 2002;36:581–8.

99. Yi ES, Kim H, Ahn H, et al. Distribution of obstructive intimal lesions and their cellular phenotypes in chronic pulmonary hypertension. A morphometric and immunohisto-chemical study. Am J Respir Crit Care Med 2000;162:1577–86.

100. Blauwet LA, Edwards WD, Tazelaar HD, et al. Surgical pathology of pulmonary thromboendarterectomy: a study of 54 cases from 1990 to 2001. Hum Pathol 2003;34:1290–8.

101. Fedullo PF, Auger WR, Channick RN, et al. Chronic thromboembolic pulmonary hypertension. Clin Chest Med 2001;22:561–81.

102. Morris TA, Marsh JJ, Chiles PG, et al. Fibrin derived from patients with chronic thromboembolic pulmonary hypertension is resistant to lysis. Am J Respir Crit Care Med 2006;173:1270–5.

103. Qi J, Kreutzer DL. Fibrin activation of vascular endothelial cells. Induction of il-8 expression. J Immunol 1995;155:867–76.

104. Martinez J, Ferber A, Bach TL, et al. Interaction of fibrin with VE-cadherin. Ann N Y Acad Sci 2001;936:386–405.
105. Tsakadze NL, Zhao Z, D'Souza SE. Interactions of intercellular adhesion molecule-1 with fibrinogen. Trends Cardiovasc Med 2002;12:101–8.
106. Barnard JW, Biro MG, Lo SK, et al. Neutrophil inhibitory factor prevents neutrophil-dependent lung injury. J Immunol 1995;155:4876–81.
107. Lang I, Kerr K. Risk factors for chronic thromboembolic pulmonary hypertension. Proc Am Thorac Soc 2006;3:568–70.
108. Morris TA, Marsh JJ, Chiles PG, et al. High prevalence of dysfibrinogenemia among patients with chronic thromboembolic pulmonary hypertension. Blood 2009;114:1929–36.
109. Linenberger ML, Kindelan J, Bennett RL, et al. Fibrinogen bellingham: a gamma-chain R275C substitution and a beta-promoter polymorphism in a thrombotic member of an asymptomatic family. Am J Hematol 2000;64:242–50.
110. Varma MR, Varga AJ, Knipp BS, et al. Neutropenia impairs venous thrombosis resolution in the rat. J Vasc Surg 2003;38:1090–8.
111. Myers D Jr, Farris D, Hawley A, et al. Selectins influence thrombosis in a mouse model of experimental deep venous thrombosis. J Surg Res 2002;108:212–21.
112. Furie B, Furie BC, Flaumenhaft R. A journey with platelet p-selectin: the molecular basis of granule secretion, signalling and cell adhesion. Thromb Haemost 2001;86:214–21.
113. Andre P. P-selectin in haemostasis. Br J Haematol 2004;126:298–306.
114. Ley K. The role of selectins in inflammation and disease. Trends Mol Med 2003;9:263–8.
115. Inami N, Nomura S, Kikuchi H, et al. P-selectin and platelet-derived microparticles associated with monocyte activation markers in patients with pulmonary embolism. Clin Appl Thromb Hemost 2003;9:309–16.
116. Celi A, Pellegrini G, Lorenzet R, et al. P-selectin induces the expression of tissue factor on monocytes. Proc Natl Acad Sci U S A 1994;91:8767–71.
117. Hidari KI, Weyrich AS, Zimmerman GA, et al. Engagement of P-selectin glycoprotein ligand-1 enhances tyrosine phosphorylation and activates mitogen-activated protein kinases in human neutrophils. J Biol Chem 1997;272:28750–6.
118. Palabrica T, Lobb R, Furie BC, et al. Leukocyte accumulation promoting fibrin deposition is mediated in vivo by P-selectin on adherent platelets. Nature 1992;359:848–51.
119. Thanaporn P, Myers DD, Wrobleski SK, et al. P-selectin inhibition decreases post-thrombotic vein wall fibrosis in a rat model. Surgery 2003;134:365–71.
120. Wang L, Brown JR, Varki A, Esko JD. Heparin's anti-inflammatory effects require glucosamine 6-O-sulfation and are mediated by blockade of L- and P-selectins. J Clin Invest 2002;110:127–36.
121. Koenig A, Norgard-Sumnicht K, Linhardt R, et al. Differential interactions of heparin and heparan sulfate glycosaminoglycans with the selectins. Implications for the use of unfractionated and low molecular weight heparins as therapeutic agents. J Clin Invest 1998;101:877–89.

Major Pulmonary Embolism

Kenneth E. Wood, DO[a,b,*]

KEYWORDS

- Pulmonary embolism • Shock
- Thrombolytic therapy • Embolectomy • Pathophysiology

The scope and spectrum of pulmonary embolism (PE) that are likely to challenge the Intensivist are dominantly confined to 2 scenarios; first, a patient presenting with undifferentiated shock or respiratory failure and, second, an established intensive care unit (ICU) or hospital patient who develops PE after admission. In either scenario, the diagnostic approach and therapeutic options are challenging. Differentiating PE from other life-threatening cardiopulmonary disorders can be exceedingly challenging, as logistic constraints can impair definitive diagnostic testing and the therapeutic approach can be appreciably altered given the hemorrhagic risks of the critically ill when anticoagulated or considered for thrombolytic therapy. This article will review a structured pathophysiologic approach to the diagnostic, resuscitative and management strategies related to PE in the ICU.

The incidence of PE causing, contributing, or associated with death in hospitalized patients has remained relatively constant at approximately 15% for the past 40 years. This is contemporarily illustrated by a recent autopsy case series of 600 ICU deaths where all patients received thromboprophylaxis for a reported overall PE incidence of 14.3%.[1] Of the 33 patients with clinically suspected PE, PE was confirmed at autopsy in only 39%. In 73 patients, PE was not suspected and was clinically discovered only at autopsy, where it was considered the cause of death in 45% of those patients. Recent abdominal surgery and the presence of renal failure were identified as factors associated with a higher risk of a misdiagnosis. The authors concluded that in an era dominated by thromboprophylaxis, critically ill patients remain at high risk for PE and consequent to the difficulties in establishing a diagnosis, the incidence of PE is higher than previously appreciated in critically ill patients. Contemporary estimates have suggested that PE occurs in more than 600,000 patients per year and is reported to cause or contribute to the death of between 50,000 and 200,000 patients. Large, contemporary observational studies of PE and similar registry studies have reported unexpectedly high mortality rates. In the Management Strategies and Determinants of Outcome in Acute PE (MAPPET) series, an overall 3-month mortality of 17% was reported in patients with PE and an in-hospital mortality of 31% when PE was

The author has nothing to disclose.

[a] Temple University School of Medicine, 3400 North Broad Street, Philadelphia, PA 19140, USA
[b] Geisinger Medical Center, 100 North Academy Avenue, Danville, PA 17822, USA
* Geisinger Medical Center, 100 North Academy Avenue, Danville, PA 17822.
E-mail address: kewood@geisinger.edu

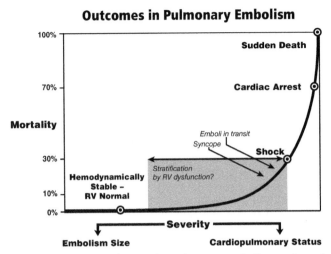

Fig. 1. Outcomes in PE. (*From* Wood KE. Major pulmonary embolism: review of a pathophysiologic approach to the golden hour of hemodynamically significant pulmonary embolism. Chest 2002;121;877–905; with permission.)

associated with hemodynamic instability. Mortality attributed to PE was 45% and 91% in the respective groups.[2] In the International Cooperative Pulmonary Embolism Registry (ICOPER), the 3-month mortality rate was 14.5% in the patients with hemodynamic stability and rose to 51.9% in those patients presenting with hemodynamic instability. Similar to the MAPPET report, PE-attributed mortality was 34% and 62.5% in the respective groups.[3]

In fatal cases of PE, it is long been recognized that approximately two-thirds of the deaths related to PE will occur within 1 hour of presentation and that anatomically massive PE will account for only half of the deaths, with the remainder attributed to nonmassive or recurrent PE. These observations have several important implications. First, using an evidence-based approach is almost impossible for the hemodynamically unstable patient, as a substantial number of these patients will die in the first hour and not undergo significant diagnostic studies. Second, it is reasonable to propose that patient outcomes from PE are related to the magnitude of the embolic obstruction against the background of the patient's underlying cardiopulmonary function. Given the dynamic interplay between a patient's underlying cardiopulmonary status and the magnitude of the embolus, similar hemodynamic presentations and clinical outcomes will manifest from an anatomically massive PE in a patient with normal cardiopulmonary function and an anatomically submassive embolus in a patient with impaired cardiopulmonary function. Third, an understanding of the pathophysiology of PE will enable the application of a physiologic risk stratification that can be used for the diagnostic evaluation and therapy of acute PE. **Fig. 1** illustrates a proposed risk stratification model defined by mortality on the ordinate and severity characterized by the cardiopulmonary status on the abscissa. Although not well appreciated, the combination of embolism size and underlying cardiopulmonary status that results in cardiac arrest is associated with a predictive mortality of 70%.[2] Given that 30% of patients with PE sustaining cardiac arrest will survive, this necessitates continued use of chest compressions to potentially mechanically fracture the PE and consideration of thrombolytic therapy or embolectomy occasionally in the absence of a definitive diagnosis when there is a high pre-test probability of PE. The combination of embolism size and cardiopulmonary status that fails to precipitate right ventricular (RV) dilatation is associated with a very low mortality, provided therapeutic anticoagulation is adequately achieved. Between these 2 extremes, a combination of embolism size and cardiopulmonary status that precipitates hemodynamic instability or shock is associated with a 30% mortality. As a consequence, the presence of shock has been traditionally defined as the threshold for thrombolytic therapy. As illustrated in **Fig. 1**, there is a broad spectrum of PE patients who have RV dysfunction and are hemodynamically stable. This ranges from a group with a minimal embolic burden and a low predicted mortality to patients with incipient shock and a predicted mortality similar to those patients presenting in shock. Thrombolytic therapy in this group of patients with hemodynamic stability with RV dysfunction is controversial, as the characteristics of patients residing in the incipient shock category are only recently being defined. Based on reported case series, syncope represents an intermediary position between shock and cardiac arrest. In patients who recover consciousness after PE-induced syncope, there is a significantly higher incidence of hemodynamic instability.[4] Recent reports have suggested that the mortality outcome in patients associated with emboli in transit and a patent foramem ovale (PFO) are likely to have a higher mortality.[5]

The prevailing orthodoxy related to risk stratification and treatment of PE for the past 40 years has focused on the anatomic size of the embolus, beginning in 1967 with James Dalen's classic review entitled, "Massive Pulmonary Embolism."[6] Contemporaneously, the purported association between the anatomic embolus burden and hemodynamic instability/outcomes continues to dominate the medical literature as the 2011 American Heart Association (AHA) scientific statement on the management of PE chose to use this traditional orthodoxy by defining massive PE as "sustained hypotension."[7] The term "massive" and the association with hemodynamic instability and outcome likely originated in an era when the diagnosis of PE by clinical findings and autopsy was supplanted by pulmonary angiography. However, it is imperative to recognize that when one partitions the mortality data by clot size and hemodynamics, there is no significant relationship between the underlying clot size and patient outcome unless the clot size represents a greater than 70% outflow obstruction. In fact, several large case series report that the vast majority of patients with anatomically massive embolus do not present with hemodynamic instability, underscoring the dynamic relationship between underlying clot size and cardiopulmonary status.[8-11] Recognizing that anatomically massive clot is not necessarily an outcome determinant, it has been suggested that the term "major" be used to describe the patient with hemodynamically unstable PE rather than "massive."[12,13]

PATHOPHYSIOLOGY

The contemporary approach to PE is defined by physiologic risk stratification for diagnosis, resuscitation, and treatment, which requires a fundamental understanding of the pathophysiology of PE. The impaction of embolic material on the pulmonary outflow track and the subsequent pathophysiologic sequence of events are depicted in **Fig. 2**. Mechanical obstruction secondary to the embolus conspires with neurohumoral factors against the background of the patient's underlying cardiopulmonary status to precipitate a significant increase in pulmonary vascular impedance and a corresponding increase in the pressure load on the RV. The mechanical obstruction secondary to embolus has been well described and is generally appreciated, although the effects of neurohumoral elements remain substantially underappreciated. Serotonin,

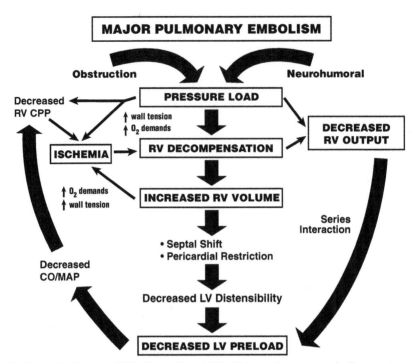

Fig. 2. Pathophysiology of PE. (*From* Wood KE. Major pulmonary embolism: review of a pathophysiologic approach to the golden hour of hemodynamically significant pulmonary embolism. Chest 2002;121;877–905; with permission.)

adenosine diphosphate (ADP), and thrombin are factors that are released from the platelets in the embedded clot that precipitate vasoconstriction in the pulmonary arteries, contributing to the increase in mean pulmonary artery pressure (MPAP).[14] An escalating RV pressure overload precipitates RV decompensation, resulting in decreased RV output. Given that the right and left hearts are hydraulically aligned in series, impaired output from the RV will significantly decrease left ventricular (LV) preload with a corresponding decrement in cardiac output and mean arterial pressure (MAP). The perfusion pressure gradient for the RV subendocardium is the gradient between the MAP and the RV end-diastolic pressure. With PE-induced increases in RV end-diastolic pressure consequent to RV pressure overload and coincident with the loss of MAP, there is impaired RV subendocardial perfusion resulting in myocardial ischemia of the RV. These events conspire to further impair RV function and output. Compensatory use of the Starling curve increases RV volume, which results in a leftward septal shift of the interventricular septum, which further impairs LV filling, distensibility, and preload resulting in decreased LV output and further decreased MAP. Integration of the preceding results in a vicious cycle of cardiac dysfunction manifesting as hemodynamic instability/shock, which has long been recognized as the discriminator for outcome. The clinical correlates of this pathophysiologic sequence are illustrated in **Fig. 3**.

The care of the critically ill patient with undifferentiated shock often proceeds along 2 pathways: a structured physiologic resuscitation combined with the development of a differential diagnosis eventuating in a definitive diagnosis and treatment. A standard

Major Pulmonary Embolism

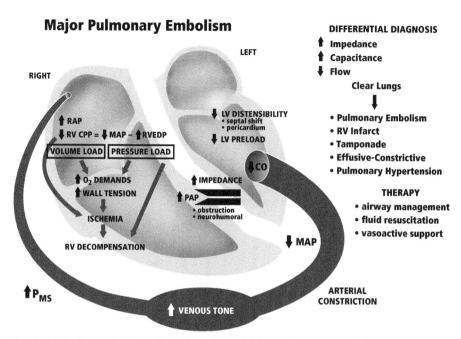

Fig. 3. Clinical correlations. (*From* Wood KE. Major pulmonary embolism: review of a pathophysiologic approach to the golden hour of hemodynamically significant pulmonary embolism. Chest 2002;121;877–905; with permission.)

and universally applicable model of the circulation to characterize the physiologic abnormalities is useful for assisting in resuscitation and differential diagnosis generation. A 3-compartment model of the circulation defined by 2 hydraulic pumps linked in series is presented in **Fig. 4**. Each hydraulic pump (RV and LV) has its own capacitance volume reservoir and impedance (resistive component) system. Given the series alignment, the output of the RV can never exceed the output of the LV and vice versa. As a consequence, both hydraulic pumps may be viewed as a single hydraulic unit. In this model, the circulatory system can be conceptualized as a venous capacitance reservoir that provides volume to a hydraulic pump that generates flow into a resistive bed. As illustrated in **Fig. 4**, any hemodynamic abnormality may be characterized by aberrations of one or more of the variables in the 3-compartment model. Clinically applicable surrogates for venous capacitance, hydraulic pump function, and resistance are the right atrial pressure (RAP), cardiac output (CO), and systemic vascular resistance (SVR). In many scenarios, invasive monitoring or echocardiographic assessment is neither in place nor available on initial presentation, and it is necessary to develop model assessments from the initial physical exam. The right internal jugular pressure is a surrogate for the venous capacitance reservoir and assessment of the pulse pressure and temperature of the extremities can be used to approximate arterial resistance. Physiologically, there is an almost uniformly reciprocal relationship between flow and resistance in most disease states. A wide pulse pressure associated with warm extremities indicates a low vascular resistance with an associated high flow state. A narrow pulse pressure with cool, clamped extremities suggests a state of high vascular resistance that results from the compensatory increase in catecholamines to maintain pressure in a low flow

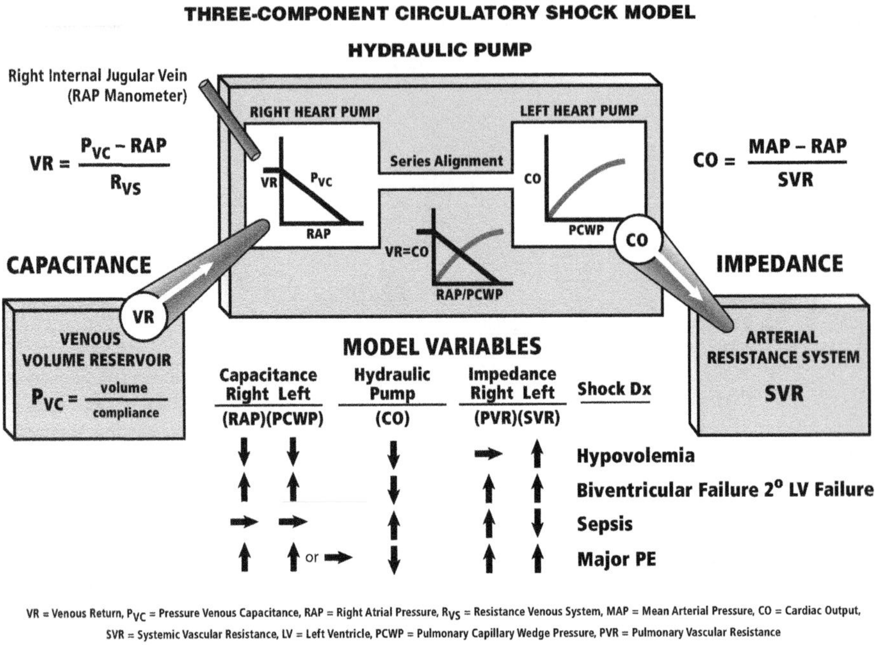

Fig. 4. Shock model. (*From* Wood KE. Major pulmonary embolism: review of a pathophysiologic approach to the golden hour of hemodynamically significant pulmonary embolism. Chest 2002;121;877–905; with permission.)

state. Appreciating that flow and resistance are almost uniformly reciprocal, it is possible to exploit this relationship to assist with the diagnostic evaluation of shock patients. The initial assessment of resistance allows for one to infer the flow status or cardiac function; cool and hypoprofused extremities reflect a catecholamine excess, high resistance, and a low flow state. With 2 hydraulic pumps aligned in series, the presence of an elevated RAP with relatively clear lungs defines the hydraulic lesion in the RV with a differential diagnosis of acute PE, RV infarction, pericardial tamponade, and decompensated pulmonary hypertension. In association with significant impairment of gas exchange, the preceding physiologic pattern is highly suggestive of PE. It is also important to recognize that PE represents a broad spectrum of presentations and that the shock presentation reflects the failure of all of the above compensatory mechanisms to maintain perfusion pressure gradients. These physical exam findings are instrumental in the initial evaluation along with the readily available diagnostic studies to ensure that PE is appropriately considered in the differential diagnosis of the undifferentiated shock patient.

Review of the clinical manifestations of PE in patients without underlying cardiopulmonary disease allows for the direct assessment of the effects of the embolic event and specific physiologic compensation. In this population, the size of the embolism directly correlates with the clinical and physiologic implications of PE.[15–17] In this population, the MPAP, RAP, PaO_2, and pulse are all correlative with the magnitude of the angiographic obstruction. These studies noted that a decrease in oxygen saturation is common and can manifest with a minimal degree of angiographic obstruction (13%), frequently being the only clinical manifestation when the degree of angiographic obstruction is less than 25%.[17] Pulmonary artery hypertension begins to occur when the extent of vascular obstruction exceeds 25% to 35%. This is in excess of experimental nonembolic obstruction illustrating the potential contributions of the neurohumoral mechanisms to pulmonary constriction. An anatomic obstruction of greater than 50% is required to precipitate RV failure as a normal RV cannot generate an MPAP in excess of 40 mm Hg. Correspondingly, finding an MPAP greater than 40 mm Hg signifies underlying cardiopulmonary disease or the compound effect of multiple embolic events. In patients with no underlying cardiopulmonary disease, an elevated RAP is consistently indicative of a large pulmonary vascular obstruction. The RAP is usually related to the MPAP and tends not to be elevated until the MPAP exceeds 30 mm Hg with an anatomic obstruction exceeding 35% to 40%. Given the compensatory cardiac mechanisms, RAP can be elevated without a decrease in CO.

In contradistinction to patients without underlying cardiopulmonary disease, patients with previous cardiopulmonary disease will manifest a greater degree of cardiovascular dysfunction with a lesser degree of vascular obstruction.[18] In this population with underlying cardiopulmonary disease, the MPAP is frequently disproportionately elevated relative to the degree of anatomic obstruction, strongly implying that the underlying cardiopulmonary hemodynamic pattern will dominate the presentation. An anatomic obstruction of only 23% was reported to be associated with significant elevations in MPAP in patients with underlying cardiopulmonary disease, whereas this level of anatomic obstruction would not be sufficient to produce an increase in MPAP in patients with no underlying disease. In this population, the RAP is an unreliable indicator of the magnitude of the embolic event and is of limited utility in the assessment of the extent of vascular obstruction. The preceding is illustrated in the European Pulmonary Embolism trial (the UKEP Study[19]), which reported 90% of the patients in shock as having prior cardiopulmonary disease and 56% of those with cardiopulmonary disease presenting in shock compared to only 2% of patients who did not have cardiopulmonary disease. In summary and in contrast to the population with no underlying cardiopulmonary disease, there is no distinct relationship between anatomic size and hemodynamic presentation in patients with underlying cardiopulmonary disease.

INITIAL EVALUATION

The generation of a differential diagnosis in patients with undifferentiated shock or respiratory failure is usually determined from elements that are derived from the history, physical findings, and the immediately available diagnostic studies such as the chest radiograph, arterial blood gases, and electrocardiogram. Recognizing the physiologic footprint that PE embeds upon these readily available studies is necessary to ensure that PE is appropriately incorporated into the differential diagnosis of the undifferentiated shock or respiratory failure patient. In critical care units, it is frequently difficult to obtain a comprehensive history, coexisting disease jeopardizes the interpretation of existing laboratory variables, and the injured critically ill patient has multiple comorbidities that may mask physical findings. All patients in a critical care unit should be considered high risk for venous thromboembolic disease and/or PE and individual case-specific risk factors should be assessed in patients from whom a complete history cannot be elicited. Using the hydraulic model of circulation to define the physiologic abnormality, hemodynamically unstable PE usually reveals an elevation of the RAP with hypoperfused extremities suggestive of low cardiac flow against the background of relatively clear lungs and the absence of significant chest radiographic abnormalities that would isolate the hemodynamic lesion to the RV with a limited differential diagnosis as suggested in **Fig. 3**. In the rare occasion that invasive hemodynamic monitoring is available, the variables usually suggest elevated RAP with a low CO and a low pulmonary capillary wedge pressure with a high SVR.

In 1935, McGinn and White described the classic $S_1Q_3T_3$ pattern of electrocardiographic cor pulmonale in a series of patients presenting with a clinical diagnosis of PE.[20] In the subsequent 75 years, multiple ECG manifestations of PE have been described. Several caveats from large PE trials and registries are important to recognize. A normal ECG is uncommon and was only appreciated in 14% of patients in UPET (6% massive and 23% submassive).[21] Similarly, only 30% of the patients in PIOPED Trial had a normal ECG.[22] In the above reported trials, rhythm disturbances were noted to be uncommon with atrial fibrillation/flutter appearing in only 0% to 5% of the patients and blocks or ventricular dysrhythmias rarely reported. Evidence of electrocardiographic cor pulmonale suggested by right axis, right bundle branch block, or $S_1Q_3T_3$ appears to be suggestive of embolic size in patients without underlying cardiopulmonary disease.[21] However, the most common ECG abnormalities in UPET and PIOPED were nonspecific ST-T segment changes appearing in 42% and 49% of patients, respectively.[22] Recently, T-wave inversion in the anterior precordial leads has been reported to be the most common ECG abnormality with PE appearing in 68% of patients. This study reported that the ECG sign that best correlated with PE severity was the anterior T-wave inversion that appeared in 90% of patients with a Miller index signifying an obstruction of greater than 50% and was evident in 81% of patients with a mean MPAP greater than 37 mm Hg. The authors stressed that the early appearance of the anterior T-wave inversion was a strong marker of severity and that normalization of the anterior T-wave that occurred after thrombolytic therapy was correlative with a resultant obstruction of less than 20% and a corresponding decrement in the MPAP to less than 20 mm Hg. T-wave reversibility by the sixth day correlated with therapeutic efficacy and a good outcome.[23]

Although the sensitivity and specificity of a chest radiograph for PE remain quite low, the chest radiograph may be useful in the diagnostic assessment by facilitating the exclusion of diseases mimicking PE, defining radiographic abnormalities that warrant further pursuit and may provide a crude severity assessment.[24] As with ECG reports in UPET and PIOPED, a normal chest radiograph is unusual with angiographically documented PE. In UPET and PIOPED, a normal chest radiograph was reported in 34% and 16% of patients, respectively. Pulmonary parenchymal abnormalities dominated the chest radiograph appearance in the UPET study and occurred in 67% of patients, with an elevated hemidiaphragm in 46%, consolidation in 39%, pleural effusion in 30%, and atelectasis in 28%. Vascular abnormalities were present in 37% of patients consisting of decreased vascularity in 22% and a prominent central pulmonary artery in 86%. In the PIOPED report, atelectasis/bronchial abnormalities were present in 68% of patients and a pleural effusion was reported in 48% of patients. Interestingly, there appears to be a correlation between the severity of the PE event, radiographic findings, the MPAP, and PaO_2 when the patients with normal chest radiographs were viewed in comparison to those with bronchial and vascular abnormalities.[24] Other findings that may be suggestive of PE on the chest radiograph include relative oligemia in the area of the embolic impaction, an abrupt cut-off of the pulmonary artery associated with relative oligemia and pulmonary artery distention reflective of pulmonary hypertension.

Despite the multiple physiologic factors that are responsible for hypoxia in patients with PE, it is important to recognize that hypoxia in PE is not uniform as a PaO_2 of 80 mm Hg or greater was reported in 12% of UPET patients and 19% of PIOPED patients.[25,26] Similarly, a normal $P(A-a)O_2$ does not effectively exclude PE.[22] In PIOPED, among patients with reported PaO_2 values of 80 mm Hg or greater and

$Paco_2$ values greater than 35 mm Hg and a normal $P/P(A-a)o_2$, 38% of the patients without underlying cardiopulmonary disease and 14% of the patients with cardiopulmonary disease had documented PE. In a population without underlying cardiopulmonary disease, the preceding values were likely representative of low levels of embolic burden. As with hemodynamic correlates, there does not appear to be a significant correlation between PE severity and Pao_2, and the degree of anatomic obstruction in patients with cardiopulmonary disease. Insofar as many critically ill patients have preexisting gas impairment and are mechanically ventilated, changes in oxygen saturation or increasing oxygen requirements should prompt consideration toward a PE evaluation. In a recent study of critically ill patients that included ARDS patients on mechanical ventilation, dead space (V_d/V_+) measurements had a sensitivity of 100% and a specificity of 89%, correlated with a degree of vascular obstruction and the extent of resolution with thrombolytic therapy.[27,28]

DIAGNOSTIC THERAPEUTIC APPROACH

The presence of hemodynamic deterioration or shock in a patient with PE either as a consequence of an anatomically massive embolus in a patient without underlying cardiopulmonary disease or as a consequence of a submassive PE in a patient with underlying cardiopulmonary disease defines a failure of the available compensatory mechanism to maintain hemodynamic stability and has traditionally been defined as the discriminator for outcome and the use of thrombolytic therapy. Classic PE studies first reported that the presence of shock was associated with a significant increase in mortality.[29,30] Given the failure of compensatory mechanisms, shock defines an early, readily available and reliable discriminator between survivors and nonsurvivors. As previously discussed, it is important to recognize that the vast majority of patients with anatomically massive PE do not present in shock.[29,30] Meneveau reported that only 3% of patients without underlying cardiopulmonary disease and anatomically massive PE necessitated vasoactive support and that CO was normal in 97% of these patients.[31] It is equally important to recognize that hemodynamically stable patients who have been reported with submassive or massive PE have similar mortality rates and that an anatomically massive PE unless associated with physiologic decompensation resulting in shock does not appear to have an associated increased mortality.[29,30]

Fig. 5 presents an algorithmic diagnostic/therapeutic approach to the patient with suspected PE based upon the presence or absence of shock. In all patients presenting with possible PE, therapeutic anticoagulation should be undertaken in the absence of any contra-indications. As critically ill patients are frequently at risk for hemorrhagic complications of anticoagulation, unfractionated heparin is preferable because of the shorter half-life and the ability to antagonize its effects with protamine sulfate. In the population with no significant hemodynamic instability, spiral CT scan has evolved as the standard for diagnostic evaluation supplanting ventilation perfusion scans. Currently, ventilation perfusion scanning is predominantly reserved for a population that is unable to tolerate a CT scan or has elevated creatinine placing the patient at jeopardy for renal failure with CT scan contrast. In either case, establishing pre-test probability is crucial for the diagnostic evaluation of PE. Pre-test probability can be accomplished through the use of scoring systems or by clinical judgment. In either case, the combination of a high pre-test probability and a high probability V/Q scan or spiral CT scan effectively confirms the diagnosis of PE. Correspondingly, a low pre-test probability and a low probability V/Q scan effectively excludes PE. The combination of a high pre-test probability for PE and a negative spiral CT scan warrants ongoing diagnostic evaluation.[32] Currently, spiral CT scanning is ostensibly

Major Pulmonary Embolism Diagnostic/Therapeutic Approach

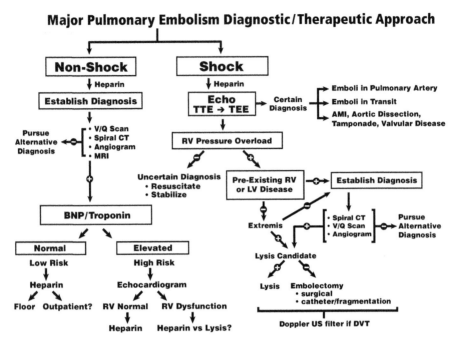

Fig. 5. Diagnostic-therapeutic mode. (*From* Wood KE. Major pulmonary embolism: review of a pathophysiologic approach to the golden hour of hemodynamically significant pulmonary embolism. Chest 2002;121;877–905; with permission.)

used to define the presence or absence of PE. Recent literature suggests that significant information may be obtained from the spiral CT scan to assist with PE risk stratification. Although gadolinium magnetic resonance angiography (MRA) is appealing, a recent large clinical trial concluded that MRA should only be done at centers where it is performed frequently and only when standard studies are contraindicated. In this study, MRA was technically inadequate in 25% of patients and identified only 57% of PE's in all patients compared to reference tests. Technically adequate MRA had a sensitivity of 78% and a specificity of 99%. Given the time constraints and need for patient transfer, it is unlikely that MRA will play a significant role in the diagnostic evaluation of unstable patients.[33,34]

Contemporaneously, CT scan is predominantly used to exclude or confirm the diagnosis of PE. However, over a decade ago, severity assessments of acute PE were proposed using spiral CT.[35–37] There are multiple measurements that may be obtained from the spiral CT scan in PE patients: calculation of the RV-short axis, the LV-short axis, and the RV/LV-short access ratio, diameters of the superior vena cava and azygos vein; embolic clot load scores; PA diameter measurements; positioning of the interventricular septum; and reflux of contrast medium into the inferior vena cava.[38] In a study that divided acute PE patients into three clinical categories consisting of pulmonary infarction, prominent dyspnea, and circulatory failure, spiral CT scanning was used to assess the pulmonary artery obstruction index and CT findings of right heart overload. The mortality rate in the above groups was noted to be 0%, 13.8%, and 25%, respectively. Consistent with previous data from the angiographic era, neither the pulmonary obstruction index nor the pulmonary artery pressure were predictive of patient outcome. CT scan findings that were correlative with outcome included an increased right-to-left ventricular ratio, proximal superior vena cava diameter, azygos vein diameter, and presence of contrast regurgitating into the inferior vena cava. Several other studies have reported associations between ventricular septal bowing and PE severity and short-term death.[39,40] However, this relationship has not been reported consistently in all studies.[38,41,42] Although the increased ratio of RV/LV diameter has been reportedly associated with RV dysfunction, the geometry of the RV makes this measurement challenging and difficult to reproduce. Recognizing that CT scanning has supplanted ventilation-perfusion scanning in the diagnosis of acute PE, it is highly likely that in the future, significant risk stratification will be derived from the multiple indices available on spiral CT that will assist with patient disposition and therapy.

In the hemodynamically stable patient with PE, brain natriueretic peptide (BNP) and troponin levels have been used to risk-stratify patients.[43,44] In patients with hemodynamic stability, the absence of an elevated BNP or troponin level signifies a patient population at low risk and opportunities for outpatient treatment of PE. An isolated, elevated BNP level is correlative with RV dilatation and places the patient at higher risk. The combination of an elevated BNP indicative of RV dilatation and an elevated troponin level suggestive of myocardial ischemia and RV damage places the patient at a higher level of risk for adverse outcomes. In a consecutive case report series of patients with acute PE, patients were stratified according to the BNP and troponin levels. Consistent with previous literature, the patients that were hemodynamically unstable had the highest mortality approximating 30%. In the group of hemodynamically stable patients with a composite 8% mortality, patients with a normal BNP level had a 0% mortality and those with an elevated BNP had an 11% mortality. Among the patients with an elevated BNP level, those with a normal troponin level had a 3.7% mortality compared to those with an elevated troponin level, which manifest a 30% mortality, almost identical to those patients presenting in shock. The preceding suggests that there is a subset of patients who present with hemodynamic stability and elevated BNP and troponin levels who are at risk for mortality similar to patients presenting in shock.[45] Many other composite studies using multiple factors to define prognostic assessment for PE are available for review and beyond the scope of this article.[46–49]

Patients presenting with suspected PE and hemodynamic instability are at a high risk for sudden death and clinical deterioration, which necessitates an expeditious approach to the diagnostic evaluation and rapid initiation of resuscitation and definitive therapeutics. Given the inherent difficulties in transporting patients to diagnostic radiology, it is ideal for the diagnostic evaluation to begin in an area where the patient may be optimally resuscitated and stabilized. Initial evaluation with duplex venous ultrasound is frequently undertaken because it is readily available and has an excellent specificity and sensitivity for DVT in symptomatic patients. A positive finding can allow for the exploitation of the identical treatment for DVT and PE.[50] Although it has been reported that venogram recognized DVT occurs in up to 90% of PE patients, DVT documentation by ultrasound is noted to occur in less than 50% of known PE patients.[51,52] Consequently, the presence of DVT does not necessarily confirm PE, nor does the absence of DVT preclude the diagnosis of PE.

As ultrasound expertise develops in critical care medicine, echocardiography is ideal for the initial diagnostic assessment of the hemodynamically unstable patient because it is readily available, useful in the recognition and differentiation of PE, and capable of assessing the severity of the hemodynamic event along with the subsequent response to therapy. Although dominantly used to define the presence and characterization of the RV pressure overload, transthoracic (TTE) or transesophageal echocardiography (TEE) is capable of detecting emboli in transit in addition to providing alternative diagnoses such as acute myocardial infarction, pericardial tamponade, aortic dissection, or valvular dysfunction. Characteristic findings of PE on TTE include RV dilatation with an increased RV/LV diameter, bowing of the interventricular septum, pulmonary artery dilatation, and tricuspid regurgitation. In patients without underlying cardiopulmonary disease, the presence and extent of the echocardiographic findings are reported to correlate with the magnitude of the anatomic outflow obstruction. RV dilatation is the most common finding and is reported in from 50% to 100% of PE cases. Coincident with the original data derived from the early angiographic series, it appears that an anatomic obstruction of 30% is necessary to produce echocardiographic evidence of ventricular dilatation. Obstruction of less than 30% will not precipitate RV dilatation. Although RV pressure load on echocardiography is a hallmark of acute PE, it is pivotal to appreciate that the presence of RV dysfunction is not specific for PE. Patients with underlying cardiopulmonary disease frequently manifest RV dysfunction at baseline. In this population with preexisting RV or LV disease, it is imperative to establish the diagnosis as previously discussed.[53,54] With a high pre-test probability for PE in a patient without underlying cardiovascular disease presenting in extremis, it will occasionally be necessary to consider lytic therapy. In hemodynamically unstable patients with suspected PE that is confirmed, assessment of the patient's candidacy for thrombolytic therapy or surgical embolectomy should be undertaken. Similarly, it is pivotal to appreciate that the absence of RV overload in an unstable patient in whom PE is considered will effectively exclude PE as the primary cause of hemodynamic instability.

Unless emboli-in-transit are directly visualized, TTE is only able to provide indirect evidence of PE. When RV dilatation is noted on TTE, PE is frequently bilateral and in up to 90% of the cases the embolus is noted to be either central or proximal.[55,56] In several series, patients with suspected PE and TTE documented RV dilatation immediately underwent TEE. Compared to definitive confirmatory studies, TEE had a sensitivity range of 80% to 96.7% and a specificity range between 84% and 100%.[57,58] Although appealing to migrate immediately from TTE to TEE to establish a diagnosis in the early resuscitative period, this approach is handicapped by the nonuniform availability of echocardiography, which will continue to necessitate transfer of patients to diagnostic radiology areas.

RESUSCITATION AND STABILIZATION

During the period of diagnostic evaluation, hemodynamically unstable patients with suspected PE frequently require aggressive resuscitation and ongoing stabilization. In these patients, marginal hemodynamic stability is frequently maintained by intense catecholamine surges. With refractory hypoxia and/or escalating oxygen requirements, patients with suspected PE frequently require intubation and mechanical ventilation, which can precipitate further deterioration in cardiovascular function for multiple reasons. First, sedatives used to facilitate intubation can antagonize the catecholamine surge upon which the patient is dependent for vasoconstriction to maintain blood pressure, as well as independently precipitate vasodilatation impairing hemodynamic stability. Second, excessive hand bagging after intubation with initial lung inflation can further impair venous return while the initiation of mechanical ventilation can increase the pulmonary vascular resistance, further contributing to further RV decompensation. As a consequence of the preceding, intubation and initiation and mechanical ventilation should be undertaken cautiously, with emphasis placed upon a conscious awake technique with topical and/or local anesthesia, a rapid sequence approach with neuromuscular paralysis and/or fiber-optic intubation. Traditionally, intravascular volume expansion with 1 to 2 L of fluid is the initial recommended treatment for hemodynamically unstable patients with undifferentiated shock. In a group of patients with anatomically massive clot associated with impaired cardiac output who were normotensive at presentation and not requiring vasoactive support, one study reported an increase in cardiac output with 500 ml dextran fluid challenge. The increase in cardiac output was proportionate to the degree of baseline RV end-diastolic volume.[59] However, in the hemodynamically unstable patient with PE and echocardiographic evidence of RV dilatation and pressure overload, caution should be exercised regarding excessive volume resuscitation. Administration of excess fluid resuscitation will further dilate the RV, increase end systolic wall stress, and further precipitate RV dysfunction. Consequently, when there is clear echocardiographic evidence of significant RV dilatation with bowing of the interventricular septum, fluids should be used with caution and early consideration toward the use of vasopressor support should be entertained. Vasoactive support facilitates the generation of a perfusion pressure gradient to enhance oxygen delivery to the RV subendocardium, which augments ventricular function. Although there is no consensus on which vasoactive agent is most appropriate, it appears that norepinephrine with its alpha vascoconstrictive effects on the arterial and venous system is recommended as it has been shown to abolish RV ischemia in animal models.[60] Given the previously described contribution of pulmonary vasoconstriction secondary to neurohumoral effects, it is appealing to consider unloading the RV with pulmonary vasodilators in patients with insipient or overt RV failure, as an adjunct to thrombolytic therapy or in patients in whom thrombolytic therapy is contraindicated awaiting embolectomy. Nitric oxide has been shown to improve pulmonary function with hemodynamically unstable PE and has been used as an adjunct to suction thombectomy for PE.[61,62] Other vasodilators that have been reported to increase cardiac output, decrease pulmonary artery pressures, and improve gas exchanges include inhaled prostacylin and sildenafil.[63,64]

DEFINITIVE THERAPY

The presence of shock or hemodynamic instability in patients with confirmed PE is an indication for either medical embolectomy with thrombolytic therapy or surgical embolectomy. PIOPED investigators considered thrombolytic therapy a standard of care for patients with shock or major disability. The investigators considered it unethical to treat patients in shock related to PE with heparin alone and consequently no randomization of this population was conducted in the initial PIOPED trial.[65] Thrombolytic therapy for acute PE has been recently reviewed, is discussed elsewhere in this clinics edition and will only be reviewed briefly.[66] Several important points regarding the use of thrombolytic therapy in PE patients warrant emphasis. First, in virtually all studies that were assessed by angiography, perfusion scans, hemodynamic measurements, or echocardiography, thrombolytic therapy has almost uniformly been shown to improve clot lysis more rapidly when compared to heparin therapy and no trial has reported any difference in the magnitude of embolic resolution after 5 to 7 days. The UPET trial conducted in 1970 is illustrative of this phenomenon. With comparable baseline angiographic obstructions in the heparin group (25%) and urokinase group (25%), the degree of angiographic resolution in the heparin group was 8.1%, and 22.1% in the urokinase-treated group in the first 24 hours. At the time of reassessment on day 5, the extent of the angiographic resolution in the heparin group and urokinase groups was virtually equivalent at 36% and 40%, respectively. In follow-up study at 1 year, the magnitude of the angiographic resolution was 77% in the heparin group and 78% in the urokinase group.[29] Recognizing that the hyperbolic relationship between pulmonary vascular resistance and vascular obstruction, a slight decrease in the magnitude of obstruction to less than 60% would be expected with thrombolysis, which can significantly reduce pulmonary vascular resistance and mitigate RV stress.[67] However appealing the rapidity of resolution of the embolic obstruction may be, there are limited data to uniformly apply thrombolytic therapy to patients with acute PE. Current recommendations from the American College of Chest Physicians support a Grade IB level of evidence in support of thrombolytic therapy administration to hemodynamically unstable acute PE patients.[68] In a subgroup analysis of randomized trials that included hemodynamically unstable patients, thrombolytic therapy when compared with heparin was associated with a significant reduction in death and recurrent PE (94% vs 19%, or 0.45).[69] Second, all clinically available thrombolytic agents appeared to be equally effective, provided that they are administered in equivalent doses over a equivalent time period.[11,70] Third, bleeding complications are far more common with thrombolytic therapy than heparin therapy. Pulled data from 11 randomized trials comparing thrombolytic therapy and heparin for acute PE reported a nonsignificant increase in major bleeding between thrombolytic therapy and heparin (9.1% vs 6.1%, or 1.42) and a significant increase in nonmajor bleeding (22.7% vs 10.0%, or 2.63).[69] Other pooled data suggest the overall incidence of major hemorrhage associated with PE with thrombolytic therapy in PE is approximately 12% and is similar among thrombolytic agents.[71] Fatal hemorrhage is reported to occur in 1% to 2% of patients with an intracranial hemorrhage rate between 1.2% and 2.1% and reported to be fatal in 50% of cases.[72,73]

Limited literature exists to assess the efficacy and response to thrombolytic therapy over the first several hours. Traditionally, a period of 4 to 6 hours is used to define the need for potential surgical embolectomy. TTE studies performed in acute PE patients prior to the initiation of thrombolytic therapy have characterized 2 distinct morphologic types of emboli, which have variant responses to thrombolytic therapy and may be of assistance in prospectively defining the likelihood of successful thrombolysis. Pulmonary emboli that were multiple with long mobile parts and appeared hypoechoic/heterogeneous on echocardiography tended to have a better response to thrombolytic therapy with improved cardiac output, central venous pressure, and pulmonary vascular resistance within the first 12 hours. In contrast, emboli visualized with echocardiography that were immobile and hyperechoic/homogeneous had a blunted response to thrombolytic therapy without a significant improvement noted in hemodynamic parameters. In the latter group, the mortality was 30% compared to 0% in the former. When available, pre-thrombolytic therapy echocardiography may assist in determining the likelihood of successful thrombolysis and facilitate planning for embolectomy.[74] Although frequently available but infrequently used, monitoring of thrombolysis with end-tidal CO_2 has been reported to be useful in assessing the efficacy of thrombolytic therapy. Presumably consequent to clot lysis and decreased PE induced dead space, end-tidal CO_2 values in patients who received thrombolytic therapy were significantly higher in survivors compared to nonsurvivors and correlated with decrements in MPAP, improvement in cardiac index, and a higher Pao_2/Fio_2 ratio.[75] Together with ongoing assessments of hemodynamic parameters, gas exchange, and echocardiography when available, end-tidal CO_2 may assist in the decision to define failed thrombolysis and migrate toward either surgical or catheter embolectomy. Although there are limited data, unsuccessful thrombolysis has been reported to occur in approximately 8.2% of patients, which was defined by persistent clinical instability and/or residual echocardiographic evidence of RV dysfunction. In this population with failed thrombolytic therapy, it appears that surgical embolectomy is preferable to repeating thrombolysis as the mortality rate and deaths attributable to PE was significantly lower in the group that underwent surgical embolectomy. Repeat thrombolysis was associated with a mortality rate of 38% compared to 7% in patients undergoing surgical embolectomy. Albeit inferior vena cava filters were placed in all patients undergoing surgical embolectomy, the incidence of recurrent PE was zero in that population compared to 35% in the group receiving repeat thrombolysis. Similarly, the hospital course was significantly less eventful in the embolectomy group.[76] As there has been a limited number of randomized, controlled trials with thrombolysis incorporating hemodynamically unstable patients conducted over the past decade, information regarding contemporary outcomes are sparse in the medical literature. In a report of patients that included those with cardiogenic shock, a vascular obstruction of greater than 50% (averaging 64%), an elevated MPAP, and evidence of RV dysfunction, 66% of those receiving thrombolytic therapy had an uneventful course. Mortality was reported at 8% with the incidence of major bleeding of 9.6% and recurrent PE occurring in 7.6%. Mean vascular obstruction decreased from 64% to 29% over a 24- to 48-hour period, which was associated with a significant decrease in pulmonary artery systolic pressure by 34% from 56 mm Hg to 37 mm Hg. RV function improved within 48 hours in 88% of patients while a lung scan improvement of 45% was noted within 6 to 8 days.[77]

PE patients with hemodynamic instability who have contraindications to thrombolytic therapy are candidates for either surgical or catheter embolectomy. Although traditionally reserved for patients with contraindications or rescue therapy in patients who have failed thrombolytic therapy, an evolving literature of contemporary case reports suggests that consideration should be given to broadening the use of embolectomy.[78–80] Almost 40 years ago, failure of thrombolytic therapy was defined as "unyielding hypertension" despite maximal medical therapy for greater than 1 hour or ongoing/intermittent cardiac arrest, which defined the need for surgical embolectomy.[81] In a review of the outcomes of pulmonary embolectomy that assessed pooled data from 46 reported case series of patients operated on during the past 50 years, the average mortality was reported to be 30%. In the era prior to 1985, the average mortality was 32% in contrast to a 20% mortality rate in patients operated on between 1985 and 2005. The presence of cardiac arrest prior to embolectomy was a significant risk factor for poor outcome in virtually all series with an inoperative mortality of 59% reported in this population compared to 29% in patients who did not experience a preoperative cardiac arrest.[32] Recent case report series illustrate the dramatic improvement in embolectomy outcomes over the past 50 years. Over a 7- year period, 25 patients underwent emergent embolectomy for central PE. Seventy-two percent presented in cardiogenic shock and 32% sustained a cardiac arrest requiring CPR prior to embolectomy. Surgery was performed with mild hypothermic cardiopulmonary bypass. A 30-day mortality of 8% was reported, with all patients surviving the procedure and 2 patients subsequently dying on postoperative day 1 and 1.[79] Several other modern case series have reported excellent outcomes, although these series liberalized the inclusion criteria to include patients with significant embolic burden who were hemodynamically stable. In a case series of 47 patients over 6 years, indications for surgical intervention were defined as a contraindication to thrombolysis (45%), failed medical treatment (10%), and RV dysfunction (32%). Importantly, only 26% of patients were in cardiogenic shock prior to embolectomy. The authors reported a mortality rate of 6% and concluded that surgical embolectomy should not be limited to patients with large central clot burden and hemodynamic instability but should include hemodynamically stable patients with RV dysfunction documented by echocardiography.[78] Similar outstanding outcomes were reported in a case series of 29 consecutive patients undergoing embolectomy over a 2-year time period with a survival rate of 89%.[80] Enhanced survivorship was attributed to improved surgical technique, rapidity of diagnosis, triage, and careful patient selection. Other factors that were indentified included the routine placement of the vena cava filter perioperatively, recognition that no patient with an out-of-hospital cardiac arrest survived emergency embolectomy in the absence of a spontaneous heart rate restoration, and the exclusion of octigenarians as suitable for embolectomy if relative contraindications existed in addition to age.

Assessment of the potential embolectomy patient can be challenging given that the vast majority of the patients will be hemodynamically unstable and a significant proportion will have sustained a cardiac arrest. Traditionally, angiographic imaging has been required prior to the surgical procedure to ensure that there is a confirmed diagnosis and establish the proximal nature of the embolism which would be amenable to surgical removal. However, it has been recognized that a commitment to confirmatory diagnostic studies in shock patients can delay definitive treatment and potentially contribute to an increased mortality.[82] Several large series have reported making an operative decision on clinical grounds and reported that angiography was performed in only 14% to 67% of patients.[83,84] Cardiopulmonary bypass with mild hypothermia has largely supplanted venous inflow occlusion with normothermic circulatory arrest and may be used for hemodynamic support in patients where angiography is mandated.[85] Preparation of the patient for pulmonary embolectomy requires careful evaluation and precise management, given the reported deteriorations in cardiovascular function with the induction of anesthesia consequent to vasodilatation in the presence of RV dysfunction.[86] Using an operational definition of hemodynamic collapse after general anesthesia induction that included hypotension refractory to vasopressors, inotrope or fluid administration, and the requirement of cardiopulmonary resuscitation followed by urgent institution of cardiopulmonary bypass, hemodynamic collapse was reported in 19% of patients. The development of hemodynamic instability and cardiovascular collapse was not predicted by any of the risk factors evaluated. The authors concluded that given the unpredictable nature of hemodynamic deterioration, all patients proposed for embolectomy should be prepared and draped before general anesthesia induction with the immediate availability of the cardiac surgery team for the emergent initiation of cardiopulmonary bypass.[87] Frequently, patients considered for embolectomy have previously received thrombolytic therapy. A limited literature suggests that previous failed thrombolytic therapy does not significantly affect the operative risk, and although postoperative complications are common, survivors have a functional outcome.[88,89]

Catheter-directed therapy or a catheter embolectomy has been traditionally reserved for patients with contraindications to both systemic thrombolytic therapy and surgical embolectomy. Assessing the efficacy of catheter directed therapy is difficult because of the absence of large clinical trials and the low likelihood of any clinical trials comparing catheter therapy to thrombolytic therapy or embolectomy.[90–92] Indications for catheter embolectomy have been defined as an acute PE with hemodynamic instability with a systolic pressure of 90 mm Hg or less or a drop in systolic arterial blood pressure greater than 40 mm Hg for 15 minutes, ongoing administration of vasoactive support for hypotension, subtotal or total filling defects in the left and/or right pulmonary artery as visualized on spiral CT scan or pulmonary angiogram, and a contraindication to thrombolytic therapy.[92] A recent comprehensive review of the literature of reported case series using catheter-directed therapy that included 594 patients from 35 studies (6 perspective and 29 retrospective) evaluated outcomes from the procedure. Using a stringent definition of clinical success to include stabilization of hemodynamics, resolution of hypoxia, and survival to hospital discharge, the authors reported that the pooled clinical success for modern catheter-directed therapy was 86.5%. Risks of minor and major procedural complications were 7.9%. In the vast majority of patients in this comprehensive review, 95% were treated with catheter-directed therapy as a first adjunct to heparin and did not receive thrombolytic therapy intravenously. The authors concluded that the current status of catheter-directed therapy represents a safe and effective treatment for major PE and, in centers with significant experience, should be considered as first-line therapy.[91] The preceding outcomes were achieved via mechanical fragmentation and/or aspiration of embolic material, including the use of rheologic thrombectomy and intraembolus thrombolytic injection. Reported advantages of catheter-directed therapy are the ability to perform diagnostic and therapy concurrently with real-time monitoring via angiography. Physiologically, the mechanical fragmentation and the ability to remove embolic fragments facilitate the rapidity of hemodynamic resolution via fragmentation and immediate minimization of the proximal embolus. Consequent to the fragmentation, there is a greater surface area of embolus that would be exposed and amenable to thrombolytic therapy. Although appealing to use intraembolus thrombolytic therapy, it is important to recognize that one-third of the patients in the compilated review with a success rate of 86.5% did not receive thrombolytic therapy and success was accomplished via mechanical fragmentation and embolus aspiration.[91]

SUMMARY

In summary, major PE remains a significant challenge to the practicing intensivist because of the logistical issues involved in making the diagnosis, masking of signs and symptoms by coexisting disease processes, and the significant risk of bleeding complications with anticoagulation and thrombolytic therapy. A pathophysiological model can be used to assist with the generation of a differential diagnosis, facilitate resuscitation, and define definitive therapy. Echocardiography is evolving a significant role in the assessment of hemodynamically unstable patients and will play a greater role in the diagnostic assessment and therapeutic evaluation of patients. Major PE is a medical/surgical emergency and all patients should be considered for medical embolectomy with thrombolytic therapy or surgical/catheter embolectomy. Expertise is evolving at select centers for surgical/catheter embolectomy and future studies will assist in defining the appropriate candidates for these therapies, which have traditionally been reserved for those either failing or with contraindications to thrombolytic therapy.

REFERENCES

1. Berlot G, Calderan C, Vergolini A, et al. Pulmonary embolism in critically ill patients receiving antithrombotic prophylaxis: a clinical-pathologic study. J Crit Care 2011; 26(1):28–33.
2. Kasper W, Konstantinides S, Geibel A, et al. Management strategies and determinants of outcome in acute major pulmonary embolism: results of a multicenter registry. J Am Coll Cardiol 1997;30(5):1165–71.
3. Goldhaber SZ, Visani L, De Rosa M. Acute pulmonary embolism: clinical outcomes in the International Cooperative Pulmonary Embolism Registry (ICOPER). Lancet 1999; 353(9162):1386–9.
4. Thames MD, Alpert JS, Dalen JE. Syncope in patients with pulmonary embolism. JAMA 1977;238(23):2509–11.

5. Konstantinides S, Geibel A, Kasper W, et al. Patent foramen ovale is an important predictor of adverse outcome in patients with major pulmonary embolism. Circulation 1998;97(19):1946–51.

6. Dalen JE, Dexter L. Diagnosis and management of massive pulmonary embolism. Dis Mon 1967:1–34.

7. Jaff MR, McMurtry MS, Archer SL, et al. Management of massive and submassive pulmonary embolism, iliofemoral deep vein thrombosis, and chronic thromboembolic pulmonary hypertension: A scientific statement from the american heart association. Circulation 2011;123(16):1788–830.

8. Diehl JL, Meyer G, Igual J, et al. Effectiveness and safety of bolus administration of alteplase in massive pulmonary embolism. Am J Cardiol 1992;70(18):1477–80.

9. Verstraete M, Miller GA, Bounameaux H, et al. Intravenous and intrapulmonary recombinant tissue-type plasminogen activator in the treatment of acute massive pulmonary embolism. Circulation 1988;77(2):353–60.

10. Tilsner V. Thrombolytic therapy in fulminant pulmonary thromboembolism. Thorac Cardiovasc Surg 1991;39(6):357–9.

11. Meneveau N, Schiele F, Metz D, et al. Comparative efficacy of a two-hour regimen of streptokinase versus alteplase in acute massive pulmonary embolism: Immediate clinical and hemodynamic outcome and one-year follow-up. J Am Coll Cardiol 1998;31(5):1057–63.

12. Hoagland P. Massive pulmonary embolism. In: Goldhaber SZ, editor. Pulmonary embolism and deep venous thrombosis. Philadelphia (PA): WB Saunders Company; 1985. p. 179.

13. Wood KE. Major pulmonary embolism: review of a pathophysiologic approach to the golden hour of hemodynamically significant pulmonary embolism. Chest 2002;121(3): 877–905.

14. Stratmann G, Gregory GA. Neurogenic and humoral vasoconstriction in acute pulmonary thromboembolism. Anesth Analg 2003;97(2):341–54.

15. Dalen JE, Banas JS Jr, Brooks HL, et al. Resolution rate of acute pulmonary embolism in man. N Engl J Med 1969;280(22):1194–9.

16. McDonald IG, Hirsh J, Hale GS, et al. Major pulmonary embolism, a correlation of clinical findings, haemodynamics, pulmonary angiography, and pathological physiology. Br Heart J 1972;34(4):356–64.

17. McIntyre KM, Sasahara AA. The hemodynamic response to pulmonary embolism in patients without prior cardiopulmonary disease. Am J Cardiol 1971;28(3):288–94.

18. McIntyre KM, Sasahara AA. Determinants of right ventricular function and hemodynamics after pulmonary embolism. Chest 1974;65(5):534–43.

19. The UKEP Study Research Group. The UKEP Study: Multicentre clinical trial on two local regimens of urokinase in massive pulmonary embolism. Eur Heart J 1987;8(1): 2–10.

20. McGinn S. Acute cor pulmonale resulting from pulmonary embolism. JAMA 1935; 104:1473–80.

21. Stein PD, Dalen JE, McIntyre KM, et al. The electrocardiogram in acute pulmonary embolism. Prog Cardiovasc Dis 1975;17(4):247–57.

22. Stein PD, Terrin ML, Hales CA, et al. Clinical, laboratory, roentgenographic, and electrocardiographic findings in patients with acute pulmonary embolism and no pre-existing cardiac or pulmonary disease. Chest 1991;100(3):598–603.

23. Ferrari E, Imbert A, Chevalier T, et al. The ECG in pulmonary embolism. predictive value of negative T waves in precordial leads— 80 case reports. Chest 1997;111(3): 537–43.

24. Stein PD, Athanasoulis C, Greenspan RH, et al. Relation of plain chest radiographic findings to pulmonary arterial pressure and arterial blood oxygen levels in patients with acute pulmonary embolism. Am J Cardiol 1992;69(4):394–6.
25. The urokinase pulmonary embolism trial. A national cooperative study. Circulation 1973;47(2 Suppl):1–108.
26. Stein PD, Goldhaber SZ, Henry JW, et al. Arterial blood gas analysis in the assessment of suspected acute pulmonary embolism. Chest 1996;109(1):78–81.
27. Anderson JT, Owings JT, Goodnight JE. Bedside noninvasive detection of acute pulmonary embolism in critically ill surgical patients. Arch Surg 1999;134(8):869–74.
28. Rodger MA, Jones G, Raymond F, et al. Dead space ventilation parallels changes in scintigraphic vascular obstruction at recurrence of pulmonary embolism and after thrombolytic therapy: a case report. Can Respir J 1998;5(3):215–8.
29. Urokinase pulmonary embolism trial. phase 1 results: a cooperative study. JAMA 1970;214(12):2163–72.
30. Alpert JS, Smith R, Carlson J, et al. Mortality in patients treated for pulmonary embolism. JAMA 1976;236(13):1477–80.
31. Meneveau N, Schiele F, Metz D, et al. Comparative efficacy of a two-hour regimen of streptokinase versus alteplase in acute massive pulmonary embolism: immediate clinical and hemodynamic outcome and one-year follow-up. J Am Coll Cardiol 1998;31(5):1057–63.
32. Stein PD, Alnas M, Beemath A, et al. Outcome of pulmonary embolectomy. Am J Cardiol 2007;99(3):421–3.
33. Stein PD, Chenevert TL, Fowler SE, et al; PIOPED III (Prospective Investigation of Pulmonary Embolism Diagnosis III) Investigators. Gadolinium-enhanced magnetic resonance angiography for pulmonary embolism: A multicenter prospective study (PIOPED III). Ann Intern Med 2010;152(7):434–43.
34. Hochhegger B, Ley-Zaporozhan J, Marchiori E, et al. Magnetic resonance imaging findings in acute pulmonary embolism. Br J Radiol 2011;84(999):282–7.
35. Bankier AA, Janata K, Fleischmann D, et al. Severity assessment of acute pulmonary embolism with spiral CT: evaluation of two modified angiographic scores and comparison with clinical data. J Thorac Imaging 1997;12(2):150–8.
36. Qanadli SD, El Hajjam M, Vieillard-Baron A, et al. New CT index to quantify arterial obstruction in pulmonary embolism: comparison with angiographic index and echocardiography. AJR Am J Roentgenol 2001;176(6):1415–20.
37. Mastora I, Remy-Jardin M, Masson P, et al. Severity of acute pulmonary embolism: evaluation of a new spiral CT angiographic score in correlation with echocardiographic data. Eur Radiol 2003;13(1):29–35.
38. Ghaye B, Ghuysen A, Bruyere PJ, et al. Can CT pulmonary angiography allow assessment of severity and prognosis in patients presenting with pulmonary embolism? what the radiologist needs to know. Radiographics 2006;26(1):23–39.
39. Schoepf UJ, Costello P. CT angiography for diagnosis of pulmonary embolism: State of the art. Radiology 2004;230(2):329–37.
40. Collomb D, Paramelle PJ, Calaque O, et al. Severity assessment of acute pulmonary embolism: evaluation using helical CT. Eur Radiol 2003;13(7):1508–14.
41. van der Meer RW, Pattynama PM, van Strijen MJ, et al. Right ventricular dysfunction and pulmonary obstruction index at helical CT: prediction of clinical outcome during 3-month follow-up in patients with acute pulmonary embolism. Radiology 2005;235(3):798–803.
42. Lim KE, Chan CY, Chu PH, et al. Right ventricular dysfunction secondary to acute massive pulmonary embolism detected by helical computed tomography pulmonary angiography. Clin Imaging 2005;29(1):16–21.

43. Bova C, Pesavento R, Marchiori A, et al. Risk stratification and outcomes in hemodynamically stable patients with acute pulmonary embolism: a prospective, multicentre, cohort study with three months of follow-up. J Thromb Haemost 2009;7(6):938–44.
44. Vuilleumier N, Le Gal G, Verschuren F, et al. Cardiac biomarkers for risk stratification in non-massive pulmonary embolism: a multicenter prospective study. J Thromb Haemost 2009;7(3):391–8.
45. Kostrubiec M, Pruszczyk P, Bochowicz A, et al. Biomarker-based risk assessment model in acute pulmonary embolism. Eur Heart J 2005;26(20):2166–72.
46. Sanchez O, Trinquart L, Caille V, et al. Prognostic factors for pulmonary embolism: The prep study, a prospective multicenter cohort study. Am J Respir Crit Care Med 2010;181(2):168–73.
47. Masotti L, Righini M, Vuilleumier N, et al. Prognostic stratification of acute pulmonary embolism: focus on clinical aspects, imaging, and biomarkers. Vasc Health Risk Manag 2009;5(4):567–75.
48. Laporte S, Mismetti P, Decousus H, et al. Clinical predictors for fatal pulmonary embolism in 15,520 patients with venous thromboembolism: findings from the registro informatizado de la enfermedad TromboEmbolica venosa (RIETE) registry. Circulation 2008;117(13):1711–6.
49. Aujesky D, Roy PM, Le Manach CP, et al. Validation of a model to predict adverse outcomes in patients with pulmonary embolism. Eur Heart J 2006;27(4):476–81.
50. Kearon C, Ginsberg JS, Hirsh J. The role of venous ultrasonography in the diagnosis of suspected deep venous thrombosis and pulmonary embolism. Ann Intern Med 1998;129(12):1044–9.
51. Girard P, Musset D, Parent F, et al. High prevalence of detectable deep venous thrombosis in patients with acute pulmonary embolism. Chest 1999;116(4):903–8.
52. Turkstra F, Kuijer PM, van Beek EJ, et al. Diagnostic utility of ultrasonography of leg veins in patients suspected of having pulmonary embolism. Ann Intern Med 1997; 126(10):775–81.
53. Mookadam F, Jiamsripong P, Goel R, et al. Critical appraisal on the utility of echocardiography in the management of acute pulmonary embolism. Cardiol Rev 2010;18(1):29–37.
54. Stawicki SP, Seamon MJ, Meredith DM, et al. Transthoracic echocardiography for suspected pulmonary embolism in the intensive care unit: unjustly underused or rightfully ignored? J Clin Ultrasound 2008;36(5):291–302.
55. Pruszczyk P, Torbicki A, Pacho R, et al. Noninvasive diagnosis of suspected severe pulmonary embolism: transesophageal echocardiography vs spiral CT. Chest 1997; 112(3):722–8.
56. Steiner P, Lund GK, Debatin JF, et al. Acute pulmonary embolism: Value of transthoracic and transesophageal echocardiography in comparison with helical CT. AJR Am J Roentgenol 1996;167(4):931–6.
57. Wittlich N, Erbel R, Eichler A, et al. Detection of central pulmonary artery thromboemboli by transesophageal echocardiography in patients with severe pulmonary embolism. J Am Soc Echocardiogr 1992;5(5):515–24.
58. Pruszczyk P, Torbicki A, Kuch-Wocial A, et al. Transoesophageal echocardiography for definitive diagnosis of haemodynamically significant pulmonary embolism. Eur Heart J 1995;16(4):534–8.
59. Mercat A, Diehl JL, Meyer G, et al. Hemodynamic effects of fluid loading in acute massive pulmonary embolism. Crit Care Med 1999;27(3):540–4.
60. Vlahakes GJ, Turley K, Hoffman JI. The pathophysiology of failure in acute right ventricular hypertension: hemodynamic and biochemical correlations. Circulation 1981;63(1):87–95.

61. Szold O, Khoury W, Biderman P, et al. Inhaled nitric oxide improves pulmonary functions following massive pulmonary embolism: a report of four patients and review of the literature. Lung 2006;184(1):1–5.

62. Faintuch S, Lang EV, Cohen RI, et al. Inhaled nitric oxide as an adjunct to suction thrombectomy for pulmonary embolism. J Vasc Interv Radiol 2004;15(11):1311–5.

63. Dias-Junior CA, Vieira TF, Moreno H Jr, et al. Sildenafil selectively inhibits acute pulmonary embolism-induced pulmonary hypertension. Pulm Pharmacol Ther 2005; 18(3):181–6.

64. Webb SA, Stott S, van Heerden PV. The use of inhaled aerosolized prostacyclin (IAP) in the treatment of pulmonary hypertension secondary to pulmonary embolism. Intensive Care Med 1996;22(4):353–5.

65. Tissue plasminogen activator for the treatment of acute pulmonary embolism. A collaborative study by the PIOPED investigators. Chest 1990;97(3):528–33.

66. Todd JL, Tapson VF. Thrombolytic therapy for acute pulmonary embolism: a critical appraisal. Chest 2009;135(5):1321–9.

67. Petitpretz P, Simmoneau G, Cerrina J, et al. Effects of a single bolus of urokinase in patients with life-threatening pulmonary emboli: a descriptive trial. Circulation 1984; 70(5):861–6.

68. Kearon C, Kahn SR, Agnelli G, et al. Antithrombotic therapy for venous thromboembolic disease: American college of chest physicians evidence-based clinical practice guidelines (8th edition). Chest 2008;133(6 Suppl):454S–545S.

69. Wan S, Quinlan DJ, Agnelli G, et al. Thrombolysis compared with heparin for the initial treatment of pulmonary embolism: A meta-analysis of the randomized controlled trials. Circulation 2004;110(6):744–9.

70. Goldhaber SZ, Kessler CM, Heit JA, et al. Recombinant tissue-type plasminogen activator versus a novel dosing regimen of urokinase in acute pulmonary embolism: a randomized controlled multicenter trial. J Am Coll Cardiol 1992;20(1):24–30.

71. Arcasoy SM, Kreit JW. Thrombolytic therapy of pulmonary embolism: a comprehensive review of current evidence. Chest 1999;115(6):1695–707.

72. Levine MN. Thrombolytic therapy for venous thromboembolism. complications and contraindications. Clin Chest Med 1995;16(2):321–8.

73. Dalen JE, Alpert JS, Hirsh J. Thrombolytic therapy for pulmonary embolism: is it effective? is it safe? when is it indicated? Arch Intern Med 1997;157(22):2550–6.

74. Podbregar M, Krivec B, Voga G. Impact of morphologic characteristics of central pulmonary thromboemboli in massive pulmonary embolism. Chest 2002;122(3): 973–9.

75. Wiegand UK, Kurowski V, Giannitsis E, et al. Effectiveness of end-tidal carbon dioxide tension for monitoring thrombolytic therapy in acute pulmonary embolism. Crit Care Med 2000;28(11):3588–92.

76. Meneveau N, Seronde MF, Blonde MC, et al. Management of unsuccessful thrombolysis in acute massive pulmonary embolism. Chest 2006;129(4):1043–50.

77. Meneveau N, Ming LP, Seronde MF, et al. In-hospital and long-term outcome after sub-massive and massive pulmonary embolism submitted to thrombolytic therapy. Eur Heart J 2003;24(15):1447–54.

78. Leacche M, Unic D, Goldhaber SZ, et al. Modern surgical treatment of massive pulmonary embolism: results in 47 consecutive patients after rapid diagnosis and aggressive surgical approach. J Thorac Cardiovasc Surg 2005;129(5):1018–23.

79. Kadner A, Schmidli J, Schonhoff F, et al. Excellent outcome after surgical treatment of massive pulmonary embolism in critically ill patients. J Thorac Cardiovasc Surg 2008;136(2):448–1.

80. Aklog L, Williams CS, Byrne JG, et al. Acute pulmonary embolectomy: a contemporary approach. Circulation 2002;105(12):1416–9.
81. Sasahara AA, Barsamian EM. Another look at pulmonary embolectomy. Ann Thorac Surg 1973;16(3):317–20.
82. Stulz P, Schlapfer R, Feer R, et al. Decision making in the surgical treatment of massive pulmonary embolism. Eur J Cardiothorac Surg 1994;8(4):188–93.
83. Doerge HC, Schoendube FA, Loeser H, et al. Pulmonary embolectomy: review of a 15-year experience and role in the age of thrombolytic therapy. Eur J Cardiothorac Surg 1996;10(11):952–7.
84. Schmid C, Zietlow S, Wagner TO, et al. Fulminant pulmonary embolism: symptoms, diagnostics, operative technique, and results. Ann Thorac Surg 1991;52(5):1102–5.
85. Mattox KL, Feldtman RW, Beall AC Jr, et al. Pulmonary embolectomy for acute massive pulmonary embolism. Ann Surg 1982;195(6):726–31.
86. Satter P. Pulmonary embolectomy with the aid of extracorporeal circulation. Thorac Cardiovasc Surg 1982;30(1):31–5.
87. Rosenberger P, Shernan SK, Shekar PS, et al. Acute hemodynamic collapse after induction of general anesthesia for emergent pulmonary embolectomy. Anesth Analg 2006;102(5):1311–5.
88. Meyer G, Tamisier D, Sors H, et al. Pulmonary embolectomy: a 20-year experience at one center. Ann Thorac Surg 1991;51(2):232–6.
89. Lund O, Nielsen TT, Ronne K, et al. Pulmonary embolism: long-term follow-up after treatment with full-dose heparin, streptokinase or embolectomy. Acta Med Scand 1987;221(1):61–71.
90. Todoran TM, Sobieszczyk P. Catheter-based therapies for massive pulmonary embolism. Prog Cardiovasc Dis 2010;52(5):429–37.
91. Kuo WT, Gould MK, Louie JD, et al. Catheter-directed therapy for the treatment of massive pulmonary embolism: systematic review and meta-analysis of modern techniques. J Vasc Interv Radiol 2009;20(11):1431–40.
92. Kucher N. Catheter embolectomy for acute pulmonary embolism. Chest 2007;132(2):657–63.

Epidemiology and Incidence: The Scope of the Problem and Risk Factors for Development of Venous Thromboembolism

Paul D. Stein, MD[a,b],*, Fadi Matta, MD[a,b]

KEYWORDS

- Epidemiology • Incidence • Venous thromboembolism
- Pulmonary embolism

PREVALENCE OF PULMONARY EMBOLISM

Pulmonary embolism (PE) is the third most common acute cardiovascular disease after myocardial infarction and stroke.[1] In 2006, 828,000 patients were hospitalized in short-stay non-Federal hospitals in the United States with acute myocardial infarction[2] and 564,000 with stroke (F. Matta and P.D. Stein, unpublished data from the National Hospital Discharge Survey, 2010). In 2006, 247,000 adults were hospitalized with acute PE.[2] The number and proportion of hospitalized patients with PE is increasing (**Figs. 1** and **2**).[3] As many as 25% may die before admission.[4] Patients with acute PE in 2006 represented 0.77% of hospitalized patients 18 years of age or older, and 110 patients/100,000 adult population.[2] In 2006, 467,000 patients were hospitalized with deep venous thrombosis (DVT).[2] This represented 1.5% of hospitalized adults and 208/100,000 adult population.[2]

The reported incidence of postthrombotic syndrome after symptomatic DVT varies and depends on the severity of the postthrombotic syndrome. Some reported that by the end of 1 month, among 347 patients with DVT, 34% developed mild postthrombotic syndrome, 10% moderate, and 4% severe.[5] Among patients with DVT who did not

---

A version of this article originally appeared in *Clinics in Chest Medicine*, 31:4.

Support: none.

Conflicts of interest: neither of the authors has any financial or other potential conflicts of interest relative to the data in this manuscript.

[a] Department of Research, St. Mary Mercy Hospital, Livonia, MI, USA

[b] Department of Internal Medicine, College of Osteopathic Medicine, Michigan State University, East Lansing, MI, USA

* Corresponding author. St. Mary Mercy Hospital, 36475 Five Mile Road, Livonia, MI 48154.

E-mail address: steinp@trinity-health.org

Crit Care Clin 27 (2011) 907–932

doi:10.1016/j.ccc.2011.09.006

0749-0704/11/$ – see front matter © 2011 Elsevier Inc. All rights reserved.

criticalcare.theclinics.com

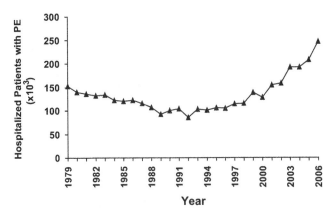

Fig. 1. Number of adults (aged ≥18 years) with PE hospitalized in short-stay hospitals in the United States from 1979 to 2006. Based on data from the National Hospital Discharge Survey.

wear compression stockings, 20% to 82% developed postthrombotic syndrome of any severity.[6–10] There is no universal agreement on a definition of postthrombotic syndrome.[7] However, all definitions include chronic complaints of the legs following DVT.[11] Symptoms may include pain, heaviness, pruritus, and paresthesia, and signs may include pretibial edema, erythema, induration, hyperpigmentation, new venous ectasia, pain during calf compression, and ulceration.[11]

GENDER

The risk of PE and DVT imparted by gender remains uncertain. PE has been reported to occur more frequently in women than in men because of estrogen use, childbearing, and a higher frequency of DVT.[12–16] The largest investigation was based on data from the National Hospital Discharge Survey, which reported on 139,000 patients who were discharged from short-stay hospitals in the United States in 1999 with a

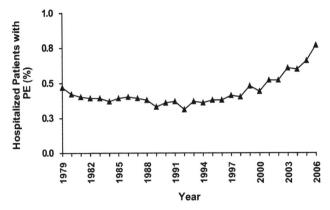

Fig. 2. Proportion of hospitalized adults (aged ≥18 years) with PE hospitalized in short-stay hospitals in the United States from 1979 to 2006. Based on data from the National Hospital Discharge Survey.

diagnosis of PE. The rate of diagnosis of PE in 1999, not adjusted for age, was higher in women (60 PE/100,000 women/y) than men (42 PE/100,000 men/y).[17] The age-adjusted rate of diagnosis of PE/100,000 population in men and women was similar.[17] The Worcester DVT Study showed higher rates of PE in men than women.[18] The French Multicenter Registry showed no differences between the sexes.[19] The Olmsted County study and the Minneapolis St Paul Metropolitan Area Study showed higher age-adjusted rates of PE among men.[20,21] The Tecumseh Community Health Study showed 4.5 PE/10,000 women/y compared with 1.75 PE/10,000 men/y.[15] In smaller investigations, results varied. Some showed a higher prevalence among women[22] and others among men[1,23] and older men.[24] Postmortem study of PE showed PE in 11% of women and 7% of men.[25] On the other hand, the prevalence of PE among 61 patients at autopsy in the Framingham Study was also higher in men.[26] Data from the Prospective Investigation of Pulmonary Embolism Diagnosis (PIOPED) showed a higher prevalence of PE in men.[27]

Contrary to PE, both the unadjusted rate of diagnosis of DVT/100,000 population/y and the age-adjusted rate of diagnosis of DVT/100,000 population/y were higher in women.[17] In 1999, among 369,000 patients discharged from non-Federal short-stay hospitals with a diagnosis of DVT, the unadjusted rate of diagnosis was 115 DVT/100,000 men/y and 154 DVT/100,000 women/y.[17] Most previous literature[19,24,28] also showed higher rates of diagnosis of DVT in women, but objectively diagnosed rates of DVT also have been reported to be higher in men.[18]

RACE

The rate of diagnosis of PE/100,000 population, not adjusted for age, was comparable among blacks and whites.[29] In 1999, the rate of diagnosis among blacks was 41 PE/100,000 population/y and among whites it was 42 PE/100,000 population. In 1999, the age-adjusted rate of diagnosis of PE among blacks was 56/100,000/y and among whites it was 40/100,000/y.[29]

As with PE, the rate of diagnosis of DVT/100,000 population/y, not adjusted for age, was comparable among blacks and whites.[29] In 1999, the rate of diagnosis among blacks was 110 DVT/100,000 population and among whites it was 115 DVT/100,000 population. In 1999, the age-adjusted rate of diagnosis of DVT among blacks was 146/100,000/y and among whites it was 111/100,000/y.[29] Caution has been recommended in the use of race as a variable when comparing blacks and whites. We must distinguish between race and socioeconomic status. An emphasis on ethnic groups, rather than on race, implies an appreciation of cultural and behavioral attitudes, beliefs, lifestyle patterns, diet environmental living conditions, and other factors.[30]

The prevalence of PE in hospitalized patients was also lower among Asians/Pacific Islanders (0.1/100 hospitalizations) than among whites (0.4/100 hospitalizations) and African Americans (0.4/100 hospitalizations).[31] The prevalence of DVT among hospitalized Asians/Pacific Islanders (0.4/100 hospitalizations) was also lower than among African Americans (1.1/100 hospitalizations) and whites (1.1/100 hospitalizations).[31]

A lower prevalence of heritable predispositions to venous thromboembolism (VTE), such as factor V Leiden, has been speculated to contribute to the lower incidence of VTE in Asians.[32] Factor V Leiden is the most common genetic mutation predisposing to VTE.[33,34] It has been found in 4% to 5% of whites in North America and Europe,[35,36] 0.9% to 1.2% of African Americans, and in only 0% to 0.5% of Asians.[35–37] Blood levels of factor VIIc and factor VIIIc were also lower in rural and urban Japanese patients than in whites and Japanese Americans.[38] Some differences of coagulation factors between Asians and whites are attributable to environmental factors, especially diet and smoking, as well as genetic differences.[34,38] Asians may have a more efficient inactivation of coagulation by activated protein C or more fibrinolytic activity than non-Asians.[32] Asians also seem to be more sensitive to warfarin than whites.[39] The target range of the International Normalized Ratio for patients with nonvalvular atrial fibrillation is 1.5 to 2.1 in Japanese patients,[40] and for mechanical prosthetic heart valves it is 1.5 to 2.5 in Japanese patients.[41]

The incidence of PE and of DVT was also lower in American Indians and Alaskan Natives than in African Americans and whites.[42] Archaeological studies suggest that Native Americans may be descended from Asians who crossed the Bering Straits thousands of years ago. A lower prevalence of Factor V Leiden in American Indians/Alaskan Natives populations (1.25%) compared with whites (5.3%) has been observed.[35] From 1996 to 2001 the rate of diagnosis of VTE in American Indians/Alaskan Natives, based on combined data from the National Hospital Discharge Survey and the Indian Health Service, was 71/100,000/y, compared with 155/100,000/y in African Americans and 131/100,000 in whites.[42] The incidence of PE in American Indians/Alaskan Natives was too low to give an accurate estimate of the rate of diagnosis. Only 1 patient with PE was hospitalized in Indian Health Service hospitals between 1996 and 2001. During this interval, an estimated 420,000 patients were hospitalized.[42] The rate of diagnosis of VTE among patients discharged from Indian Health Service hospital care from 1980 to 1996 was reported as 33/100,000/y in American Indians/Alaskan Natives.[43]

AGE

The incidence of PE and DVT increases sharply with age, probably exponentially[18,21,44] (**Fig. 3**). The diagnosis of PE in patients 70 years or older was 6.2 times the rate in younger patients. DVT was diagnosed 12.7 times more frequently in patients aged 70 to 79 years than in younger patients aged 20 to 29 years.[44]

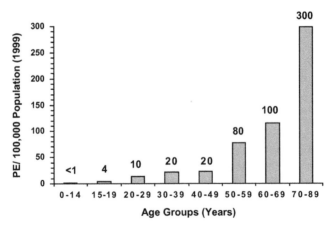

Fig. 3. PE/100,000 population, diagnosed at hospital discharge, shown according to age for the year 1999. (*Data from* Stein PD, Hull RD, Kayali F, et al. Venous thromboembolism according to age: the impact of an aging population. Arch Intern Med 2004;164:2260–5; Stein PD, Kayali F, Olson RE. Incidence of pulmonary thromboembolism in infants and children. J Pediatrics 2004;145:563–5.) (*Reproduced from* Stein PD. Pulmonary embolism. 2nd edition. Oxford (UK): Blackwell Future; 2007; with permission.)

The data relating the incidence of PE to age fit a smooth exponential curve.[18,21,44] There is no cutoff age at which there is no risk of VTE. Even children may suffer a PE or DVT.[45] From 1979 to 2001, PE was diagnosed at discharge from short-stay non-Federal hospitals throughout the United States in 13,000 infants and children 17 years of age or younger and DVT was diagnosed in DVT in 64,000.[45] Rates of diagnosis were 0.9 PE/100,000 children/y, 4.2 DVT/100,000 children/y, and 4.9 VTE/100,000 children/y.[45]

A double peaked curve was shown, with the highest rates of diagnosis in infants less than 1 year old and a second peak in teenagers.[45,46] The rates in infants were comparable with the rates in teenagers. Teenage girls had twice the rates of DVT and VTE as teenage boys, although in younger children the frequencies were comparable in boys and girls.

Abortion and/or contraceptives were shown to be risk factors in 75% of female adolescents who had PE.[47] Teenage users of oral contraceptives did not seem to be at an increased risk of VTE compared with older users.[48] Teenage girls with DVT had an associated pregnancy in 27% of cases.[45] The rate of DVT in nonpregnant teenage girls was 10 DVT/100,000 teenage girls/y, and the rate of pregnancy-associated DVT was 109 DVT/100,000 teenage girls/y.[45] The rate of DVT in nonpregnant teenage girls did not differ significantly from the rate for teenage boys.

Indwelling catheter use was the most common predisposing factor for PE or DVT in children and adolescents, followed by surgery and trauma.[49] Neonatal thrombosis, with the exception of spontaneous renal vein thrombosis, was associated with indwelling catheters in 89%.[50] Lower-extremity DVT in children, when unrelated to venous catheterization or surgery, seemed to be related to local infection of the involved extremity, trauma, or immobilization.[51] One or more coagulopathies were reported in 65% of children with venous thrombosis who had an evaluation for a deficiency of protein C, protein S, or antithrombin III and assessment for a lupus anticoagulant.[52]

SEASON

An analysis of data from the National Hospital Discharge Survey based on 2,457,000 patients with PE and 5,767,000 patients with DVT obtained over 21 years showed no seasonal difference.[53] An absence of seasonal variation was shown in all regions of the United States, including the southern region, where winters are mild, and the northeastern and midwestern regions, where seasons are sharply defined.[53]

REGIONAL RATES OF DIAGNOSIS OF PE AND DVT

The Western region of the United States showed lower rates of DVT and PE from 1979 to 2001 than any other region (**Fig. 4**).[54] Other regional differences were shown as well. Rate ratios of the diagnosis of DVT and PE comparing the Western region with other regions ranged from 0.65 to 0.87.[54]

The mortality from PE was 40% to 45% lower in the Western region of the United States than any other region.[54] A younger population in the Western region does not explain the difference because lower rates were also observed in patients 65 years or older. A higher percentage of Asian Americans and/or Pacific Islanders living in the Western region might be considered to explain the difference because incidences of PE and of DVT are lower in Asian Americans than in African Americans or whites.[31,55,56] However, lower rates of PE and DVT were also shown in whites in the Western region. The observed difference in regional rates of diagnosis of DVT and VTE is not likely to be related to differences in climate. No seasonal variation was

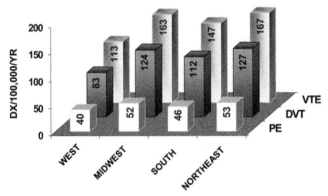

Fig. 4. Rates of diagnosis (Dx)/100,000 population/y of PE, DVT, and VTE according to region from 1979 to 2001. (*Reprinted from* Stein PD, Kayali F, Olson RE. Regional differences in rates of diagnosis and mortality of pulmonary thromboembolism. Am J Cardiol 2004;93:1194–7; with permission.)

observed in the rate of diagnosis of DVT, PE, or VTE in any of the regions, including the Southern region, where winters are mild, and the Northeastern and Midwestern regions, where seasons are sharply defined.[53]

POPULATION MORTALITY RATES FROM PE

The number of patients who died of PE in 1998 based on death certificates was 24,947.[57] This amounts to 9 PE deaths/100,000 population in 1 year. Assuming that death certificates are only 26.7% accurate for the diagnosis of fatal PE,[58] the estimated number of deaths from PE in 1998 may have been 93,000 and the death rate may have been 34 PE deaths/100,000 population.

In the last 2 decades the population mortality from PE (deaths from PE/100,000 population/y) decreased.[57,59] This finding could be a consequence of a declining incidence of PE (diagnoses of PE/100,000 population/y) or a declining case fatality rate from PE (deaths from PE/100 cases of PE) or the combination. From 1979 to 1989, there was no decline in the case fatality rate, which suggests that the declining population mortality from PE was largely due to a declining incidence of PE (**Fig. 5**). From 1979 to 1999 the incidence of diagnosis has decreased.[17]

CASE FATALITY RATE

In untreated patients with clinically apparent DVT, the incidence of fatal PE was 37%.[60] In patients with clinically apparent PE, 37% died of the initial PE and an additional 36% died of a recurrent PE, total mortality being 73%.[61] The applicability of these results to the present era of early diagnosis of mild disease is questionable. The mortality from PE of patients with untreated silent DVT, found by radioactive fibrinogen scintiscans, was 5%.[62] Among patients with mild PE who inadvertently were untreated because the diagnosis was not made from the ventilation-perfusion (V/Q) lung scan, 1 of 20 (5%) died of the initial or recurrent PE.[63]

The estimated case fatality rate (deaths/100 cases of PE) between 1979 and 1998 ranged from 6.7% to 10.5% (see **Fig. 5**).[64] This rate is higher than has been reported in diagnostic trials and in pharmaceutical investigations. The case fatality rate in the PIOPED was 2.5%.[65] In PIOPED, which was an investigation of the accuracy of V/Q

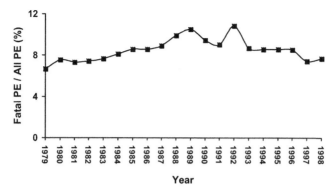

Fig. 5. Estimated case fatality rate for PE from 1979 to 1998. (*Reprinted from* Stein PD, Kayali F, Olson RE. Estimated case fatality rate of pulmonary embolism, 1979–1998. Am J Cardiol 2004;93:1197–9; with permission.)

lung scans, patients were excluded if they were too ill to participate. In addition, most deaths from PE occur within the first 2.5 hours after the diagnosis is made,[66] thereby excluding another group of patients from such studies. For similar reasons, case fatality rates in trials of treatment with low-molecular-weight heparin (LMWH) were only 0.6% to 1.0%.[67,68] The case fatality rate from PE increased exponentially with age from 3.6% in patients aged 25 to 34 years to 17.4% in patients older than 85 years (**Fig. 6**).[64]

RISK FACTORS

Among all patients with PE in the PIOPED II trial 94% had 1 or more of the following assessed risk factors: bed rest within the last month of 3 days or more, travel within the last month of 4 hours or more, surgery within 3 months, malignancy, past history

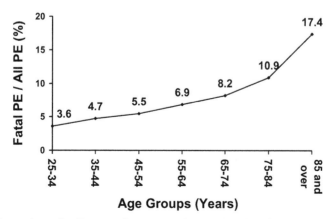

Fig. 6. Estimated case fatality rates for PE according to decades of age. The estimated case fatality rates are the average of yearly values over a 20-year period. (*Reprinted from* Stein PD, Kayali F, Olson RE. Estimated case fatality rate of pulmonary embolism, 1979–1998. Am J Cardiol 2004;93:1197–9; with permission.)

of DVT or PE, trauma of lower extremities or pelvis, central venous instrumentation within 3 months, stroke, paresis or paralysis, heart failure or chronic obstructive pulmonary disease (COPD).[69] Immobilization of only 1 or 2 days may predispose to PE, and 65% of those who were immobilized were immobilized for 2 weeks or less.[70]

Obesity and Height

Investigations that reported an increased risk for VTE caused by obesity have been criticized because they failed to control for hospital confinement or other risk factors.[71] High proportions of patients with VTE have been found to be obese,[18,72] but the importance of the association is diminished because of the high proportion of obesity in the general population.[73] Some investigations showed an increased risk ratio for DVT or PE in obese women,[26,74–76] but data in men were less compelling. The Nurses' Health Study showed that the age-adjusted risk ratio for PE women with a body mass index (BMI, calculated as weight in kilograms divided by the square of height in meters) 29.0 kg/m^2 or higher was 3.2 compared with the leanest category of less than 21.0 kg/m^2.[74] The Framingham Heart Study showed that metropolitan relative weight was significantly and independently associated with PE among women, but not men.[77] However, the Study of Men Born in 1913 showed that men in the highest decile of waist circumference ($\geq$100 cm) had an adjusted relative risk for VTE of 3.92 compared with men with a waist circumference less than 100 cm.[78] Among 1272 outpatients (men and women), the odds ratio for DVT, comparing obese (BMI> 30 kg/m^2) with nonobese patients, was 2.39.[79] Others showed a similar odds ratio for DVT of 2.26 compared with nonobese patients.[75] BMI correlated linearly with the development of PE in women.[80] On the other hand, the Olmsted County, Minnesota case-control study found no evidence that current BMI was an independent risk factor for VTE in men or women.[71,81] Others did not show obesity to be a risk for VTE in men.[26,76]

Analysis of the huge database of the National Hospital Discharge Survey[82] showed compelling evidence that obesity is a risk factor for VTE.[83] Among patients hospitalized in short-term hospitals throughout the United States, in whom obesity was coded among the discharge diagnoses but not defined, 91,000 of 12,015,000 (0.8%) had PE.[83] Among hospitalized patients who were not diagnosed with obesity, PE was diagnosed in 2,366,000 of 691,000,000 (0.3%). DVT was diagnosed in 243,000 of 12,015,000 (2.0%) of patients diagnosed with obesity, and in 5,524,000 of 691,000,000 (0.8%) who were not diagnosed with obesity.

The relative risk of PE, comparing obese patients with nonobese patients, was 2.18 and for DVT it was 2.50.[83] The relative risks for PE and DVT were age dependent. Obesity had the greatest effect on patients less than 40 years of age, in whom the relative risk for PE in obese patients was 5.19 and the relative risk for DVT was 5.20.[83] The higher relative risk of obesity in younger patients may have reflected that younger patients uncommonly have multiple confounding associated risk factors, which make the risk of obesity inapparent.

Previous investigators used several indices of obesity including a BMI greater than 35 kg/m^2 as well as BMI 30 to 35 kg/m^2,[84] BMI 29 kg/m^2 or greater,[74] weight more than 20% of median recommended weight for height,[18] and for men, waist circumference 100 cm or greater.[78] It is likely that all patients diagnosed with obesity in the National Hospital Discharge Survey database were obese, irrespective of the criteria used. However, some obese patients may not have had a listed discharge diagnosis of obesity, and they would have been included in the nonobese group. This situation would have tended to reduce the relative risk of obesity in VTE.

Various abnormalities of hemostasis have been described in obesity, in particular increased plasminogen activator inhibitor-1 (PAI-1).[85–87] Other abnormalities of coagulation have been reported as well,[87] including increased platelet activation,[77] increased levels of plasma fibrinogen, factor VII, factor VIII, and von Willebrand factor.[88] Fibrinogen, factor VIIc, and PAI-1 correlated with BMI.[89]

Regarding height, in the study of Swedish men, those taller than 179 cm (5' 10") had a 1.5 times higher risk of VTE than men shorter than 172 cm.[90] The Physicians' Health Study of male physicians also showed that taller men had a significantly increased risk of VTE.[91]

Air Travel

The possibility of VTE after travel is not unique to air travel.[92–94] Prolonged periods in cramped quarters, irrespective of travel, can lead to PE.[95] The term economy class syndrome was introduced in 1988,[96] but has since been replaced with flight-related DVT in recognition that all travelers are at risk, irrespective of the class of travel.[97]

Rates of development of PE with air travel lasting 12 to 18 hours have been calculated as 2.6 PE/million travelers.[98] With air travel of 8 hours or longer, 1.65/million passengers had acute PE on arrival.[99] With 6 to 8 hours of air travel the rate of acute PE on arrival was 0.25/million and among those who traveled for 6 hours or less none developed acute PE on arrival.[99] The trend showing increasing rates of PE with duration of travel is compelling, but the incidence of DVT was about 3000 times higher in a prospective investigation.[100] In a prospective investigation of travelers who traveled for 10 hours or longer, 4 of 878 (0.5%) developed PE and 5 of 878 (0.6%) developed DVT.[100]

Varicose Veins

Varicose veins were found by some to be an age-dependent risk factor for VTE.[81] Among patients aged 45 years the odds ratio for VTE was 4.2.[81] In patients aged 60 years the odds ratio was 1.9 and at aged 75 years, varicose veins were not associated with an increased risk of VTE.[81] However, others did not find varicose veins to be a risk factor for DVT[101] or PE found at autopsy.[26]

Oral Contraceptives

Although the risk of VTE is higher among users of oral estrogen-containing contraceptives than nonusers,[102,103] the absolute risk is low.[104] An absolute risk of VTE of less than 1/10,000 patients/y increased to only 3 to 4/10,000 patients/y during the time oral contraceptives were used.[104]

The relative risk for VTE in women using oral contraceptives containing 50 μg of estrogen, compared with users of oral contraceptives that contained less than 50 μg was 1.5.[105] The relative risk for VTE in women using oral contraceptives containing more than 50 μg of estrogen, compared with users of oral contraceptives that contained less than 50 μg was 1.7.[105] No difference in the risk of VTE was found with various levels of low doses of 20, 30, 40, and 50 μg/d.[106] With doses of estrogen of 50 μg/d, the rate of VTE was 7.0/10,000 contraceptive users/y and with more than 50 μg/d, the rate of VTE was 10.0/10,000 oral contraceptive users/y (**Fig. 7**).[105] However, some found no appreciable difference in the relative risk of VTE in relation to low or higher estrogen doses.[107]

Reports of the risk of VTE in relation to the duration of use of oral contraceptives are inconsistent. Some showed relative risks increased as the duration of use of estrogen-containing oral contraceptives increased.[108] The relative risks were 0.7 in

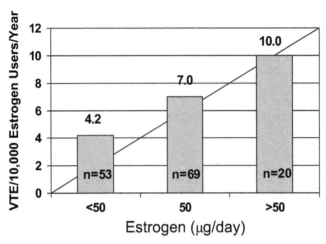

Fig. 7. VTE per 10,000 estrogen-using patients per year according to daily dose. (*Data from* Gerstman BB, Piper JM, Tomita DK, et al. Oral contraceptive estrogen dose and the risk of deep venous thromboembolic disease. Am J Epidemiol 1991;133:32–7.) (*Reproduced from* Stein PD. Pulmonary embolism. 2nd edition. Oxford (UK): Blackwell Future; 2007; with permission.)

women who used oral contraceptives for less than 1 year, 1.4 for those who used oral contraceptives for 1 to 4 years and 1.8 in those who used it for 5 years or longer.[108] Others showed the opposite effect, with a decreasing relative risk with duration of use.[106] The relative risk for DVT or PE was 5.1 with use for less than 1 year, 2.5 with use for 1 to 5 years, and 2.1 with use for longer than 5 years.[106] Some showed the risk to be unaffected by the duration of use.[107]

A synergistic effect of oral contraceptives with obesity has been shown.[109–111] The odds ratio of DVT in obese women (BMI $\geq$30 kg/m^2) who were users of oral contraceptives ranged from 5.2 to 7.8 compared with obese women who did not use oral contraceptives[75,109,110] and among women with a BMI 35 kg/m^2 or higher, the odds ratio was 3.1 compared with similarly obese nonusers of oral contraceptives.[111]

Tamoxifen

Tamoxifen is a selective estrogen-receptor modulator used for treatment of breast cancer and for prevention of breast cancer in high-risk patients.[112–114] Among women with breast cancer currently being treated with tamoxifen, compared with previous users or those who never used it, the odds ratio was 7.1.[114] Others found a lower odds ratio of 2.7.[81] The odds ratio for VTE in women at high risk of breast cancer who received tamoxifen to prevent breast cancer was 2.1.[113] Others found a hazard ratio of 1.63.[112]

Hormonal Replacement Therapy

There is a 2- to 3-fold increased risk of VTE with the use of hormone replacement therapy in postmenopausal women.[115–119] Among postmenopausal women who had coronary artery disease and received estrogen plus progestin, the relative hazard of VTE was 2.7 compared with nonusers.[120] Review showed that the risk of VTE is highest in the first year of hormone replacement therapy.[121] The risk of VTE is increased for oral estrogen alone, oral estrogen combined with progestin, and probably for transdermal hormone replacement therapy.[121]

Hypercoagulable Syndrome

Hypercoagulable syndromes include inherited and acquired thrombophilias. The former is discussed in detail in the article by Weitz in this issue. The latter includes the antiphospholipid syndrome, heparin-induced thrombocytopenia, acquired dysfibrinogenemia, myeloproliferative disorders, and malignancy. Myeloproliferative disorders and malignancy are described elsewhere in this article.

Regarding the antiphospholipid syndrome, antiphospholipid antibodies are associated with both arterial and venous thrombosis.[122] The most commonly detected subgroups of antiphospholipid antibodies are lupus anticoagulant antibodies, anticardiolipin antibodies and anti-β_2 -glycoprotein I antibodies.[123] DVT, the most common manifestation of the antiphospholipid syndrome, occurs in 29% to 55% of patients with the syndrome, and about half of these patients have pulmonary emboli.[124–126]

The risk of heparin-associated thrombocytopenia is more duration related than dose related. Heparin-associated thrombocytopenia occurs more frequently with unfractionated heparin when used for an extended duration than with LMWH used for an extended duration.[127] When used for prophylaxis, there was a higher prevalence of heparin-associated thrombocytopenia in those receiving unfractionated heparin (1.6%, 57 of 3463) than in those receiving LMWH (0.6%, 23 of 3714).[127] However, treatment resulted in only a small difference in the prevalence of heparin-associated thrombocytopenia comparing unfractionated heparin (0.9%, 22 of 2321) with LMWH (0.6%, 18 of 3126).[127]

Acquired dysfibrinogenemia occurs most often in patients with severe liver disease.[128] The impairment of the fibrinogen is a structural defect caused by an increased carbohydrate content impairing the polymerization of the fibrin, depending on the degree of abnormality of the fibrinogen molecule.[128]

Heart Failure

Congestive heart failure (CHF) is considered a major risk factor for VTE.[18,79,101,129–131] Among patients with established CHF, those with lower ejection fractions had a higher risk of thromboembolic event.[132,133] However, some investigators did not evaluate CHF among the risk factors for VTE.[134] The reported frequency of PE in patients with heart failure has ranged widely from 0.9% to 39% of patients.[18,132,133,135–138] The reported frequency of DVT in patients with CHF also ranged widely from 10% to 59%.[18,79,101] The largest investigation was from the National Hospital Discharge Survey.[139] Among 58,873,000 patients hospitalized with heart failure in short-stay hospitals from 1979 to 2003, 1.63% had VTE (relative risk [RR] = 1.47).[139] The relative risk for VTE was highest in patients less than 40 years old (RR = 6.91). Some showed the lower the ejection fraction, the greater the risk of VTE.[140] Among 755,807 adults older than 20 years with heart failure who died from 1980 to 1998, PE was listed as the cause of death in 20,387 (2.7%).[141] Assuming that the accuracy of death certificates was only 26.7%,[58] the rate of death from PE in these patients may have been as high as 10.1%. Therefore, the estimated death rate from PE in patients who died with heart failure was 3% to 10%. CHF seems to be a stronger risk factor in women. Dries and colleagues[132] reported a higher proportion of PE in women (24%) compared with men (14%). We too showed a higher relative risk of PE and of DVT in women with CHF than in men.[139] Although these data seem compelling, multivariate logistic analysis failed to identify CHF as an independent risk factor for DVT or PE.[81] However, it was a risk factor for postmortem VTE that was not a cause of death.[81]

COPD

Hospitalized patients with exacerbations of COPD, when routinely evaluated, showed PE in 25% to 29%.[142,143] From 1979 to 2003, 58,392,000 adults older than 20 years were hospitalized with COPD in short-stay hospitals in the United States.[144] PE was diagnosed in 381,000 (0.65%) and DVT in 632,000 (1.08%).[144] The relative risk for PE in adults hospitalized with COPD was 1.92 and for DVT it was 1.30. Among those aged 20 to 39 years with COPD, the relative risk for PE was 5.34. Among patients with COPD aged 40 to 59 years, the relative risk for PE decreased to 2.02, and among patients aged 60 to 79 years the relative risk for PE was 1.23.[144] The relative risk for DVT was also higher in patients with COPD aged 20 to 39 years (RR = 2.58) than in patients aged 40 years or older (RR 0.92–1.17, depending on age).[144] In young adults, other risk factors in combination with COPD are uncommon, so the contribution of COPD to the risk of PE becomes more apparent than in older patients. Although these data strongly suggest that COPD is a risk factor for PE and DVT, multivariate logistic analysis did not identify it as an independent risk factor.[81] Others, with univariate analysis, did not identify COPD as a risk factor.[101]

Stroke

Patients with stroke are at particular risk of developing DVT and PE because of limb paralysis, prolonged bed rest, and increased prothrombotic activity.[145] Among 14,109,000 patients with ischemic stroke hospitalized in short-stay hospitals from 1979 to 2003, VTE was diagnosed in 165,000 (1.17%).[146] Among 1,606,000 patients with hemorrhagic stroke, the incidence of VTE was higher (1.93%).

Among patients with ischemic stroke who died from 1980 to 1998, PE was the listed cause of death in 11,101 of 2,000,963 (0.55%).[147] Based on an assumed sensitivity of death certificates for fatal PE of 26.7% to 37.2%,[58,148] the corrected rate of fatal PE was 1.5% to 2.1%. Death rates from PE among patients with ischemic stroke decreased from 1980 to 1998, suggesting effective use of antithrombotic prophylaxis.

Cancer

From 1979 to 1999, among 40,787,000 patients hospitalized in short-stay hospitals with any of 19 malignancies studied, 827,000 (2.0%) had VTE.[149] This was twice the incidence in patients without these malignancies.[149] The highest incidence of VTE was in patients with carcinoma of the pancreas (4.3%) and the lowest incidences were in patients with carcinoma of the bladder and carcinoma of the lip, oral cavity, or pharynx (<0.6% to 1.0%). Incidences with cancer were not age dependent.[149] Myeloproliferative disease and lymphoma were associated with relative risks for VTE of 2.9 and 2.5, respectively (**Fig. 8**).[149] Leukemia was associated with a lower relative risk (1.7).

Based on death certificates from 1980 to 1998 among patients who died with cancer, PE was the listed cause of death in 0.21%.[150] Adjustment of the data for the frailty of the diagnosis of fatal PE based on death certificates indicated a likely range of 0.31% to 1.97%.[150]

Pregnancy

Pregnancy-associated DVT based on data from the National Hospital Discharge Survey was diagnosed in 93,000 of 80,798,000 women (0.12%) from 1979 to 1999.[151] The rate of pregnancy-associated DVT (vaginal delivery and cesarean section) increased from 1982 to 1999, although the rate of nonpregnancy-associated DVT decreased for most of this period (**Fig. 9**). Some showed the rate of pregnancy-associated DVT was twice the

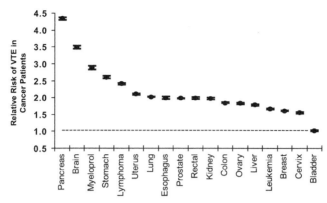

Fig. 8. Relative risks of VTE in patients hospitalized with cancer compared with those without cancer. The relative risk of VTE ranged from 1.02 to 4.34. (*Reprinted from* Stein PD, Beemath A, Meyers FA, et al. Incidence of venous thromboembolism in patients hospitalized with cancer. Am J Med 2006;119:60–8; with permission.)

rate of nonpregnancy-associated DVT.[151] A 6-fold increase in the rate of thromboembolism during pregnancy and the puerperium compared with nonpregnant women has been reported by others.[152]

Although the rate of pregnancy-associated DVT was higher than the rate of nonpregnancy-associated DVT, the rate of pregnancy-associated PE was lower than the rate of nonpregnancy-associated PE.[151] The reason for this difference is unknown and could reflect difference of the natural history of DVT in pregnancy. It also could reflect a reluctance to expose pregnant women to ionizing radiation associated with imaging for PE, resulting in a decreased frequency of diagnosis of PE.

The rate of pregnancy-associated DVT was higher among women aged 35 to 44 years than in younger women. The rate of pregnancy-associated DVT among black women was higher than among white women.[151,153,154]

DVT was more frequent among women who underwent cesarean section (104/100,000/y) than those who underwent vaginal delivery (47/100,000/y).[151] VTE in pregnancy is discussed in detail in the article by Marik elsewhere in this issue.

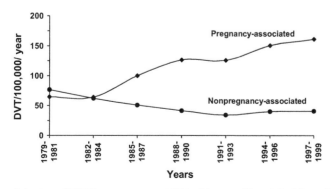

Fig. 9. Triennial rates of DVT in women aged 15 to 44 years. (*Reprinted from* Stein PD, Hull RD, Kayali F, et al. Venous thromboembolism in pregnancy: 21 year trends. Am J Med 2004;117:121–5; with permission.)

Surgery and Trauma

In PIOPED, trauma of the lower extremities was a predisposing factor in 10% of patients with PE, and in PIOPED II trauma of the lower extremities or pelvis was a predisposing factor in 14%.[69,70] Surgery within 3 months of the acute PE was a predisposing factor in 54% in PIOPED and in 23% in PIOPED II.[69,70] The prevalence of VTE following various categories of surgery and trauma has been reviewed in detail by Geerts and colleagues[155]

UPPER-EXTREMITY DVT

As the use of central venous lines and pacemaker wires has increased, their role in the cause of upper-extremity DVT has become prominent.[156–160] The incidence of upper-extremity DVT in a community teaching general hospital in adults (>20 years) was 64 of 34,567 (0.19%).[161] This prevalence of upper-extremity DVT was the same as reported by others (0.2%).[156]

All of the patients with upper-extremity DVT received therapy with anticoagulants.[161] None developed PE.[161] Others reported that 7% to 9% of patients with upper-extremity DVT had an acute PE.[162–164] Most PE (94%) in patients with upper-extremity DVT occurred in untreated patients.[165] Routine ventilation/perfusion lung scans in patients with upper-extremity DVT were high probability for PE in 13%.[164] Only 20% of patients with upper-extremity DVT who did not have a contraindication to anticoagulation were receiving anticoagulant prophylaxis at the time of diagnosis of upper-extremity DVT.[166]

MEDICAL ILLNESSES
Inflammatory Bowel Disease

The incidence of VTE among hospitalized medical patients with ulcerative colitis was 1.9% and the incidence with Crohn disease was lower (1.2%).[167] Among medical patients who had neither ulcerative colitis nor Crohn disease the incidence was 1.1%.[167] The relative risk of VTE among patients with ulcerative colitis compared with patients who did not have inflammatory bowel disease was 1.9 and with Crohn disease it was 1.2 **(Table 1)**. Among patients younger than 40 years with ulcerative colitis, the relative risk of VTE compared with patients who did not have inflammatory bowel disease was 2.96 and in patients younger than 40 years with Crohn disease the relative risk was 2.23.[167]

Liver Disease

Patients with chronic liver disease (both alcoholic and nonalcoholic) seem to have a lower risk of PE than patients without liver disease,[81,168] but data are inconsistent.[169]

Chronic liver disease may result in impaired production of vitamin-K–dependent procoagulant factors.[170] However, decreased production of vitamin-K–dependent endogenous anticoagulants, such as protein C, protein S, and antithrombin III, may counter the hypocoagulability in such patients.[170] Other prothrombotic factors may counteract the impaired production of vitamin-K–dependent procoagulant factors including lupus anticoagulant, activated protein C resistance, PT20210A mutation, Factor V Leiden, MTHFR mutation, and increased levels of factor VIII.[171]

Based on data from the National Hospital Discharge Survey, among 4,927,000 hospitalized patients with chronic alcoholic liver disease from 1979 to 2006, the prevalence of VTE was 0.6% and among 4,565,000 hospitalized patients with chronic nonalcoholic liver disease it was 0.9%.[168] The prevalence of VTE was higher in those with chronic alcoholic liver disease than with nonalcoholic liver disease, but the

Table 1
Relative risk or odds ratio of VTE in selected medical illnesses compared with hospitalized patients who do not have the indicated illness

Medical Illness	Relative Risk VTE	References
Systemic lupus erythematosus	4.3 (odds ratio)	Cogo et al[101]
Rheumatoid arthritis	2.0	Matta et al[175]
Ulcerative colitis	1.9	Saleh et al[167]
Nephrotic syndrome	1.7[a]	Kayali et al[178]
Hypothyroidism	1.6	Danescu et al[172]
Crohn disease	1.2	Saleh et al[167]
Human immunodeficiency virus	1.2	Matta et al[177]
Diabetes mellitus	1.1	Stein et al[176]
Sickle cell disease	0.8	Stein et al[179]
Nonalcoholic liver disease	0.7	Saleh et al[168]
Alcoholic liver disease	0.5	Saleh et al[168]

[a] Relative risk for DVT.

difference was small and of no clinical consequence.[168] Both showed a lower prevalence of VTE than in hospitalized patients with most other medical diseases (see **Table 1**). It may be that both chronic alcoholic liver disease and chronic nonalcoholic liver disease have protective antithrombotic mechanisms although the mechanisms differ.

Hypothyroidism
Among 19,519,000 hospitalized patients with a diagnosis of hypothyroidism from 1979 to 2005, 119,000 (0.61%) had PE (RR = 1.64) (see **Table 1**).[172] DVT was diagnosed in 1.36% of hypothyroid patients (RR = 1.62).[172] The relative risk for PE in patients with hypothyroidism was highest in patients younger than 40 years (RR = 3.99) and the relative risk for DVT was also highest in patients younger than 40 years (RR = 2.25). Hyperthyroidism was not associated with an increased risk for VTE (RR = 0.98).

Rheumatoid arthritis
Rheumatoid arthritis is not generally considered a risk factor for VTE, although abnormalities of coagulation factors have been found in patients with rheumatoid arthritis.[173,174] Among 4,818,000 patients hospitalized in short-stay hospitals from 1979 to 2005 with rheumatoid arthritis who did not have joint surgery, the incidence of PE was 2.3%, and the relative risk of VTE compared with those who did not have rheumatoid arthritis was 1.99 (see **Table 1**).[175] Among patients younger than 50 years the relative risk was higher (2.13).[175]

Diabetes mellitus
Among 92,240,000 patients with diabetes mellitus hospitalized from 1979 to 2005, 1,267,000 (1.4%) had VTE.[176] The relative risk for VTE was increased only in patients younger than 50 years and was highest in patients aged 20 to 29 years (RR = 1.73). In patients with diabetes mellitus who did not have obesity, stroke, heart failure, or cancer, compared with those who did not have diabetes mellitus and did not have any of these comorbid conditions, the relative risk for VTE was 1.52 in patients aged

20 to 29 years and 1.19 in patients 30 to 39 years. In older patients, the relative risk of VTE in patients with diabetes mellitus was not increased.[176] Among all adults with diabetes mellitus, the relative risk of VTE was 1.05 (see **Table 1**).[176]

Human immunodeficiency virus

Among 2,429,000 patients older than 18 years hospitalized in short-stay hospitals from 1990 through 2005 with human immunodeficiency virus (HIV) infection; the prevalence of VTE was 1.7% (RR = 1.21) (see **Table 1**).[177] The prevalence of VTE in patients aged 30 to 49 years was also 1.7%, but the relative risk compared with patients who did not have HIV infection was higher (1.65).[177]

Nephrotic syndrome

From 1979 to 2005, 925,000 patients were discharged from short-stay hospitals with nephrotic syndrome and 14,000 (1.5%) had DVT (RR = 1.72) (see **Table 1**).[178] In patients aged 18 to 39 years the relative risk for DVT was 6.81.[178] Renal vein thrombosis was so uncommon that too few were reported to calculate its prevalence. Therefore, PE, if it occurs, is likely to be due to emboli from the lower extremities and not the renal vein.

Sickle cell disease

Sickle cell disease does not seem to be a risk factor for DVT.[179] Among 1,804,000 patients hospitalized in short-stay hospitals with sickle cell disease from 1979 to 2003, 11,000 (0.61%) had a discharge diagnosis of DVT, which was not more than in African Americans without sickle cell disease (0.81%).[179] Among patients with sickle cell disease, a discharge diagnosis of PE was made in 0.50% compared with 0.33% who did not have sickle cell disease. Regarding patients younger than 40 years, 0.44% had PE, whereas among patients who did not have sickle cell disease, 0.12% had PE.[179] The higher prevalence of apparent PE in patients with sickle cell disease compared with African American patients the same age who did not have sickle cell disease, and the comparable prevalence of DVT in both groups, is compatible with the concept that thrombosis in situ may be present in many.

Systemic lupus erythematosus

Systemic lupus erythematosus is believed to be independently associated with the risk of developing DVT.[101] The odds ratio for DVT in patients with systemic lupus erythematosus, compared with those without it, was 4.3 (see **Table 1**).[101]

Behçet disease

Behçet disease is a rare multisystem inflammatory disorder of unknown cause.[180] VTE occurs in about one-fifth of patients with Behçet disease.[181]

Paroxysmal nocturnal hemoglobinuria

Review of 13 retrospective studies of patients with paroxysmal nocturnal hemoglobinuria showed a 30% prevalence of venous thrombotic events in patients from Western nations.[182] The majority was within the hepatic and mesenteric veins.[182]

Buerger disease

PE associated with thromboangiitis obliterans (Buerger disease) is rare, and to our knowledge, limited to a case report.[183]

SUMMARY

One-quarter of a million patients are hospitalized yearly in the United States with acute PE. Home treatment of DVT has resulted in fewer hospital admissions for DVT than PE. The incidence of PE and of DVT is lower in Asian Americans, American Indians, and Alaskan Natives than in African Americans and whites. The incidence of PE increases exponentially with age, but PE can occur at any age. The estimated case fatality rate is 7% to 11%, and it too increases exponentially with age. More than 90% of patients with PE have 1 or more risk factors, including bed rest, travel, surgery, malignancy, history of DVT or PE, trauma of lower extremities or pelvis, central venous instrumentation, stroke, paresis or paralysis, heart failure, or COPD. Compelling evidence suggests that obesity is a risk factor for VTE. Although the risk of VTE is higher among users of oral estrogen-containing contraceptives than nonusers, the absolute risk is low. There is a 2- to 3-fold increased risk of VTE with the use of hormone replacement therapy in postmenopausal women. DVT occurs in 29% to 55% of patients with the antiphospholipid syndrome, and about half of these patients have PE. Unfractionated heparin, when used for prophylaxis, was associated with a higher incidence of heparin-associated thrombocytopenia than when used for treatment. Pregnancy-associated DVT is 2 to 6 times the frequency of nonpregnancy-associated DVT. The rate of pregnancy-associated DVT has been increasing. Ulcerative colitis, rheumatoid arthritis, and nephrotic syndrome are associated with a nearly 2-fold risk of VTE. Patients with severe liver disease have about half the risk of VTE as patients without liver disease.

REFERENCES

1. Giuntini C, DiRicco G, Marini C, et al. Pulmonary embolism: epidemiology. Chest 1995;107(Suppl):3S–9.
2. Stein PD, Matta F. Acute pulmonary embolism. Curr Prob Cardiol 2010;35:314–76.
3. DeMonaco NA, Dang Q, Kapoor WN, et al. Pulmonary embolism incidence is increasing with use of spiral computed tomography. Am J Med 2008;121:611–7.
4. Heit JA, Silverstein MD, Mohr DN, et al. Predictors of survival after deep vein thrombosis and pulmonary embolism: a population-based, cohort study. Arch Intern Med 1999;159:445–53.
5. Kahn SR, Shrier I, Julian JA, et al. Determinants and time course of the postthrombotic syndrome after acute deep venous thrombosis. Ann Intern Med 2008;149:698–707.
6. Brandjes DP, Büller HR, Heijboer H, et al. Randomized trial of effect of compression stockings in patients with symptomatic proximal-vein thrombosis. Lancet 1997;349:759–62.
7. Ginsberg JS, Hirsh J, Julian J, et al. Prevention and treatment of postphlebitic syndrome: results of a 3-part study. Arch Intern Med 2001;161:2105–9.
8. Partsch H, Kaulich M, Mayer W. Immediate mobilisation in acute vein thrombosis reduces post-thrombotic syndrome. Int Angiol 2004;23:206–12.
9. Prandoni P, Lensing AW, Prins MH, et al. Below-knee elastic compression stockings to prevent the post-thrombotic syndrome: a randomized, controlled trial. Ann Intern Med 2004;141:249–56.
10. Aschwanden M, Jeanneret C, Koller MT, et al. Effect of prolonged treatment with compression stockings to prevent post-thrombotic sequelae: a randomized controlled trial. J Vasc Surg 2008;47:1015–21.
11. Kearon C, Kahn SR, Agnelli G, et al. American College of Chest Physicians. Antithrombotic therapy for venous thromboembolic disease: American College of chest physicians evidence-based clinical practice guidelines (8th edition). Chest 2008;133:454S–545.
12. Palevsky HI. Pulmonary hypertension and thromboembolic disease in women. Cardiovasc Clin 1989;19:267–83.

13. Bernstein D, Goupey S, Schonberg SK. Pulmonary embolism in adolescents. AJDC 1986;140:667–71.
14. Coon W. Epidemiology of venous thromboembolism. Ann Surg 1977;186:149–64.
15. Coon WW, Willis PW, III, Keller JB. Venous thrombosis and other venous disease in the Tecumseh Community Study. Circulation 1973;48:839–46.
16. Breckenridge RT, Ralnoff OD. Pulmonary embolism and unexpected death in supposedly normal persons. N Engl J Med 1964;270:298–9.
17. Stein PD, Hull RD, Patel KC, et al. Venous thromboembolic disease: comparison of the diagnostic process in men and women. Arch Intern Med 2003;163:1689–94.
18. Anderson FA Jr, Wheeler HB, Goldberg RJ, et al. A population-based perspective of the hospital incidence and case-fatality rates of deep vein thrombosis and pulmonary embolism. The Worcester DVT study. Arch Intern Med 1991;151:933–8.
19. Ferrari E, Baudouy M, Cerboni P, et al. Clinical epidemiology of venous thromboembolic disease. Results of a French multicentre registry. Eur Heart J 1997;18:685–91.
20. Lilienfeld DE, Godbold JH, Burke GL, et al. Hospitalization and case fatality for pulmonary embolism in the twin cities: 1979–1984. Am Heart J 1990;120:392–5.
21. Silverstein MD, Heit JA, Mohr DN, et al. Trends in the incidence of deep vein thrombosis and pulmonary embolism. A 25-year population-based study. Arch Intern Med 1998;158:585–93.
22. Stein PD, Huang H-L, Afzal A, et al. Incidence of acute pulmonary embolism in a general hospital: relation to age, sex, and race. Chest 1999;116:909–13.
23. Stein PD, Patel KC, Kalra NK, et al. Estimated incidence of acute pulmonary embolism in a community/teaching general hospital. Chest 2002;121:802–5.
24. Kniffin WD Jr, Baron JA, Barrett J, et al. The epidemiology of diagnosed pulmonary embolism and deep venous thrombosis in the elderly. Arch Intern Med 1994;154:861–6.
25. Karwinski B, Svendsen E. Comparison of clinical and postmortem diagnosis of pulmonary embolism. J Clin Pathol 1989;42:135–9.
26. Goldhaber SZ, Savage DD, Garrison RJ, et al. Risk factors for pulmonary embolism. The Framingham Study. Am J Med 1983;74:1023–8.
27. Quinn DA, Thompson BT, Terrin ML, et al. A prospective investigation of pulmonary embolism in women and men. JAMA 1992;268:1689–96.
28. Stein PD, Patel KC, Kalra NK, et al. Deep venous thrombosis in a general hospital. Chest 2002;122:960–2.
29. Stein PD, Hull RD, Patel KC, et al. Venous thromboembolic disease: comparison of the diagnostic process in blacks and whites. Arch Intern Med 2003;163:1843–8.
30. Haynes MA, Smedley BD, editors. The unequal burden of cancer: an assessment of NIH research and programs for ethnic minorities and the medically underserved. Washington, DC: National Academy Press; 1999. p. 19.
31. Stein PD, Kayali F, Olson RE, et al. Pulmonary thromboembolism in Asian-Pacific Islanders in the United States: analysis of data from the National Hospital Discharge Survey and the United States Bureau of the Census. Am J Med 2004;116:435–42.
32. White RH. The epidemiology of venous thromboembolism. Circulation 2003;107:I4–8.
33. Svensson PJ, Dahlback B. Resistance to activated protein C as a basis for venous thrombosis. N Engl J Med 1994;330:517–22.
34. Franco RF, Reitsma PH. Genetic risk factors of venous thrombosis. Hum Genet 2001;109:369–84.
35. Ridker PM, Miletich JP, Hennekens CH, et al. Ethnic distribution of factor V Leiden in 4047 men and women. Implications for venous thromboembolism screening. JAMA 1997;277:1305–7.

36. Rees DC, Cox M, Clegg JB. World distribution of factor V Leiden. Lancet 1995;346: 1133–4.
37. Gregg JP, Yamane AJ, Grody WW. Prevalence of the factor V-Leiden mutation in four distinct American ethnic populations. Am J Med Genet 1997;73:334–6.
38. Iso H, Folsom AR, Wu KK, et al. Hemostatic variables in Japanese and Caucasian men. Plasma fibrinogen, factor VIIc, factor VIIIc, and von Willebrand factor and their relations to cardiovascular disease risk factors. Am J Epidemiol 1989;130:925–34.
39. Takahashi H, Echizen H. Pharmacogenetics of CYP2C9 and interindividual variability in anticoagulant response to warfarin. Pharmacogenomics J 2003;3:202–14.
40. Yamaguchi T. Optimal intensity of warfarin therapy for secondary prevention of stroke in patients with nonvalvular atrial fibrillation: a multicenter, prospective, randomized trial. Stroke 2000;31:817–21.
41. Matsuyama K, Matsumoto M, Sugita T, et al. Anticoagulant therapy in Japanese patients with mechanical mitral valves. Circulation 2002;66:668–70.
42. Stein PD, Kayali F, Olson RE, et al. Pulmonary thromboembolism in American Indians and Alaskan Natives. Arch Intern Med 2004;164:1804–6.
43. Hooper WC, Holman RC, Heit JA, et al. Venous thrombembolism hospitalizations among American Indians and Alaska Natives. Thromb Res 2003;108:273–8.
44. Stein PD, Hull RD, Kayali F, et al. Venous thromboembolism according to age: the impact of an aging population. Arch Intern Med 2004;164:2260–5.
45. Stein PD, Kayali F, Olson RE. Incidence of pulmonary thromboembolism in infants and children. J Pediatr 2004;145:563–5.
46. Andrew M, David M, Adams M, et al. Venous thromboembolic complications (VTE) in children: first analyses of the Canadian Registry of VTE. Blood 1994;83:1251–7.
47. Bernstein D, Coupey S, Schonberg SK. Pulmonary embolism in adolescents. Am J Dis Child 1986;140:667–71.
48. Royal College of General Practitioners' Oral Contraception Study Oral contraceptives, venous thrombosis, and varicose veins. J R Coll Gen Pract 1978;28:393–9.
49. David M, Andrew M. Venous thromboembolic complications in children. J Pediatr 1993;123:337–46.
50. Schmidt B, Andrew M. Neonatal thrombosis: report of a prospective Canadian and international registry. Pediatrics 1995;96:939–43.
51. Wise RC, Todd JK. Spontaneous, lower-extremity venous thrombosis in children. Am J Dis Child 1973;126:766–9.
52. Nuss R, Hays T, Manco-Johnson M. Childhood thrombosis. Pediatrics 1995;96: 291–4.
53. Stein PD, Kayali F, Olson RE. Analysis of occurrence of venous thromboembolic disease in the four seasons. Am J Cardiol 2004;93:511–3.
54. Stein PD, Kayali F, Olson RE. Regional differences in rates of diagnosis and mortality of pulmonary thromboembolism. Am J Cardiol 2004;93:1194–7.
55. Klatsky AL, Armstrong MA, Poggi J. Risk of pulmonary embolism and/or deep venous thrombosis in Asian-Americans. Am J Cardiol 2000;85:1334–7.
56. White RH, Zhou H, Romano PS. Incidence of idiopathic deep venous thrombosis and secondary thromboembolism among ethnic groups in California. Ann Intern Med 1998;128:737–40.
57. Horlander KT, Mannino DM, Leeper KV. Pulmonary embolism mortality in the United States, 1979-1998: an analysis using multiple-cause mortality data. Arch Intern Med 2003;163:1711–7.
58. Attems J, Arbes S, Bohm G, et al. The clinical diagnostic accuracy rate regarding the immediate cause of death in a hospitalized geriatric population; an autopsy study of 1594 patients. Wien Med Wochenschr 2004;154:159–62.

59. Lilienfeld DE. Decreasing mortality from pulmonary embolism in the United States, 1979–1996. Int J Epidemiol 2000;29:465–9.
60. Byrne JJ. Phlebitis: a study of 748 cases at the Boston City Hospital. N Engl J Med 1955;253:579–86.
61. Hermann RE, Davis JH, Holden WD. Pulmonary embolism: a clinical and pathologic study with emphasis on the effect of prophylactic therapy with anticoagulants. Am J Surg 1961;102:19–28.
62. Collins R, Scrimgeour A, Yusuf S, et al. Reduction in fatal pulmonary embolism and venous thrombosis by perioperative administration of subcutaneous heparin. Overview of results of randomized trials in general, orthopedic, and urologic surgery. N Engl J Med 1988;318:1162–73.
63. Stein PD, Henry JW, Relyea B. Untreated patients with pulmonary embolism: outcome, clinical and laboratory assessment. Chest 1995;107:931–5.
64. Stein PD, Kayali F, Olson RE. Estimated case fatality rate of pulmonary embolism, 1979–1998. Am J Cardiol 2004;93:1197–9.
65. Carson JL, Kelley MA, Duff A, et al. The clinical course of pulmonary embolism. N Engl J Med 1992;326:1240–5.
66. Stein PD, Henry JW. Prevalence of acute pulmonary embolism among patients in a general hospital and at autopsy. Chest 1995;108:978–81.
67. The Columbus Investigators Low-molecular-weight heparin in the treatment of patients with venous thromboembolism. N Engl J Med 1997;337:657–62.
68. Simonneau G, Sors H, Charbonnier B, et al. A comparison of low-molecular-weight heparin with unfractionated heparin for acute pulmonary embolism. The THESSE Study Group. N Engl J Med 1997;337:663–9.
69. Stein PD, Beemath A, Matta F, et al. Clinical characteristics of patient with acute pulmonary embolism: data from PIOPED II. Am J Med 2007;120:871–9.
70. Stein PD, Terrin ML, Hales CA, et al. Clinical, laboratory, roentgenographic and electrocardiographic findings in patients with acute pulmonary embolism and no pre-existing cardiac or pulmonary disease. Chest 1991;100:598–603.
71. Heit JA, Silverstein MD, Mohr DN, et al. The epidemiology of venous thromboembolism in the community. Thromb Haemost 2001;86:452–63.
72. Anderson FA Jr, Wheeler HB, Goldberg RJ, et al. The prevalence of risk factors for venous thromboembolism among hospital patients. Arch Intern Med 1992;152:1660–4.
73. Hedley AA, Ogden CL, Johnson CL, et al. Prevalence of overweight and obesity among US children, adolescents, and adults, 1999–2002. JAMA 2004;291:2847–50.
74. Goldhaber SZ, Grodstein F, Stampfer MJ, et al. A prospective study of risk factors for pulmonary embolism in women. JAMA 1997;277:642–5.
75. Abdollahi M, Cushman M, Rosendaal FR. Obesity: risk of venous thrombosis and the interaction with coagulation factor levels and oral contraceptive use. Thromb Haemost 2003;89:493–8.
76. Coon WW, Coller FA. Some epidemiologic considerations of thromboembolism. Surg Gynecol Obstet 1959;109:487–501.
77. Basili S, Pacini G, Guagnano MT, et al. Insulin resistance as a determinant of platelet activation in obese women. J Am Coll Cardiol 2006;48:2531–8.
78. Hansson PO, Eriksson H, Welin L, et al. Smoking and abdominal obesity: risk factors for venous thromboembolism among middle-aged men: "the study of men born in 1913". Arch Intern Med 1999;159:1886–90.
79. Samama MM. An epidemiologic study of risk factors for deep vein thrombosis in medical outpatients: the Sirius study. Arch Intern Med 2000;160:3415–20.

80. Kabrhel C, Varraso R, Goldhaber SZ, et al. Prospective study of BMI and the risk of pulmonary embolism in women. Obesity (Silver Spring) 2009;17:2040–6.
81. Heit JA, Silverstein MD, Mohr DN, et al. Risk factors for deep vein thrombosis and pulmonary embolism: a population-based case-control study. Arch Intern Med 2000;160:809–15.
82. US Department of Health and Human Services. Public Health Service, National Center for Health Statistics National Hospital Discharge Survey 1979–2006 Multiyear Public-Use Data File Documentation. Available at: http://www.cdc.gov/nchs/about/major/hdasd/nhds.htm. Accessed April 28, 2010.
83. Stein PD, Beemath A, Olson RE. Obesity as a risk factor in venous thromboembolism. Am J Med 2005;118:978–80.
84. Farmer RD, Lawrenson RA, Todd JC, et al. A comparison of the risks of venous thromboembolic disease in association with different combined oral contraceptives. Br J Clin Pharmacol 2000;49:580–90.
85. Pannaciulli N, De Mitrio V, Marino R, et al. Effect of glucose tolerance status on PAI-1 plasma levels in overweight and obese subjects. Obes Res 2002;10:717–25.
86. Juhan-Vague I, Alessi MC, Mavri A, et al. Plasminogen activator inhibitor-1, inflammation, obesity, insulin resistance and vascular risk. J Thromb Haemost 2003;1:1575–9.
87. De Pergola G, Pannacciulli N. Coagulation and fibrinolysis abnormalities in obesity. J Endocrinol Invest 2002;25:899–904.
88. Mertens I, Van Gaal LF. Obesity, haemostasis and the fibrinolytic system. Obes Rev 2002;3:85–101.
89. Bara L, Nicaud V, Tiret L, et al. Expression of a paternal history of premature myocardial infarction on fibrinogen, factor VIIC and PAI-1 in European offspring–the EARS study. European Atherosclerosis Research Study Group. Thromb Haemost 1994;71:434–40.
90. Rosengren A, Fredén M, Hansson PO, et al. Psychosocial factors and venous thromboembolism: a long-term follow-up study of Swedish men. J Thromb Haemost 2008;6:558–64.
91. Glynn RJ, Rosner B. Comparison of risk factors for the competing risks of coronary heart disease, stroke, and venous thromboembolism. Am J Epidemiol 2005;162:975–82.
92. Homans J. Thrombosis of the deep leg veins due to prolonged sitting. N Engl J Med 1954;250:148–9.
93. Symington IS, Stack BH. Pulmonary thromboembolism after travel. Br J Dis Chest 1977;71:138–40.
94. Tardy B, Page Y, Zeni F, et al. Phlebitis following travel. Presse Med 1993;22:811–4.
95. Simpson K. Shelter deaths from pulmonary embolism. Lancet 1940;2:744.
96. Cruickshank JM, Gorlin R, Jennett B. Air travel and thrombotic episodes: the economy class syndrome. Lancet 1988;2:497–8.
97. Collins J. Thromboembolic disease related to air travel: what you need to know. Semin Roentgenol 2005;40:1–2.
98. Hertzberg SR, Roy S, Hollis G, et al. Acute symptomatic pulmonary embolism associated with long haul air travel to Sydney. Vasc Med 2003;8:21–3.
99. Perez-Rodriguez E, Jimenez D, Diaz G, et al. Incidence of air travel-related pulmonary embolism at the Madrid-Barajas airport. Arch Intern Med 2003;163:2766–70.
100. Hughes RJ, Hopkins RJ, Hill S, et al. Frequency of venous thromboembolism in low to moderate risk long distance air travellers: the New Zealand Air Traveller's Thrombosis (NZATT) study. Lancet 2003;362:2039–44.

101. Cogo A, Bernardi E, Prandoni P, et al. Acquired risk factors for deep-vein thrombosis in symptomatic outpatients. Arch Intern Med 1994;154:164–8.
102. Lewis MA. The epidemiology of oral contraceptive use: a critical review of the studies on oral contraceptives and the health of young women. Am J Obstet Gynecol 1998;179:1086–97.
103. Realini JP, Goldzieher JW. Oral contraceptives and cardiovascular disease: a critique of the epidemiologic studies. Am J Obstet Gynecol 1985;152:729–98.
104. Vandenbroucke JP, Rosing J, BloemenkampK W, et al. Oral contraceptives and the risk of venous thrombosis. N Engl J Med 2001;344:1527–35.
105. Gerstman BB, Piper JM, Tomita DK, et al. Oral contraceptive estrogen dose and the risk of deep venous thromboembolic disease. Am J Epidemiol 1991;133:32–7.
106. Lidegaard O, Edstrom B, Kreiner S. Oral contraceptives and venous thromboembolism. A case-control study. Contraception 1998;57:291–301.
107. World Health Organization Collaborative Study of Cardiovascular Disease and Steroid Hormone ContraceptionVenous thromboembolic disease and combined oral contraceptives: results of international multicentre case-control study. Lancet 1995;346:1575–82.
108. Helmrich SP, Rosenberg L, Kaufman DW, et al. Venous thromboembolism in relation to oral contraceptive use. Obstet Gynecol 1987;69:91–5.
109. Pomp ER, le Cessie S, Rosendaal FR, et al. Risk of venous thrombosis: obesity and its joint effect with oral contraceptive use and prothrombotic mutations. Br J Haemotol 2007;139:289–96.
110. Lidegaard O, Edstrom B, Kreiner S. Oral contraceptives and venous thromboembolism: a five-year national case-control study. Contraception 2002;65:187–96.
111. Nightingale AL, Lawrenson RA, Simpson EL, et al. The effects of age, body mass index, smoking and general health on the risk of venous thromboembolism in users of combined oral contraceptives. Eur J Contracept Reprod Healthcare 2000;5:265–74.
112. Decensi A, Maisonneuve P, Rotmensz N, et al. Italian Tamoxifen Study Group. Effect of tamoxifen on venous thromboembolic events in a breast cancer prevention trial. Circulation 2005;111:650–6.
113. Duggan C, Marriott K, Edwards R, et al. Inherited and acquired risk factors for venous thromboembolic disease among women taking tamoxifen to prevent breast cancer. J Clin Oncol 2003;21:3588–93.
114. Meier CR, Jick H. Tamoxifen and risk of idiopathic venous thromboembolism. Br J Clin Pharmacol 1998;45:608–12.
115. Daly E, Vessey MP, Hawkins MM, et al. Risk of venous thromboembolism in users of hormone replacement therapy. Lancet 1996;348:977–80.
116. Jick H, Derby LE, Myers MW, et al. Risk of hospital admission for idiopathic venous thromboembolism among users of postmenopausal oestrogens. Lancet 1996;348:981–3.
117. Grodstein F, Stampfer MJ, Goldhaber SZ, et al. Prospective study of exogenous hormones and risk of pulmonary embolism in women. Lancet 1996;348:983–7.
118. Perez Gutthann S, García Rodriguez LA, Castellsague J, et al. Hormone replacement therapy and risk of venous thromboembolism: population based case-control study. BMJ 1997;314:796–800.
119. Varas-Lorenzo C, García-Rodriguez L, Cattaruzzi C, et al. Hormone replacement therapy and the risk of hospitalization for venous thromboembolism: a population-based study in southern Europe. Am J Epidemiol 1998;147:387–90.

120. Grady D, Wenger NK, Herrington D, et al. Postmenopausal hormone therapy increases risk for venous thromboembolic disease. The Heart and Estrogen/progestin Replacement Study. Ann Intern Med 2000;132:689–96.

121. Peverill RE. Hormone therapy and venous thromboembolism. Best Pract Res Clin Endocrinol Metab 2003;17:149–64.

122. Greaves M. Antiphospholipid antibodies and thrombosis. Lancet 1999;353: 1348–53.

123. Levine JS, Branch DW, Rauch J. The antiphospholipid syndrome. N Engl J Med 2002;346:752–63.

124. Asherson RA, Khamashta MA, Ordi-Ros J, et al. The "primary" antiphospholipid syndrome: major clinical and serological features. Medicine (Baltimore) 1989;68: 366–74.

125. Alarcon-Segovia D, Perez-Vazquez ME, Villa AR, et al. Preliminary classification criteria for the antiphospholipid syndrome within systemic lupus erythematosus. Semin Arthritis Rheum 1992;21:275–86.

126. Vianna JL, Khamashta MA, Ordi-Ros J, et al. Comparison of the primary and secondary antiphospholipid syndrome: a European Multicenter Study of 114 patients. Am J Med 1994;96:3–9.

127. Stein PD, Hull RD, Matta F, et al. Incidence of thrombocytopenia in hospitalized patients with venous thromboembolism. Am J Med 2009;122:919–30.

128. Brick W, Burgess R, Faguet GB. Dysfibrinogenemia. WebMD. Available at: www.webmd.com. Accessed March 19, 2010.

129. Shively BK. Deep venous thrombosis prophylaxis in patients with heart disease. Curr Cardiol Rep 2001;3:56–62.

130. Isnard R, Komajda M. Thromboembolism in heart failure, old ideas and new challenges. Eur J Heart Fail 2001;3:265–9.

131. Jafri SM, Ozawa T, Mammen E, et al. Platelet function, thrombin and fibrinolytic activity in patients with heart failure. Eur Heart J 1993;14:205–12.

132. Dries DL, Rosenberg YD, Waclawiw MA, et al. Ejection fraction and risk of thromboembolic events in patients with systolic dysfunction and sinus rhythm: evidence for gender differences in the studies of left ventricular dysfunction trials. J Am Coll Cardiol 1997;29:1074–80.

133. Kyrle PA, Korninger C, Gossinger H, et al. Prevention of arterial and pulmonary embolism by oral anticoagulants in patients with dilated cardiomyopathy. Thromb Haemost 1985;54:521–3.

134. Nordström M, Lindblad B, Bergqvist D, et al. A prospective study of the incidence of deep-vein thrombosis within a defined urban population. J Intern Med 1992;232: 155–60.

135. Segal JP, Harvey WP, Gurel T. Diagnosis and treatment of primary myocardial disease. Circulation 1965;32:837–44.

136. Dunkman WB, Johnson GR, Carson PE, et al. Incidence of thromboembolic events in congestive heart failure. The V-HeFT VA Cooperative Studies Group. Circulation 1993;87(Suppl 6):VI94–101.

137. Kinsey D, White P. Fever in congestive heart failure. Arch Intern Med 1940;65: 163–70.

138. Roberts WC, Siegel RJ, McManus BM. Idiopathic dilated cardiomyopathy: analysis of 152 necropsy patients. Am J Cardiol 1987;60:1340–55.

139. Beemath A, Stein PD, Skaf E, et al. Risk of venous thromboembolism in patients hospitalized with heart failure. Am J Cardiol 2006;98:793–5.

140. Howell MD, Geraci JM, Knowlton AA. Congestive heart failure and outpatient risk of venous thromboembolism: a retrospective, case-control study. J Clin Epidemiol 2001;54:810–66.
141. Beemath A, Skaf E, Stein PD. Pulmonary embolism as a cause of death in adults who died with heart failure. Am J Cardiol 2006;98:1073–5.
142. Mispelaere D, Glerant JC, Audebert M, et al. Pulmonary embolism and sibilant types of chronic obstructive pulmonary disease decompensations. Rev Mal Respir 2002; 19:415–23.
143. Tillie-Leblond I, Marquette CH, Perez T, et al. Pulmonary embolism in patients with unexplained exacerbation of chronic obstructive pulmonary disease: prevalence and risk factors. Ann Intern Med 2006;144:390–6.
144. Stein PD, Beemath A, Meyers FA, et al. Pulmonary embolism and deep venous thrombosis in patients hospitalized with chronic obstructive pulmonary disease. J Cardiovasc Med 2007;8:253–7.
145. Harvey RL. Prevention of venous thromboembolism after stroke. Topics Stroke Rehab 2003;10:61–9.
146. Skaf E, Stein PD, Beemath A, et al. Venous thromboembolism in patients with ischemic and hemorrhagic stroke. Am J Cardiol 2005;96:1731–3.
147. Skaf E, Stein PD, Beemath A, et al. Fatal pulmonary embolism and stroke. Am J Cardiol 2006;97:1776–7.
148. Dismuke SE, VanderZwaag R. Accuracy and epidemiological implications of the death certificate diagnosis of pulmonary embolism. J Chronic Dis 1984;37:67–73.
149. Stein PD, Beemath A, Meyers FA, et al. Incidence of venous thromboembolism in patients hospitalized with cancer. Am J Med 2006;119:60–8.
150. Stein PD, Beemath A, Meyers FA, et al. Pulmonary embolism as a cause of death in patients who died with cancer. Am J Med 2006;119:163–5.
151. Stein PD, Hull RD, Kayali F, et al. Venous thromboembolism in pregnancy: 21 year trends. Am J Med 2004;117:121–5.
152. Anonymous Oral contraception and thrombo-embolic disease. J R Coll Gen Pract 1967;13:267–79.
153. Rochat RW, Koonin LM, Atrash HK, et al. Maternal mortality in the United States: report from the Maternal Mortality Collaborative. Obstet Gynecol 1988;72:91–7.
154. Buehler JW, Kaunitz AM, Hogue CJR, et al. Maternal mortality in women aged 35 years or older: United States. JAMA 1986;255:53–7.
155. Geerts WH, Bergqvist D, Pineo GF, et al. Preventive of venous thromboembolism. American College of Chest physicians evidence-based clinical practice guidelines (8th edition). Chest 2008;133:381S–453.
156. Kroger K, Schelo C, Gocke C, et al. Colour Doppler sonographic diagnosis of upper limb venous thromboses. Clin Sci 1998;94:657–61.
157. Timsit JF, Farkas JC, Boyer JM, et al. Central vein catheter-related thrombosis in intensive care patients: incidence, risks factors, and relationship with catheter-related sepsis. Chest 1998;114:207–13.
158. Haire WD, Lieberman RP, Edney J, et al. Hickman catheter-induced thoracic vein thrombosis. Frequency and long-term sequelae in patients receiving high-dose chemotherapy and marrow transplantation. Cancer 1990;66:900–8.
159. Ryan JA Jr, Abel RM, Abbott WM, et al. Catheter complications in total parenteral nutrition. A prospective study of 200 consecutive patients. N Engl J Med 1974;290: 757–61.
160. Dollery CM, Sullivan ID, Bauraind O, et al. Thrombosis and embolism in long-term central venous access for parenteral nutrition. Lancet 1994;344:1043–5.

161. Mustafa S, Stein PD, Patel KC, et al. Upper extremity deep venous thrombosis. Chest 2003;163:1213–9.
162. Hingorani A, Ascher E, Lorenson E, et al. Upper extremity deep venous thrombosis and its impact on morbidity and mortality rates in a hospital-based population. J Vasc Surg 1997;26:853–60.
163. Becker DM, Philbrick T, Walker FBIV. Axillary and subclavian venous thrombosis. Prognosis and treatment. Arch Intern Med 1991;151:1934–43.
164. Monreal M, Lafoz E, Ruiz J, et al. Upper-extremity deep venous thrombosis and pulmonary embolism. A prospective study. Chest 1991;99:280–3.
165. Horattas MC, Wright DJ, Fenton AH, et al. Changing concepts of deep venous thrombosis of the upper extremity–report of a series and review of the literature. Surgery 1988;104:561–7.
166. Joffe HV, Kucher N, Tapson VF, et al. Upper-extremity deep vein thrombosis: a prospective registry of 592 patients. Circulation 2004;110:1605–11.
167. Saleh T, Matta F, Yaekoub AY, et al. Risk of venous thromboembolism with inflammatory bowel disease. Clin Appl Thromb Hemost 2011;17(3):254–8.
168. Saleh T, Matta F, Alali F, et al. Liver disease and risk of venous thromboembolism. Submitted for publication.
169. Søgaard KK, Horváth-Puhó E, Grønbaek H, et al. Risk of venous thromboembolism in patients with liver disease: a nationwide population-based case-control study. Am J Gastroenterol 2009;104:96–101.
170. Northup PG, McMahon MM, Ruhl AP, et al. Coagulopathy does not fully protect hospitalized cirrhosis patients from peripheral venous thromboembolism. Am J Gastroenterol 2006;101:1524–8.
171. Tripodi A, Primignani M, Chantarangkul V, et al. An imbalance of pro- vs anti-coagulation factors in plasma from patients with cirrhosis. Gastroenterology 2009; 137:2105–11.
172. Danescu L, Badshah A, Danescu SC, et al. Venous thromboembolism in patients hospitalized with thyroid dysfunction. Clin Appl Thromb Hemost 2009;15: 676–80.
173. Seriolo B, Accardo S, Garnero A, et al. Anticardiolipin antibodies, free protein S levels and thrombosis: a survey in a selected population of rheumatoid arthritis patients. Rheumatology 1999;38:675–8.
174. McEntegart A, Capell HA, Creran D, et al. Cardiovascular risk factors, including thrombotic variables, in a population with rheumatoid arthritis. Rheumatology 2001; 40:640–4.
175. Matta F, Singala R, Yaekoub AY, et al. Risk of venous thromboembolism with rheumatoid arthritis. Thromb Haemost 2009;101:134–8.
176. Stein PD, Goldman J, Matta F, et al. Diabetes mellitus and risk of venous thrombo-embolism. Am J Med Sic 2009;337:259–64.
177. Matta F, Yaekoub AY, Stein PD. Human immunodeficiency virus infection and risk of venous thromboembolism. Am J Med Sci 2008;336:402–6.
178. Kayali F, Najjar R, Aswad F, et al. Venous thromboembolism in patients hospitalized with nephrotic syndrome. Am J Med 2008;121:226–30.
179. Stein PD, Beemath A, Meyers FA, et al. Deep venous thrombosis and pulmonary embolism in patients hospitalized with sickle cell disease. Am J Med 2006;119:897–901.
180. Navarro S, Ricart JM, Medina P, et al. Activated protein C levels in Behçet's disease and risk of venous thrombosis. Br J Haematol 2004;126:550–6.

181. Gül A, Ozbek U, Oztürk C, et al. Coagulation factor V gene mutation increases the risk of venous thrombosis in behçet's disease. Br J Rheumatol 1996;35: 1178–80.
182. Ray JG, Burows RF, Ginsberg JS, et al. Paroxysmal nocturnal hemoglobinuria and the risk of venous thrombosis: review and recommendations for management of the pregnant and nonpregnant patient. Haemostasis 2000;30:103–17.
183. Fischer MD, Hopewell PC. Recurrent pulmonary emboli and Buerger's disease. West J Med 1981;135:238–41.

Hypercoagulable States

Julia A.M. Anderson, MD[a,b], Jeffrey I. Weitz, MD[c,]*

KEYWORDS

- Thrombophilia • Hypercoagulable state • Thrombosis
- Thromboprophylaxis • Anticoagulation

Arterial thrombosis and venous thrombosis are common problems facing clinicians. Some patients with thrombosis have an underlying hypercoagulable state. These states can be divided into 3 categories: inherited disorders, acquired disorders, and those that are mixed in origin.[1,2]

Inherited hypercoagulable states, also known as thrombophilic disorders, can be caused by loss of function of natural anticoagulant pathways or gain of function in procoagulant pathways (**Table 1**). Acquired hypercoagulable states represent a heterogeneous group of disorders in which the risk of thrombosis is higher than that in the general population. The spectrum covers such diverse risk factors as a prior history of thrombosis, obesity, pregnancy, cancer and its treatment, antiphospholipid antibody syndrome, heparin-induced thrombocytopenia, and myeloproliferative disorders. The pathogenesis of thrombosis in these situations is largely unknown and, in many cases, is likely multifactorial in origin. Finally, mixed disorders are those with both an inherited and an acquired component such as hyperhomocysteinemia.[2]

Genetic hypercoagulable states and acquired risk factors combine to establish an intrinsic risk of thrombosis for each individual.[3,4] This risk can be modified by extrinsic or environmental factors such as surgery, immobilization, or hormonal therapy, all of which increase the risk of thrombosis. When the intrinsic and extrinsic forces exceed a critical threshold, thrombosis occurs (**Fig. 1**). Appropriate thromboprophylaxis can prevent the thrombotic risk from exceeding this critical threshold, but breakthrough thrombosis can occur if procoagulant stimuli overwhelm protective mechanisms.

Focusing on hypercoagulable states, this article (a) details the inherited, acquired, and mixed hypercoagulable states, (b) explains how these disorders trigger thrombosis, (c) discusses the laboratory evaluation of hypercoagulable states, (d) identifies those patients who deserve laboratory evaluation for an underlying hypercoagulable state, and (e) outlines the treatment of patients with hypercoagulable states.

A version of this article originally appeared in *Clinics in Chest Medicine*, 31:4.

[a] Department of Clinical and Laboratory Hematology, Royal Infirmary of Edinburgh, Scotland EH16 4SA, UK

[b] Department of Medicine, McMaster University, Hamilton, Ontario L8N 3Z5, Canada

[c] Departments of Medicine, Biochemistry and Biomedical Sciences, Thrombosis & Atherosclerosis Research Institute, McMaster University, 237 Barton Street East, Hamilton, ON L8L 2X2, Canada

* Corresponding author.

E-mail address: weitzj@taari.ca

Crit Care Clin 27 (2011) 933–952

doi:10.1016/j.ccc.2011.09.007

0749-0704/11/$ – see front matter © 2011 Elsevier Inc. All rights reserved.

criticalcare.theclinics.com

Table 1
Classification of hypercoagulable states

Hereditary	Mixed	Acquired
Loss of Function		
Antithrombin deficiency	Hyperhomocysteinemia	Previous venous thromboembolism
Protein C deficiency		Obesity
Protein S deficiency		Cancer
		Pregnancy, puerperium
		Drug-induced:
		Heparin-induced thrombocytopenia
		Prothrombin complex concentrates
		L-Asparaginase
		Hormonal therapy
Gain of Function		
Factor V Leiden		Postoperative
Prothrombin F11G20210A		Myeloproliferative disorders
Elevated factor VIII, IX, or XI		

INHERITED HYPERCOAGULABLE STATES

Inherited disorders are found in up to half of the patients who present with venous thromboembolism before the age of 45 years, particularly those whose event occurred in the absence of well-recognized risk factors, such as surgery or immobilization, or with minimal provocation, such as after a long-distance flight or after taking estrogens. Patients with inherited thrombophilic disorders often have a family history of thrombosis. Of greatest significance is a family history of sudden death due to pulmonary embolism or a history of multiple family members requiring long-term anticoagulation therapy because of recurrent thrombosis. Patients who present with venous thrombosis in unusual sites, such as the cerebral venous sinuses or

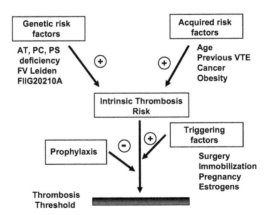

Fig. 1. Thrombosis threshold. Genetic and acquired risk factors determine the intrinsic risk of thrombosis for each individual. This risk is increased by extrinsic triggering factors and decreased by thromboprophylaxis. If the intrinsic and extrinsic forces exceed a critical threshold where thrombin generation overwhelms the protective mechanisms, thrombosis will result. AT, antithrombin; PC, protein C; PS, protein S.

Table 2
Causes of acquired antithrombin deficiency

Decreased Synthesis	Increased Consumption	Enhanced Clearance
Hepatic cirrhosis	Major surgery	Heparin
Severe liver disease	Acute thrombosis	Nephrotic syndrome
L-Asparaginase	Disseminated intravascular coagulation	
	Severe sepsis	
	Multiple trauma	
	Malignancy	
	Prolonged extracorporeal circulation	

mesenteric veins, those with recurrent thrombosis, and patients who develop skin necrosis on initiation of warfarin therapy also should be suspected of having an inherited hypercoagulable state.[5,6]

Loss of Function of Endogenous Anticoagulants

This group of disorders includes deficiency of antithrombin, protein C, or protein S.

Antithrombin deficiency

Antithrombin, a member of the serine protease inhibitor (serpin) superfamily, is synthesized in the liver. Antithrombin plays a critical role in regulating coagulation by forming a 1:1 covalent complex with thrombin, factor Xa, and other activated clotting factors. The rate of antithrombin interaction with its target proteases is accelerated by heparin.[7]

Antithrombin deficiency can be inherited or acquired. Acquired antithrombin deficiency can reflect decreased antithrombin synthesis, increased consumption, or enhanced clearance (**Table 2**). Inherited antithrombin deficiency is relatively rare, occurring in about 1 in 2000, and can be one of two types (**Table 3**), both of which are inherited in an autosomal dominant fashion.[8,9] Type I deficiency is the result of reduced synthesis of biologically normal antithrombin.[10] More than 250 mutations have been identified as causes of Type I antithrombin deficiency, including non-sense mutations, small deletions, insertions, single base deletions, and gene deletions.[8]

Type II antithrombin deficiencies are characterized by normal levels of antithrombin with reduced functional activity. This condition is caused by mis-sense mutations that result in single amino acid substitutions. The clinical consequences of Type II antithrombin deficiency depend on the location of the mutation.[11]

Protein C deficiency

The protein C pathway is a natural anticoagulant "on demand" pathway that is activated when thrombin is generated (**Fig. 2**). Protein C deficiency can be inherited

Table 3
Types of inherited antithrombin deficiency

Type	Antigen	Activity (No Heparin)	Activity (With Heparin)
I (decreased protein)	Low	Low	Low
II (active site defect)	Normal	Low	Low
II (heparin-binding site defect)	Normal	Normal	Low

Protein C Pathway

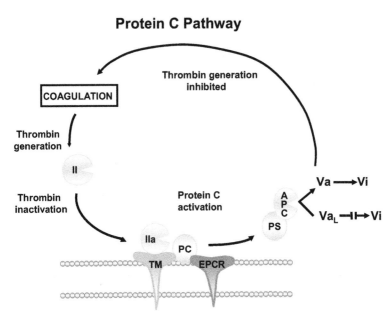

Fig. 2. Protein C pathway. Activation of coagulation triggers thrombin (IIa) generation. Excess thrombin binds to thrombomodulin (TM) on the endothelial cell surface. Once bound, the substrate specificity of thrombin is altered so that it no longer acts as a procoagulant but becomes a potent activator of protein C (PC). Endothelial protein C receptor (EPCR) binds protein C and presents it to thrombomodulin-bound thrombin where it is activated. Activated protein C (APC), together with its cofactor, protein S (PS), binds to the activated platelet-surface and protolytically degrades factor Va (Va) into inactive fragments (Vi). Because factor Va is a critical component of the prothrombinase complex, factor Va inactivation by activated protein C attenuates thrombin generation. Factor Va_{Leiden} (FVa_L) is resistant to inactivation by activated protein C. Consequently, patients with the factor V_{Leiden} mutation have reduced capacity to regulate thrombin generation.

or acquired. Like antithrombin deficiency, protein C deficiency is inherited in an autosomal dominant fashion.[12] Heterozygous protein C deficiency can be found in up to 1 in 200 of the adult population,[13] but many of these individuals do not have a history of thrombosis. Thus, the phenotypic expression of hereditary protein C deficiency is highly variable and may depend on other, as yet unrecognized, modifying factors. In contrast to antithrombin deficiency where the homozygous state is embryonic lethal, homozygous or doubly heterozygous protein C deficiency can occur. Newborns with these disorders often present with purpura fulminans characterized by widespread thrombosis. Individuals with heterozygous protein C deficiency can develop skin necrosis on initiation of warfarin therapy.[14–16]

As outlined in **Table 4**, hereditary protein C deficiency can be further delineated into 2 subtypes using immunologic and functional assays.[17] The most common form of hereditary protein C deficiency is the classic or type I deficiency state. This disorder reflects reduced synthesis of a normal protein, and is characterized by a parallel reduction in protein C antigen and activity. Type II protein C deficiency, which reflects synthesis of a dysfunctional protein, is characterized by normal protein C antigen with reduced functional activity. Most Type II protein C deficiency states are caused by point mutations.[6,18]

Table 4
Types of inherited protein C deficiency

Type	Antigen	Activity
I	Low	Low
II	Normal	Low

Acquired protein C deficiency can be caused by decreased synthesis or increased consumption. Decreased synthesis can occur in patients with liver disease or in those given warfarin.[19] Warfarin decreases functional activity more than immunologic activity. Newborns have protein C levels 20% to 40% lower than those of adults, and premature infants have even lower levels.[20] Protein C consumption can occur with severe sepsis, with disseminated intravascular coagulation, or after surgery.

Protein S deficiency

Protein S serves as a cofactor for activated protein C (APC) and enhances its capacity to inactivate factors Va and VIIIa. In addition, protein S may have direct anticoagulant activity by inhibiting prothrombin activation through its capacity to bind factor Va or factor Xa, components of the prothrombinase complex. The importance of the direct anticoagulant activity of protein S is uncertain.[12] In the circulation, about 60% of total protein S is bound to C4b-binding protein, a complement component. Only the 40% of the protein S that is free is functionally active.[6] Diagnosis of protein S deficiency, therefore, requires measurement of both free and bound forms of protein S.[21,22]

Protein S deficiency can be inherited or acquired. As outlined in **Table 5**, based on measurements of total and free protein S antigen and protein S activity, 3 types of inherited protein S deficiency have been identified. Type I or classic deficiency results from decreased synthesis of a normal protein, and is characterized by reduced levels of total and free protein S antigen together with reduced protein S functional activity. Type II protein S deficiency is characterized by normal levels of total and free protein S, associated with reduced protein S activity. Type III protein S deficiency is characterized by normal levels of total protein S, but low levels of free protein S associated with reduced protein S activity. The molecular basis of Type III deficiency appears to be similar to that of Type I deficiency states, and the 2 types are likely part of the spectrum of the same disorder.

Acquired protein S deficiency can be caused by decreased synthesis, increased consumption, and loss or shift of free protein S to the bound form. Patients with nephrotic syndrome can lose free protein S in their urine, causing decreased protein S activity.[23] Total protein S levels in these patients are often normal because the levels of C4b-binding protein increase, shifting more protein S to the bound form. C4b-binding protein levels also increase in pregnancy and with the use of oral

Table 5
Types of inherited protein S deficiency

Type	Total Protein S	Free Protein S	Protein S Activity
I	Low	Low	Low
II	Normal	Normal	Low
III	Normal	Low	Low

contraceptives. This process shifts more protein S to the bound form, and lowers the levels of free protein S and protein S activity.[24] The pathophysiological consequences of this phenomenon are uncertain.

Gain of Function Mutations

Gain of function mutations include factor V Leiden, FIIG20210A, and elevated levels of procoagulant proteins.

Factor V Leiden

In 1993, Dahlbäck and colleagues[25,26] described 3 families with a history of venous thromboembolism. Affected family members exhibited limited prolongation of the activated partial thromboplastin time (aPTT) when APC was added to their plasma. Accordingly, this phenotype was designated APC resistance (APCR). Bertina and colleagues[27] demonstrated that APCR cosegregated with the factor V gene and was caused by a single base substitution, guanine to adenine at position 1691, that produced an Arg 506 Gln mutation at one of the APC cleavage sites on factor Va.[27–29] This mutation, which is designated Factor V_{Leiden}, endows activated Factor V_{Leiden} with a 10-fold longer half-life in the presence of APC than its wild-type counterpart.

The Factor V_{Leiden} mutation is responsible for most cases of APCR.[30] Other causes are mutations at Arg 306, another APC cleavage site. Arg 306 is replaced by a Gly residue in $FV_{Hong\ Kong}$[31] and by a Thr residue in $FV_{Cambridge}$[32]; neither mutation is associated with thrombosis.

The Factor V_{Leiden} mutation is inherited in an autosomal dominant fashion. The prevalence of the mutation ranges from 2% to 5% in Caucasians, but is rare in Asians and Africans. The prevalence of Factor V_{Leiden} homozygosity is about 1 in 2500.[6] Patients with Factor V Leiden are at lower risk for thrombotic complications than those with deficiencies of antithrombin, protein C, or protein S.[33–35] Heterozygotes with the Factor V_{Leiden} mutation have an annual risk of thrombosis of 0.1% to 0.3%, whereas the risk with deficiencies of antithrombin, protein C, or protein S ranges from 0.5% to 1.5% per year.

A diagnosis of APCR is established using a functional assay based on the ratio of the aPTT after APC addition divided by that determined before APC addition.[36] The use of Factor V–deficient plasma renders the test more specific, but questionable results can be confirmed with a genetic test for the Factor V_{Leiden} mutation.[37]

Prothrombin Gene Mutation

After extensive screening of 28 families with unexplained venous thromboembolism, Poort and colleagues[38] identified a heterozygous G to A nucleotide transition at position 20210 in the 3'-untranslated region of the prothrombin gene in 5 of the probands. This mutation, FIIG20210A, results in elevated levels of prothrombin. Elevated levels of prothrombin, in turn, may increase the risk of thrombosis by enhancing thrombin generation[39,40] or by inhibiting factor Va inactivation by APC.[41]

FIIG20210A is found in 1% to 6% of Caucasians. The mutation is more common in southern than in northern Europe, a gradient opposite to that of Factor V_{Leiden}.[42] Rare individuals homozygous for the FIIG20210A mutation have been identified.[43,44] Laboratory diagnosis of FIIG20210A depends on genetic screening after polymerase chain reaction (PCR) amplification of the 3'-untranslated region of the FII gene. Although FIIG20210A heterozygotes have 30% higher levels of prothrombin than noncarriers, the wide range of prothrombin levels in healthy individuals precludes the use of this phenotype to identify carriers.

Elevated Levels of Procoagulant Proteins

Elevated levels of factor VIII and other coagulation factors, including factors XI and IX, have been implicated as independent risk factors for thrombosis.[45–47] Although the molecular bases for the high levels of these coagulation factors have yet to be identified, genetic mechanisms are likely responsible because of the high heritability of these quantitative abnormalities.

ACQUIRED HYPERCOAGULABLE STATES

Acquired hypercoagulable states include antiphospholipid antibody syndrome, cancer, heparin-induced thrombocytopenia, pregnancy and estrogen therapy (oral contraception or hormone replacement therapy), and a prior history of venous thromboembolism.

Antiphospholipid Antibody Syndrome

Antiphospholipid antibodies are a heterogeneous group of autoantibodies directed against proteins that bind phospholipid.[48] Antibodies can be categorized into those that prolong phospholipid-dependent coagulation assays, known as lupus anticoagulants (LA), or anticardiolipin antibodies (ACL), that target cardiolipin. A subset of ACL recognizes other phospholipid-bound proteins, particularly β_2 -glycoprotein I.

Patients with thrombosis in association with an LA and/or ACL are diagnosed with antiphospholipid antibody syndrome (APS). APS is considered primary when it occurs in isolation and secondary when it is associated with autoimmune disorders, such as systemic lupus erythematosus or other connective tissue diseases. Thrombosis in APS patients can be arterial, venous, or placental. Placental thrombosis is hypothesized to be the cause of the pregnancy-related complications that characterize APS. These complications include fetal loss before 10 weeks' gestation and unexplained fetal death after 10 weeks' gestation.[49] Intrauterine growth retardation, preeclampsia, and eclampsia also have been associated with APS.

Laboratory diagnosis of APS requires the presence of LA or ACL on at least 2 assays with a period of at least 6 weeks between each test. LA are detected using phospholipid-dependent clotting tests. Most screening assays are based on the aPTT. aPTT reagents differ in their sensitivity for detection of LA, and many laboratories have adopted less sensitive aPTT reagents for routine aPTT testing. LA is suspected when the aPTT is prolonged and fails to correct after mixing with normal plasma. The diagnosis is confirmed by demonstrating that addition of excess hexagonal phase phospholipid normalizes the aPTT, thereby documenting the phospholipid dependence of the abnormal test result. In addition to the aPTT, a battery of phospholipid-dependent clotting tests is often used for diagnosis of LA. These tests include the dilute Russell viper venom time and kaolin clotting time.[50]

ACL antibodies are detected using immunoassays.[51] Only ACL antibodies of medium to high titer and of the IgG or IgM subclass are associated with thrombosis. Lack of standardization of ACL assays makes it difficult to compare results between laboratories. ACL antibodies are found in 3% to 10% of healthy individuals and with infections such as mycobacterial pneumonia, malaria, or parasitic disorders, and after exposure to some medications. Often, these antibodies are of low titer and are transient. ACL antibodies are detected in about 30 to 50% of patients with systemic lupus erythematosus.[52] Of these, 10% to 20% also have LA. In contrast to most hypercoagulable states, APS can be associated with spontaneous arterial thrombosis as well as with venous thromboembolism. Arterial thrombosis can manifest as a

Table 6	
Features of heparin-induced thrombocytopenia	
Feature	Details
Thrombocytopenia	Platelet count of 100,000/μL or less or a decrease in platelet count of 50% or more
Timing	Platelet count falls 5–10 days after starting heparin
Type of heparin	More common with unfractionated heparin than LMWH. Rare with fondaparinux
Type of patient	More common in surgical patients than medical patients. More common in women than in men
Thrombosis	Venous thrombosis more common than arterial thrombosis

stroke or transient ischemic attack.[53,54] Thrombosis of the sagittal sinus, a form of venous thrombosis, also can cause stroke in these patients.[55]

Heparin-Induced Thrombocytopenia

Heparin-induced thrombocytopenia (HIT) is diagnosed on the basis of clinical features (**Table 6**) and laboratory detection of HIT antibodies. The risk of HIT is higher with unfractionated heparin than with low molecular weight heparin (LMWH), is more common in surgical patients than medical patients, and more common in women than in men.[56]

Typical clinical features of HIT include thrombocytopenia and thrombosis (arterial or venous). Less common features include necrotic skin lesions at the sites of subcutaneous heparin injection, acute systemic reactions to heparin and, rarely, disseminated intravascular coagulation.[56,57] Thrombocytopenia is the most common finding, occurring in 90% of patients. The platelet count typically decreases 5 to 10 days after heparin is started. However, thrombocytopenia can occur earlier if the patient has been exposed to heparin in the past 3 months. Rarely, the onset of HIT can be delayed and occurs several days after stopping heparin.[58]

HIT is an autoimmune-like disorder and is caused by heparin-dependent, platelet-activating antibodies of the IgG subclass. These antibodies are directed against neoantigens exposed on platelet factor 4 (PF4) when it is complexed by heparin. By binding to FcγII receptors on platelets, these antibodies trigger platelet activation. Activated platelets and platelet-derived microparticles provide an anionic phospholipid surface on which coagulation factors assemble and promote thrombin generation. This process produces a hypercoagulable state and explains why 30% to 70% of HIT patients develop thrombosis.[59,60]

The diagnosis of HIT is supported by assays that capitalize on the platelet-activating properties of HIT antibodies. The platelet serotonin release assay is the gold standard for the diagnosis of HIT.[61] Enzyme immunoassays for detection of antibodies against PF4 are more sensitive, but are less specific than the serotonin release assay.[62]

When the diagnosis of HIT is established, heparin must be stopped and an alternative anticoagulant should be given (**Box 1**). Options include direct thrombin inhibitors, such as lepirudin, argatroban, or bivalirudin. Factor Xa inhibitors, such as fondaparinux, have also been used successfully, but have yet to receive regulatory approval for this indication. Treatment with these agents should be continued until the platelet count returns to baseline levels, at which point low-dose warfarin can be initiated.

Box 1
Management of heparin-induced thrombocytopenia

Stop all heparin

Give an alternative anticoagulant, such as lepirudin, argatroban, bivalirudin, or fondaparinux

Do not give platelet transfusions

Do not give warfarin until the platelet count returns to its baseline level. If warfarin was administered, give vitamin K to restore the international normalized ratio (INR) to normal

Evaluate for thrombosis, particularly deep vein thrombosis

Cancer

About 25% of patients who present with venous thromboembolism have cancer.[63] Cancer patients who develop venous thromboembolism have reduced survival compared with those who do not develop venous thromboembolism. Patients with brain tumors and advanced ovarian or prostate cancer have particularly high rates of venous thromboembolism.[64] Treatment with chemotherapy, hormonal therapy, and biologic agents, such as erythropoietin and antiangiogenic drugs, further increases the risk of venous thromboembolism.

The pathogenesis of thrombosis in cancer patients is multifactorial in origin and represents a complex interplay between the tumor, characteristics of the patient, and the hemostatic system. Tumor cells often express tissue factor or other procoagulants that can initiate coagulation.[65,66] In addition to its role in coagulation, tissue factor also acts as a cell-signaling molecule that promotes tumor proliferation and spread. Patient-related factors that contribute to venous thromboembolism include immobility and venous stasis secondary to extrinsic compression of major veins by tumor. Surgical procedures, indwelling central venous catheters, and chemotherapy can produce vessel wall injury.[67] In addition, tamoxifen and selective estrogen receptor modulators (SERM) induce an acquired hypercoagulable state by reducing the levels of natural anticoagulant proteins.[68]

Some patients who present with unprovoked venous thromboembolism have occult cancer. This observation has prompted some experts to recommend extensive screening for cancer in such patients. Any benefits of this approach, however, are offset by potential harms, including procedure-related morbidity, the psychological impact of false-positive tests, and the cost of screening. Furthermore, early detection of cancer is only of benefit if there is potentially curative therapy and only screening for breast, cervical, and possibly colon cancer has been shown to reduce mortality.[69] Small studies comparing extensive cancer screening with no screening in patients with unprovoked venous thromboembolism have yet to demonstrate that extensive screening reduces cancer-related mortality. Therefore, it is difficult to recommend extensive screening at this time. Instead, a careful history should be taken to identify any symptoms suggestive of underlying cancer. If there are no symptoms suggestive of underlying cancer, patients should be encouraged to undergo age-appropriate screening tests for breast, cervical, or colon cancer.

Pregnancy

Venous thromboembolic disease is the leading cause of maternal morbidity and mortality. About 1 in 1000 pregnancies are complicated by venous thromboembolism and about 1 in 1000 women develop venous thromboembolism in the postpartum period.[70] The individual risk of venous thromboembolism in pregnancy and the puerperium is influenced by patient-related factors; these include age older than 35 years, body mass index greater than 29 (calculated as the weight in kilograms divided by height in meters squared), Cesarean delivery, and thrombophilia, or family history of venous thromboembolism.[70,71] A personal history of venous thromboembolism, ovarian hyperstimulation, and multiparity are other risk factors.

More than 90% of deep vein thrombosis in pregnancy occurs in the left leg because the enlarged uterus further compresses the left iliac vein by placing pressure on the overlying right iliac and ovarian arteries.[72,73] A similar mechanism likely explains the isolated left iliofemoral thrombosis that can occur in pregnancy.

Hypercoagulability of the blood occurs in pregnancy, and reflects a combination of venous stasis and changes in the hemostatic system. The enlarging uterus reduces venous blood flow from the lower extremities. However, this is not the only mechanism responsible for venous stasis because blood flow from the lower extremities begins to decrease by the end of the first trimester, likely reflecting hormonally induced venous dilatation. Systemic factors also contribute to hypercoagulability. Thus, the levels of circulating procoagulant proteins, such as factor VIII, fibrinogen, and von Willebrand protein, increase in the third trimester of pregnancy.[74,75] Coincidentally, there is suppression of natural anticoagulant pathways. Thus, there is an acquired resistance to activated protein C related, at least in part, to reduced levels of free protein S.[76,77] The net effect of these changes is enhanced thrombin generation as evidenced by elevated levels of prothrombin fragments and thrombin/antithrombin complexes.[78,79]

About half of the episodes of venous thromboembolism in pregnancy occur in women with thrombophilia.[80,81] The risk of venous thromboembolism in women with thrombophilic defects depends on the type of abnormality and the presence of other risk factors The risk appears to be highest in women with antithrombin, protein C, or protein S deficiency, and lower in those with Factor V_{Leiden} or the prothrombin gene mutation.[82,83] In general, the daily risk of venous thromboembolism in these women is higher in the postpartum period than it is during pregnancy. The risk during pregnancy is similar in all 3 trimesters. Therefore, if thromboprophylaxis is given during pregnancy, it must be administered throughout the pregnancy and continued for at least 6 weeks postpartum.[84]

Hormonal Therapy

Oral contraceptives, estrogen replacement therapy, and SERM are all associated with an increased risk of thrombosis.[85,86] The relatively high risk of venous thromboembolism associated with early oral contraceptives prompted development of low-dose formulations containing reduced doses of estrogen and progestin. Currently available low-estrogen combination oral contraceptives contain 20 to 50 μg of ethinylestradiol and one of several different progestins. Even these low-dose combination contraceptives are associated with a 3- to 4-fold increased risk of venous thromboembolism compared with the risk in nonusers. In absolute terms, this translates to an incidence of 3 to 4 per 10,000 compared with 5 to 10 per 100,000 in nonusers of reproductive age.[87]

Case-control studies suggest that the risk of venous thromboembolism is 20- to 30-fold higher in women with inherited thrombophilia who use oral contraceptives than it is in nonusers with thrombophilia or users without these defects. Despite the increased risk, however, routine screening for thrombophilia is not indicated in women considering the use of oral contraceptives. Based on the estimated incidence and case fatality rate of thrombotic events, it is estimated that 400,000 women would need to be screened to detect 20,000 carriers of Factor V$_{Leiden}$. Oral contraceptives would need to be withheld in all of these women to prevent a single death.[88] For less prevalent thrombophilic defects, even large numbers of women would need to be screened. Based on these considerations, routine screening cannot be recommended. There is mounting evidence that hormonal replacement therapy with conjugated equine estrogen, with or without a progestin, increases the risk of myocardial infarction, ischemic stroke, and venous thromboembolism. Consequently, the use of hormone replacement therapy has markedly decreased.

Prior History of Venous Thromboembolism

A history of previous venous thromboembolism places patients at risk for recurrence.[89,90] Those with unprovoked venous thromboembolism have a particularly high risk of recurrence when anticoagulant treatment is stopped[91]; 10% at 1 year and 30% at 5 years. This risk appears to be independent of whether or not there is an underlying thrombophilic defect, such as Factor V$_{Leiden}$ or the prothrombin gene mutation.

The risk of recurrent venous thromboembolism is lower in patients whose incident event occurs in association with a well-recognized and transient risk factor, such as major surgery or prolonged immobilization. These patients have a risk of recurrence of about 4% at 1 year and 10% at 5 years. Patients whose venous thromboembolic event occurred against the background of minor risk factors, such as oral contraceptive use or a long-distance flight, likely have an intermediate risk of recurrence. Patients at highest risk for recurrence are those with inherited deficiencies of antithrombin, protein C or protein S, antiphospholipid antibody syndrome, advanced malignancy, or those homozygous for Factor V$_{Leiden}$ or the prothrombin gene mutation. Their risk of recurrence is likely to be at least 15% at 1 year and up to 50% at 5 years.

COMBINED INHERITED AND ACQUIRED HYPERCOAGULABLE STATES

Hyperhomocysteinemia is the prototypical hypercoagulable state that occurs due to a combination of inherited and acquired factors.[92,93] Homocysteine is an intermediate sulfur-containing amino acid that acts as a methyl group donor during the metabolism of methionine, an essential amino acid derived from the diet. The interconversion of methionine and homocysteine depends on the availability of 5-methyltetrahydrofolate, a methyl group donor, vitamin B12 and folate, cofactors in the interconversion, and the enzyme methionine synthase.[94] Increased levels of homocysteine can be the result of increased production or reduced metabolism. Severe hyperhomocysteinemia and cysteinuria are rare and are usually caused by deficiency in the enzyme, cystathione β-synthetase. More common is mild to moderate hyperhomocysteinemia, which can be caused by genetic mutations in methyltetrahydrofolate reductase (MTHFR) when they are accompanied by nutritional deficiency of folate, vitamin B12, or vitamin B6.[95] The cofactor requirements are therefore increased with these mutations.[96]

A fasting serum homocysteine level greater than 15 mmol/L is considered elevated. Although elevated levels were a common finding, routine fortification of flour with folic acid has resulted in lower homocysteine levels in the general population.[96,97] Elevated serum levels of homocysteine have been associated with an increased risk of arterial thrombosis (myocardial infarction, stroke, and peripheral arterial disease) and venous thromboembolism.

Administration of folate, along with vitamin B12 and vitamin B6, will reduce homocysteine levels.[98] Recent randomized trials, however, have shown that such therapy does not reduce the risk of recurrent cardiovascular events in patients with coronary artery disease or stroke,[99] nor does it lower the risk of recurrent venous thromboembolism. Based on these negative trials and the declining incidence of hyperhomocysteinemia, the enthusiasm for screening for hyperhomocysteinemia has rapidly declined.

TREATMENT OF THROMBOSIS IN PATIENTS WITH HYPERCOAGULABLE STATES
Initial Treatment

With few exceptions, management of initial thrombotic events in patients with hypercoagulable states is no different from the management of these events in patients without underlying hypercoagulable disorders. The exceptions are purpura fulminans in newborns with homozygous protein C or protein S deficiency and thrombosis in patients with severe antithrombin deficiency. Newborns with purpura fulminans require protein C or protein S concentrates or sufficient amounts of plasma to increase the levels of protein C or protein S.[100,101] Patients with severe antithrombin deficiency require antithrombin concentrates to increase plasma levels of antithrombin to a point where heparin or LMWH can be used for treatment.[102]

Extended Therapy

Extended treatment of thrombosis in patients with hypercoagulable states is similar to that in those without these underlying disorders. Caution is needed when starting patients with protein C or protein S deficiency on warfarin or other vitamin K antagonists to prevent skin necrosis. Warfarin should not be started in these patients until therapeutic anticoagulation has been achieved with heparin or LMWH. Once started, low doses of warfarin should be given to prevent precipitous decreases in the levels of protein C or protein S.

Recent randomized trials have shown that usual-intensity warfarin (target INR of 2.0–3.0) is as effective as higher-intensity warfarin in patients with antiphospholipid antibody syndrome. The risk of major bleeding is lower with usual-intensity warfarin than it is with higher-intensity regimens.[103,104] A target INR of 2.0 to 3.0 is appropriate for patients with other hypercoagulable states as well.

Patients with thrombosis against a background of metastatic cancer do better with extended treatment with LMWH than with warfarin. Randomized clinical trials have shown that compared with warfarin, LMWH reduces the risk of recurrent venous thromboembolism without increasing bleeding.[105] Furthermore, LMWH simplifies treatment because it can be given subcutaneously once daily without coagulation monitoring. The drug can be held before invasive procedures and the dose reduced if there is thrombocytopenia. The major drawback of LMWH is cost, although the drug has been shown to be cost-effective in patients at high risk for recurrent venous thromboembolism.[106]

Duration of Treatment

The presence of a hypercoagulable state has no influence on the duration of anticoagulant treatment in patients whose venous thromboembolic event has occurred in the setting of a well-recognized and transient risk factor, such as major surgery or prolonged immobilization due to medical illness. These patients are treated with anticoagulants for at least 3 months.[107] For those with unprovoked venous thromboembolism, lifelong anticoagulation treatment is often recommended provided that patients are not at high risk for bleeding.[91,108] An elevated D-dimer 1 month after stopping anticoagulant therapy and persistent abnormalities on compression ultrasonography may identify patients at highest risk for recurrence. Heterozygosity for Factor V$_{Leiden}$ or the prothrombin gene mutation does not influence the risk of recurrence. In contrast, patients with deficiency of antithrombin, protein C or protein S, or those homozygous for Factor V$_{Leiden}$ or the prothrombin gene mutation appear to be at higher risk for recurrence and likely require lifelong anticoagulation treatment.[109–111] Likewise, patients with APS with a persistently positive LA also are at high risk for recurrence and require lifelong treatment.

Treatment and Prevention of Thrombosis During Pregnancy

Thrombophilic disorders have no influence on the treatment of venous thrombosis during pregnancy. These women require therapeutic doses of subcutaneous heparin, LMWH, or fondaparinux throughout pregnancy.[84,112] Heparin is given once daily with the dose titrated to achieve a therapeutic mid-interval aPTT. LMWH can be given once or twice daily in a weight-adjusted fashion. Monitoring with anti–factor Xa levels is recommended, particularly in the third trimester. Fondaparinux is given once daily. It is uncertain whether monitoring is required. After delivery, LMWH or warfarin should be given for at least 4 to 6 weeks. In total, treatment should be given for 6 months from the time of diagnosis. Warfarin should be avoided in pregnancy because it crosses the placenta and can cause bone and central nervous system abnormalities, fetal hemorrhage, or placental abruption. Warfarin can be safely administered in nursing mothers, with no detectable anticoagulant effect in breast milk.[113] (See the article by Marik elsewhere in this issue).

Women with a history of unprovoked or recurrent venous thromboembolism, those with deficiencies of antithrombin, protein C, or protein S, and those homozygous for Factor V$_{Leiden}$ or the prothrombin gene mutation should receive antepartum prophylaxis with heparin or LMWH.[84] Postpartum, LMWH or warfarin should be given for 4 to 6 weeks. Postpartum treatment with LMWH or warfarin for 4 to 6 weeks is likely adequate for women with a history of venous thrombosis secondary to a well-defined risk factor.[114] Prophylaxis during pregnancy, as well as postpartum, should be considered for women who have developed venous thromboembolism after taking oral contraceptives, particularly if they have underlying thrombophilia. Women with thrombophilic defects and no prior history of venous thromboembolism likely do not require antepartum prophylaxis or postpartum treatment, but definitive data are lacking.[84] A summary of these recommendations is provided in **Table 7**.

THROMBOPHILIA SCREENING

The indications for thrombophilia screening re-main controversial.[115,116] For patients with a first episode of venous thromboembolism, thrombophilia screening is indicated if the results influence the duration of treatment or impact on family counseling regarding use of estrogen-containing compounds. It is reasonable to screen patients whose first episode of thrombosis has occurred before the age of 45 years, those with recurrent thrombosis, particularly if unprovoked, and patients with thrombosis in an unusual site,[117] such as cerebral or mesenteric veins and those with 2 or more first-degree relatives with thrombosis. It may also be reasonable to screen women with a history of 3 or more second-trimester pregnancy losses or an intrauterine death for LA and ACL.[6]

Screening should include functional assays for antithrombin and protein C, a free protein S level, testing for activated protein C resistance using the modified APC sensitivity ratio with DNA testing for the Factor V$_{Leiden}$ mutation if the screening test

Table 7
Management of women with a history of venous thrombosis during pregnancy and the puerperium

Clinical History	Thrombophilia	Antepartum	Postpartum[a]
Prior venous thrombosis secondary to a transient risk factor	No	Surveillance	Yes
Prior venous thrombosis secondary to pregnancy or estrogens	Yes or no	Prophylactic heparin or LMWH	Yes
Prior idiopathic venous thrombosis	Yes or no	Prophylactic heparin or LMWH	Yes
Recurrent venous thrombosis	Yes or no	Treatment-dose heparin or LMWH	Resume long-term anticoagulation
No prior venous thrombosis	Antithrombin deficiency; *FIIG20210A* or factor V Leiden	Prophylactic heparin or LMWH	Yes

[a] Postpartum prophylaxis involves a 4- to 6-week course of warfarin with the dose adjusted to achieve an INR of 2.0 to 3.0. Prophylactic doses of LMWH can be used as an alternative.

is equivocal, DNA testing for the prothrombin gene mutation, phospholipid-based clotting tests to detect LA, and enzyme immunoassay for ACL identification.

SUMMARY AND FUTURE DIRECTIONS

With increased understanding of the regulation of coagulation, inherited or acquired hypercoagulable states can now be identified in up to 50% of patients with venous thromboembolism. The role of these disorders in the pathogenesis of arterial thrombosis is less clear. Therefore, more work is needed to identify patients who are vulnerable to arterial thrombosis after plaque rupture.

Although our ability to diagnose hypercoagulable states has improved, the impact of this information on clinical decisions remains limited. Common congenital hypercoagulable states increase the risk of a first thrombotic episode, but have little impact on the risk of recurrence. Identification of patients at risk for recurrent thrombosis and elucidation of new hypercoagulable states are goals for the future.

REFERENCES

1. Crowther MA, Kelton JG. Congenital thrombophilic states associated with venous thrombosis: a qualitative overview and proposed classification system. Ann Intern Med 2003;138(2):128–34.
2. Jacques PF, Bostom AG, Williams RR, et al. Relation between folate status, a common mutation in methylenetetrahydrofolate reductase, and plasma homocysteine concentrations. Circulation 1996;93(1):7–9.
3. Salomon O, Steinberg DM, Zivelin A, et al. Single and combined prothrombotic factors in patients with idiopathic venous thromboembolism: prevalence and risk assessment. Arterioscler Thromb Vasc Biol 1999;19(3):511–8.
4. Vandenbroucke JP, Koster T, Briët E, et al. Increased risk of venous thrombosis in oral-contraceptive users who are carriers of factor V Leiden mutation. Lancet 1994;3449(8935):1453–7.

5. Kitchens CS. Thrombophilia and thrombosis in unusual sites. In: Colman RW, Hirsh J, Marder VJ, editors. Hemostasis and thrombosis. Basic principles and clinical practice. Philadelphia: J.B. Lippincott Company; 1994. p. 1255–73.

6. Aiach M, Emmerich J. Thrombophilia genetics. In: Colman RW, Marder VJ, Clowes AW, et al, editors. Hemostasis and thrombosis basic principles and clinical practice. 5th edition. Philadelphia: Lippincott, Williams and Wilkins; 2006. p. 779–93.

7. Olson ST, Björk I. Regulation of thrombin activity by antithrombin and heparin. Semin Thromb Hemost 1994;20(4):373–409.

8. Perry D, Carrell R. Molecular genetics of human antithrombin deficiency. Hum Mutat 1996;7(1):7–22.

9. Perry DJ. Antithrombin and its inherited deficiencies. Blood Rev 1994;8(1):37–55.

10. Ambruso DR, Leonard BD, Bies RD. Antithrombin III deficiency: decreased synthesis of a biochemically normal molecule. Blood 1982;60(1):78–83.

11. van Boven H, Lane D. Antithrombin and its inherited deficiency states. Semin Hematol 1997;34(3):188–204.

12. Griffin JH, Evatt B, Zimmerman TS. Deficiency of protein C in congenital thrombotic disease. J Clin Invest 1981;68(5):1370–3.

13. Tait RC, Walker ID, Reitsma PH, et al. Prevalence of protein C deficiency in the healthy population. Thromb Haemost 1995;73(1):87–93.

14. Monagle P, Andrew M, Halton J, et al. Homozygous protein C deficiency: description of a new mutation and successful treatment with low molecular weight heparin. Thromb Haemost 1998;79(4):756–61.

15. Alhenc-Gelas M, Emmerich J, Gandrille S, et al. Protein C infusion in a patient with inherited protein C deficiency caused by two missense mutations: Arg 178 to Gln and Arg-1 to His. Blood Coagul Fibrinolysis 1995;6(1):35–41.

16. Pescatore P, Horellou HM, Conard J, et al. Problems of oral anticoagulation in an adult with homozygous protein C deficiency and late onset of thrombosis. Thromb Haemost 1993;69(4):311–5.

17. Miletich JP. Laboratory diagnosis of protein C deficiency. Semin Throm Haemost 1990;16(2):169–76.

18. Broze GJ, Warren LA, Novotny WF, et al. The lipoprotein-associated coagulation inhibitor that inhibits the factor VII-tissue factor complex also inhibits factor Xa: insight into its possible mechanism of action. Blood 1988;71(2):335–43.

19. Weiss P, Soff GA, Halkin H, et al. Decline of protein C and S and Factors II, VII, IX and X during the initiation of warfarin therapy. Thromb Res 1987;45(6):783–90.

20. Manco-Johnson MJ, Marlar RA, Jacobson LY, et al. Severe protein C deficiency in newborn infants. J Pediatr 1988;113(2):359–63.

21. Wolf M, Boyer-Neumann C, Martinoli JL, et al. A new functional assay for human protein S activity using activated factor V as substrate. Thromb Haemost 1989;62(4):1144–5.

22. Tripodi A. A review of the clinical and diagnostic utility of laboratory tests for the detection of congenital thrombophilia. Semin Thromb Hemost 2005;31(1):25–32.

23. Vigano-D'Angelo S, d'Angelo A, Kaufman CE Jr, et al. Protein S deficiency occurs in the nephrotic syndrome. Ann Intern Med 1987;107(1):42–7.

24. Malm J, Laurell M, Dahlbäck B. Changes in the plasma levels of vitamin K-dependent proteins C and S and of C4b-binding protein during pregnancy and oral contraception. Br J Haematol 1988;68(4):437–43.

25. Dahlbäck B, Carlsson M, Svensson PJ. Familial thrombophilia due to a previously unrecognized mechanism characterized by poor anticoagulant response to activated protein C: prediction of a cofactor to activated protein C. Proc Natl Acad Sci U S A 1993;90(3):1004–8.

26. Dahlbäck B. The discovery of activated protein C resistance. J Thromb Haemost 2003;1(1):3–9.
27. Bertina RM, Koeleman BP, Koster T, et al. Mutation in blood coagulation factor V association with resistance to activated protein C. Nature 1994;369(6475):64–7.
28. Kalafatis M, Bertina RM, Rand MD, et al. Characterisation of the molecular defect in factor VR506Q. J Biol Chem 1995;270(8):4053–7.
29. Camire RM, Kalafatis M, Cushman M, et al. The mechanism of inactivation of human platelet factor Va from normal and activated protein C-resistant individuals. J Biol Chem 1995;270(35):20794–800.
30. Nicolaes G, Dahlbäck B. Activated protein C resistance (FV Leiden) and thrombosis: factor V mutations causing hypercoagulable states. Hematol Oncol Clin North Am 2003;17(1):37–61.
31. Chan WP, Lee CK, Kwong YL, et al. A novel mutation of Arg306 of factor V gene in Hong Kong Chinese. Blood 1998;91(4):1135–9.
32. Williamson D, Brown K, Luddington R, et al. Factor V: Cambridge: a new mutation (Arg306-Thr) associated with resistance to activated protein C. Blood 1998;91(4): 1140–4.
33. Rodegheiro F, Tosetto A. Activated protein C resistance and factor V Leiden mutation are independent risk factors for venous thromboembolism. Ann Intern Med 1999;130(8):643–50.
34. Martinelli I, Mannucci PM, De Stefano V, et al. Different risks of thrombosis in four coagulation defects associated with inherited thrombophilia: a study of 150 families. Blood 1998;92(7):2353–8.
35. Bucciarelli P, Rosendaal FR, Tripodi A, et al. Risks of venous thromboembolism and clinical manifestations in carriers of antithrombin, protein C, protein S deficiency, or activated protein C resistance: a multicenter collaborative family study. Arterioscler Thromb Vasc Biol 1999;19(4):1026–33.
36. Dahlback B, Hildebrand B. Inherited resistance to activated protein C is corrected by anticoagulant cofactor activity found to be a property of factor V. Proc Natl Acad Sci U S A 1994;91(4):1396–400.
37. Hertzberg MS. Genetic testing for thrombophilia mutations. Semin Thromb Hemost 2005;31(1):33–8.
38. Poort SR, Rosendaal FR, Reitsma PH, et al. A common genetic variation in the 3'-untranslated region of the prothrombin gene is associated with elevated plasma prothrombin levels and an increase in venous thrombosis. Blood 1996;88(10):3698– 703.
39. Wolberg AS, Monroe DM, Roberts HR, et al. Elevated prothrombin results in clots with an altered fiber structure: a possible mechanism of the increased thrombotic risk. Blood 2003;101(8):3008–13.
40. Kyrle PA, Mannhalter C, Beguin S, et al. Clinical studies and thrombin generation in patients homozygous or heterozygous for the G20210A mutation in the prothrombin gene. Arterioscler Thromb Vasc Biol 1998;18(8):1287–91.
41. Smirnov MD, Safa O, Esmon NL, et al. Inhibition of activated protein C anticoagulant activity by prothrombin. Blood 1999;94(11):3839–46.
42. Bauer K. Hypercoagulable states. In: Hoffman R, Benz EJ Jr, Shattil SJ, et al. editors. Hematology, basic principles and practice. 4th edition. Philadelphia (PA): Elsevier Churchill Livingstone; 2005. p. 2197–224.
43. Zawadzki C, Gaveriaux V, Trillot N, et al. Homozygous G20210A transition in the prothrombin gene associated with severe venous thrombotic disease: two cases in a French family. Thromb Haemost 1998;80(6):1027–8.

44. Kosch A, Junker R, Wermes C, et al. Recurrent pulmonary embolism in a 13-year-old homozygous for the prothrombin G20210A mutation combined with protein S deficiency and increased lipoprotein (a). Thromb Res 2002;105(1): 49–53.
45. Kraaijenhagen RA, in't Anker PS, Koopman MM, et al. High plasma concentration of factor VIIIc is a major risk factor for venous thromboembolism. Thromb Haemost 2000;83(1):5–9.
46. Meijers JC, Tekelenburg WL, Bouma BN, et al. High levels of coagulation factor XI as a risk factor for venous thrombosis. N Engl J Med 2000;342(10):696–701.
47. van Hylckama Vlieg A, van der Linden IK, Bertina RM, et al. High levels of factor IX increase the risk of venous thrombosis. Blood 2000;95(12):3678–82.
48. Lim W, Crowther MA, Eikelboom JW. Management of antiphospholipid antibody syndrome. JAMA 2006;295(9):1050–7.
49. Rai RS, Clifford K, Cohe H, et al. High prospective fetal loss rate in untreated pregnancies of women with recurrent miscarriage and antiphospholipid antibodies. Humanit Rep 1995;10(12):3301–4.
50. Brandt JT, Barna LK, Triplett DA. Laboratory identification of lupus anticoagulants: results of the Second International Workshop for Identification of Lupus Anticoagulants. Thromb Haemost 1995;74(6):1597–603.
51. Harris EN, Gharavi AE, Boey ML, et al. Anticardiolipin antibodies: detection by radioimmunoassay and association with thrombosis in systemic lupus erythematosus. Lancet 1983;2(8361):1211–4.
52. Long A, Ginsberg JS, Brill-Edwards P. The relationship of antiphospholipid antibodies to thromboembolic disease in systemic lupus erythematosus: a cross-sectional study. Thromb Haemost 1991;66(5):520–4.
53. Brey RL, Chapman J, Levine SR. Stroke and the antiphospholipid syndrome: consensus meeting Taormina 2002. Lupus 2003;12(7):508–13.
54. Brey RL, Escalante A. Neurological manifestations of antiphospholipid antibody syndrome. Lupus 1998;7(Suppl 2):S67–74.
55. Carhuapoma JR, Mitsias P, Levine SR. Cerebral venous thrombosis and anticardiolipin antibodies. Stroke 1997;28(12):2363–9.
56. Warkentin TE. Heparin-induced thrombocytopenia. In: Colman RW, Marder VJ, Clowes AW, et al. editors. Hemostasis and thrombosis basic principles and clinical practice. 5th edition. Philadelphia: Lippincott, Williams and Wilkins; 2006. p. 1649–61.
57. Warkentin TE. Heparin-induced thrombocytopenia: pathogenesis and management. Br J Haematol 2003;121(4):535–55.
58. Warkentin TE, Kelton JG. Delayed-onset heparin-induced thrombocytopenia and thrombosis. Ann Intern Med 2001;135(7):502–6.
59. Warkentin TE, Roberts RS, Hirsh J. An improved definition of immune heparin-induced thrombocytopenia in postoperative orthopedic patients. Arch Intern Med 2003;163(20):2518–24.
60. Lee DH, Warkentin TE. Frequency of heparin-induced thrombocytopenia. In: Warkentin TE, Greinacher A, editors. Heparin induced thrombocytopenia. 3rd edition. New York: Marcel Dekker Inc; 2004. p. 107–48.
61. Sheridan D, Carter C, Kelton JG. A diagnostic test for heparin-induced thrombocytopenia. Blood 1986;67(1):27–30.
62. Greinacher A, Amiral J, Dummel V, et al. Laboratory diagnosis of heparin-associated thrombocytopenia and comparison of platelet aggregation test, heparin-induced platelet activation test, and platelet factor 4/heparin enzyme-linked immunosorbent assay. Transfusion 1994;34(5):381–5.

63. Lee AY, Levine MN. Venous thromboembolism and cancer: risks and outcomes. Circulation 2003;107(23 Suppl 1):I17–121.

64. Lee AY. Management of thrombosis in cancer: primary prevention and secondary prophylaxis. Br J Haematol 2006;128:291–302.

65. Ruf W. Molecular regulation of blood clotting in tumor biology. Haemostasis 2001; 31(Suppl 1):5–7.

66. Gale AJ, Gordon SG. Update on tumor cell procoagulant factors. Acta Haematol 2001;106(1–2):25–32.

67. Bertomeu MC, Gallo S, Lauri D, et al. Chemotherapy enhances endothelial cell reactivity to platelets. Clin Exp Metastasis 1990;8(6):511–8.

68. Pritchard KI, Paterson AH, Paul NA, et al. Increased thromboembolic complications with concurrent tamoxifen and chemotherapy in a randomized trial of adjuvant therapy for women with breast cancer. J Clin Oncol 1996;14(10):2731–7.

69. Levine MN, Lee AY, Kakkar AK. Cancer and thrombosis. In: Colman RW, Marder VJ, Clowes AW, et al, editors. Hemostasis and thrombosis. basic principles and clinical practice. 5th edition. Philadelphia: Lippincott, Williams and Wilkins; 2006. p. 1251–62.

70. Greer IA. Thrombosis in pregnancy: maternal and fetal issues. Lancet 1999; 353(9160):1258–65.

71. McColl MD, Ramsay JE, Tait RC, et al. Risk factors for pregnancy associated venous thromboembolism. Thromb Haemost 1997;78(4):1183–8.

72. Cockett FB, Thomas ML. The iliac compression syndrome. Br J Surg 1965;52(10): 816–21.

73. Ginsberg JS, Brill-Edwards P, Burrows RF, et al. Venous thrombosis during pregnancy: leg and trimester of presentation. Thromb Haemost 1992;67(5):519–20.

74. Clark P. Changes of hemostasis variables during pregnancy. Semin Vasc Med 2003;3(1):13–24.

75. Bremme K. Haemostatic changes in pregnancy. Best Pract Res Clin Haematol 2003;16(2):153–68.

76. Comp P, Thurnau GR, Welsh J, et al. Functional and immunologic protein S levels are decreased during pregnancy. Blood 1986;68(4):881–5.

77. Clark P, Brennand J, Conkie JA, et al. Activated protein C sensitivity, protein C, protein S and coagulation in normal pregnancy. Thromb Haemost 1998;79(6): 1166–70.

78. Stirling Y, Woolf L, North WR, et al. Haemostasis in normal pregnancy. Thromb Haemost 1984;52:176–82.

79. Eichinger S, Weltermann A, Philipp K, et al. Prospective evaluation of hemostatic system activation and thrombin potential in healthy pregnant women with and without factor V Leiden. Thromb Haemost 1999;82(4):1232–6.

80. Martinelli I, Legnani C, Bucciarelli P. Risk of pregnancy-related venous thrombosis in carriers of severe inherited thrombophilia. Thromb Haemost 2001;86(3):800–3.

81. Greer IA. Inherited thrombophilia and venous thromboembolism. Best Pract Res Clin Obstet Gynaecol 2003;17(3):413–25.

82. Gerhardt A, Scharf R, Beckmann M, et al. Prothrombin and factor V mutations in women with a history of thrombosis during pregnancy and the puerperium. N Engl J Med 2000;342(6):374–80.

83. Friederich PW, Sanson BJ, Simioni P, et al. Frequency of pregnancy-related venous thromboembolism in anticoagulant factor-deficient women: implications for prophylaxis. Ann Intern Med 1996;125(12):955–60.

84. Bates SM, Greer IA, Hirsh J, et al. Use of antithrombotic agents during pregnancy: the Seventh ACCP Conference on antithrombotic and thrombolytic therapy. Chest 2006;126(Suppl 3):627S.
85. Vandenbroucke JP, Rosing J, Bloemenkamp KW, et al. Oral contraceptives and the risk of venous thrombosis. N Engl J Med 2001;344(20):1527–35.
86. Daly E, Vessey MP, Hawkins MM, et al. Risk of venous thromboembolism in users of hormone replacement therapy. Lancet 1996;348(9033):977–80.
87. Martinelli I. Risk factors in venous thromboembolism. Thromb Haemost 2001;86(1): 395–403.
88. Rosendaal FR. Oral contraceptives and screening for factor V Leiden. Thromb Haemost 1996;75(3):524–5.
89. Prandoni P, Lensing AW, Cogo A, et al. The long-term clinical course of acute deep venous thrombosis. Ann Intern Med 1996;125(1):1–7.
90. Heit JA, Silverstein MD, Mohr DN, et al. Risk factors for deep vein thrombosis and pulmonary embolism: a population-based case-control study. Arch Intern Med 2000;160(6):809–15.
91. Kearon C, Gent M, Hirsh J, et al. A comparison of three months of anticoagulation with extended anticoagulation for a first episode of idiopathic venous thromboembolism. N Engl J Med 1999;340(12):901–7.
92. Cattaneo M. Hyperhomocysteinemia, atherosclerosis and thrombosis. Thromb Haemost 1999;81(2):165–76.
93. Ray J. Meta-analysis of hyperhomocysteinemia as a risk factor for venous thromboembolic disease. Arch Intern Med 1998;158(19):2101–6.
94. Finkelstein JD. Methionine metabolism in mammals. J Nutr Biochem 1990;1(5): 228–37.
95. Kluijtmans LA, van den Huevel LP, Boers GH, et al. Molecular genetic analysis in mild hyperhomocysteinemia: a common mutation in the methylenetetrahydrofolate reductase gene is a genetic risk factor for cardiovascular disease. Am J Hum Genet 1996;58(1):35–41.
96. Jacques PF, Selhub J, Bostom AG, et al. The effect of folic acid fortification on plasma folate and total homocysteine concentrations. N Engl J Med 1999;340(19): 1449–54.
97. Molloy AM, Scott JM. Folates and prevention of disease. Public Health Nutr 2001; 4(2B):601–9.
98. Homocysteine Lowering Trialists' Collaboration. Lowering blood homocysteine with folic acid based supplements: meta-analysis of randomised trials. BMJ 1998;316: 894–8.
99. Lonn E, Yusuf S, Arnold MJ, et al. Homocysteine lowering with folic acid and B vitamins in vascular disease. N Engl J Med 2006;354(15):1567–77.
100. Dreyfus M, Magny JF, Bridey F, et al. Treatment of homozygous protein C deficiency and neonatal purpura fulminans with a purified protein C concentrate. N Engl J Med 1991;325(22):1565–8.
101. Monagle P, Chan A, Massicotte P, et al. Antithrombotic therapy in children: the Seventh ACCP Conference on Antithrombotic and Thrombolytic Therapy. Chest 2004;126(3):645–87.
102. Lechner K, Kyrle P. Antithrombin III concentrates—are they clinically useful?. Thromb Haemost 1995;73(3):340–8.
103. Crowther MA, Ginsberg JS, Julian J, et al. A comparison of two intensities of warfarin for the prevention of recurrent thrombosis in patients with the antiphospholipid antibody syndrome. N Engl J Med 2003;349(7):631–9.

104. Finazzi G, Marchioli R, Brancaccio V. A randomised clinical trial of high-intensity warfarin versus conventional antithrombotic therapy for the prevention of recurrent thrombosis in patients with the antiphospholipid antibody syndrome. J Thromb Haemost 2005;3(5):848–53.

105. Lee AYY, Levine MN, Baker RI, et al. Low-molecular-weight heparin versus a coumarin for the prevention of recurrent venous thromboembolism in patients with cancer. N Engl J Med 2003;349(2):146–53.

106. Marchetti M, Pistorio A, Barone M, et al. Low-molecular-weight heparin versus warfarin for secondary prophylaxis of venous thromboembolism: a cost-effectiveness analysis. Am J Med 2001;111(2):130–9.

107. Levine MN, Hirsh J, Gent M, et al. Optimal duration of oral anticoagulant therapy: a randomized trial comparing four weeks with three months of warfarin in patients with proximal deep venous thrombosis. Thromb Haemost 1995;74(2):606–11.

108. Agnelli G, Prandoni P, Santamaria MG, et al. Three months versus one year of oral anticoagulant therapy for idiopathic deep vein thrombosis. N Engl J Med 2001; 345(3):165–9.

109. Buller HR, Agnelli G, Hull RD, et al. Antithrombotic therapy for venous thromboembolic disease: the Seventh ACCP Conference on Antithrombotic and Thrombolytic Therapy. Chest 2004;126(3):401S–28.

110. Ridker PM, Goldhaber SZ, Danielson E, et al. Long-term, low-intensity warfarin therapy for the prevention of recurrent venous thromboembolism. N Engl J Med 2003;348(15):1425–34.

111. Gallus AS. Management options for thrombophilias. Semin Thromb Hemost 2005; 31(1):118–26.

112. Mazzolai L, Hohlfeld P, Spertini F, et al. Fondaparinux is a safe alternative in case of heparin intolerance during pregnancy. Blood 2006;108(5):1569–70.

113. McKenna R, Cole ER, Vasan U. Is warfarin sodium contraindicated in lactating mothers?. J Pediatr 1983;103(2):325–7.

114. Brill-Edwards P, Ginsberg JA, Gent M, et al. Safety of withholding heparin in pregnant women with a history of venous thromboembolism. N Engl J Med 2000; 343(20):1439–44.

115. Greaves M, Baglin T. Laboratory testing for heritable thrombophilia; impact on clinical management of thrombotic disease. Br J Haematol 2000;109(4):699–703.

116. Mannucci PM. Genetic hypercoagulability: prevention suggests testing family members. Blood 2001;98(1):21–2.

117. Heron E, Lozinguez O, Alhenc-Gelas M, et al. Hypercoagulable states in primary upper-extremity deep vein thrombosis. Arch Intern Med 2000;160(3):382–6.

Mortality Risk Assessment and the Role of Thrombolysis in Pulmonary Embolism

Mareike Lankeit, MD[a], Stavros Konstantinides, MD[b],*

KEYWORDS
- Pulmonary embolism • Thrombolysis • Risk assessment
- Mortality risk

Acute venous thromboembolism remains a frequent disease, with an incidence that ranges between 23 and 69 cases per 100,000 population per year.[1,2] Of these patients, approximately one-third present with clinical symptoms of acute pulmonary embolism (PE) and two-thirds with deep venous thrombosis (DVT).[3] Unfortunately, morbidity and mortality associated with acute PE remain high despite the recent advances in noninvasive imaging modalities, notably computed tomographic pulmonary angiography, and of the highly effective therapeutic options currently available. Case fatality rates vary widely depending on the clinical severity of the thromboembolic episode,[4–7] but large recent registries and cohort studies suggest that approximately 10% of all patients with acute PE die during the first 1 to 3 months after diagnosis.[8,9] In the United States, venous thromboembolism may contribute to as many as 100,000 deaths each year.[10] Overall, 1% of all patients admitted to hospitals die of acute PE, and 10% of all hospital deaths are PE-related.[11–13] These facts emphasize the need to better implement our knowledge on the pathophysiology of the disease, recognize the determinants of death or major adverse events in the early phase of acute PE, and most importantly, identify those patients who necessitate prompt medical, surgical, or interventional treatment to restore the patency of the pulmonary vasculature.

DEFINING HIGH-RISK PE

Acute PE is not universally life threatening, but rather covers a wide spectrum of clinical severity and death risk. In various studies, early (30-day or in-hospital)

A version of this article originally appeared in *Clinics in Chest Medicine*, 31:4.
[a] Department of Cardiology and Pulmonology, Georg August University of Göttingen, Germany
[b] Department of Cardiology, Democritus University of Thrace, University General Hospital, 68100 Alexandroupolis, Greece
* Corresponding author.
E-mail address: skonst@med.duth.gr

mortality rates were reported to range between less than 1% and well over 50%, mostly depending on the baseline clinical profile of the patients studied.[4–9,14]

It is now well established that the principal pathophysiological factor that determines disease severity and consequently the patients' clinical course and risk of death over the short term is the presence or absence of right ventricular (RV) dysfunction and failure resulting from acute pressure overload.[15] Almost 4 decades ago, it was found that increased pulmonary artery pressure may develop in up to 60% to 70% of patients who suffer acute PE, particularly when the emboli obstruct more than one-third of the area of the pulmonary vasculature. It has repeatedly been emphasized, however, that the magnitude of pulmonary artery hypertension and, as a result, the extent of RV pressure overload, is only roughly (and unreliably) related to thrombus burden and the severity of anatomic obstruction.[16–18] This complexity is due to the involvement of numerous pathophysiological variables, which include platelet activation, pulmonary vasoconstriction, and sympathetic (inotropic) stimulation of the heart. Once the patient develops RV pressure overload, persistent myocardial ischemia (even in the absence of maintained coronary flow to the right ventricle), preexisting cardiovascular disease or other serious comorbidity, and the presence of a patent foramen ovale with right to left shunt and serious arterial hypoxemia, may further enhance the hemodynamic impact of the thromboembolic event.[19–23] The interplay of all these factors, each one of which, if present, may be more or less pronounced in the individual patient, determines the development and extent of acute RV dysfunction. This latter event may in turn initiate a vicious circle of increased myocardial oxygen demand, myocardial ischemia or even infarction, leftward septal displacement, and left ventricular preload reduction, which ultimately lead to cardiogenic shock and death.[15]

Based on these pathophysiological mechanisms and their impact on the patients' prognosis, it has been proposed that clinical assessment of PE severity should focus on PE-related early death risk rather than reflect the volume, shape, or distribution of intrapulmonary emboli as determined by various imaging modalities. Accordingly, the recently updated guidelines of the European Society of Cardiology have introduced the terms high-risk and non-high-risk (the latter including intermediate-risk and low-risk) PE in an attempt to replace potentially confusing definitions such as "massive," "nonmassive" or "submassive" PE, which may be used in a different sense among pathologists, radiologists, and clinicians caring for the patient.[24,25] According to this updated nomenclature, "clinically massive" high-risk PE indicates overt RV failure that results in refractory arterial hypotension and shock (ie, systolic blood pressure <90 mm Hg, or a pressure drop ≥40 mm Hg for at least 15 minutes). This condition accounts for almost 5% of all cases of acute PE and is associated with a high risk of in-hospital death, particularly during the first hours after admission.[5,26,27] On the other hand, in the absence of hemodynamic instability, patients are generally thought to have a favorable clinical outcome provided that the disease is diagnosed correctly and anticoagulation can be instituted without delay.[14,28]

RISK-ADJUSTED DIAGNOSTIC APPROACH TO PE

Numerous multistep algorithms have been proposed and prospectively validated for the diagnostic workup of normotensive patients with suspected PE. Recent algorithms are based on the superior diagnostic sensitivity and specificity of multidetector-row computed tomography (MDCT)/pulmonary angiography, and its ability to confirm and in particular safely exclude PE without the need for venous ultrasound as an intermediate step.[25,29–31] On the other hand, management of the hemodynamically unstable, hypotensive patient with suspected high-risk PE should, as in all emergency situations, direct the focus not on perfect diagnostic accuracy but rather on immediate availability of the diagnostic modality, and on whether it offers the ability to begin life-saving treatment as rapidly as possible. The latter treatment consists of recanalization of the pulmonary vasculature with thrombolytic agents or surgery/intervention to reverse RV pressure overload and failure. Clinical probability is usually high in this setting, and there is no rationale for performing a time-consuming D-dimer test in such a life-threatening situation. Thus, according to the algorithm proposed in recent guidelines,[25] if MDCT pulmonary angiography is not readily available or the transfer to the Radiology Department is deemed unsafe for the unstable patient, a bedside echocardiogram is the quickest and thus most appropriate imaging test for confirming the presence of acute RV failure. Additional information that can be obtained from ultrasound imaging includes the presence of large floating intracardiac thrombi, which indicate an imminent threat of recurrent, potentially fatal PE.[32] Finally, if RV dysfunction can be excluded, echocardiography may provide alternative explanations for the patient's hypotension and shock such as left ventricular failure due to cardiomyopathy or large myocardial infarction, critical valvular disease, pericardial tamponade, or aortic dissection. In mechanically ventilated patients, transesophageal echocardiography is a useful alternative to transthoracic imaging, permitting direct visualization of possible thrombi in the right atrium, foramen ovale, right ventricle, or the proximal segments of the common and right pulmonary artery.

Conventional pulmonary angiography is rarely necessary in acute high-risk PE. However, it may be a valuable diagnostic option in selected cases, particularly when the patient is already in the catheterization laboratory due, for example, to suspected myocardial infarction, or if catheter-based aspiration or fragmentation of the pulmonary thrombus is being considered.[33,34]

BENEFITS OF THROMBOLYSIS IN ACUTE PE

In view of the high early mortality and complication risk associated with high-risk PE,[5,26,27] existing guidelines[25,35] and the overwhelming majority of experts and clinicians agree that patients who present with persistent arterial hypotension or shock are in need of immediate pharmacologic or mechanical recanalization of the occluded pulmonary arteries.

In early reports dating back to 1971, streptokinase infusion over 72 hours resulted in a significant reduction of systolic pulmonary artery pressure, total pulmonary resistance, and the angiographic index of PE severity; in comparison, conventional heparin anticoagulation appeared to have no appreciable effect on these parameters during the first 3 days.[36] Subsequently, several randomized trials[37–44] published between 1973 and 1993 showed that thrombolytic therapy with urokinase, streptokinase, or alteplase was capable of reducing thromboembolic obstruction, as assessed by pulmonary angiography, more rapidly than endogenous thrombolysis aided by heparin anticoagulation. The short-term benefits of thrombolytic agents also extended to hemodynamic parameters and the improvement of RV function as determined by right heart catheterization or echocardiography. On the other hand, these trials were unable to show that thrombolysis may also improve the short- or long-term clinical outcome of patients with acute PE. Although this may partly be due to the small size of most of them,[38–43] the explanation probably lies in that they did not focus on patients at high risk of early PE-related death as possible candidates for thrombolytic treatment. In this regard, the hemodynamic benefits of thrombolysis over heparin alone are confined to the first few days after acute PE, and studies performed in the late 1960s indicated that endogenous thrombolysis supported by heparin anticoagulation was (also) capable of reversing pulmonary artery hypertension within a 3-week (or longer) period in most cases.[45] More recently, trials directly comparing thrombolysis with heparin and including follow-up angiographic or echocardiographic studies showed that 1 week after treatment, the improvement in the severity of vascular obstruction[37,43] and the reversal of RV dysfunction[46] no longer differed between thrombolysis-treated and heparin-treated patients. Thus, it is important to consider thrombolysis only in those cases in which a high probability of early (ie, within the first few hours or days after presentation) PE-related death is anticipated.

POTENTIAL RISKS OF THROMBOLYSIS

Pooled data from controlled thrombolysis trials in PE, which either compared thrombolysis with heparin alone or different thrombolytic regimens with each other,[37,41,43,47–54] revealed a 13% cumulative rate of major bleeding and a 1.8% rate of intracranial/fatal hemorrhage.[55] Major hemorrhage has been less common in the most recent (and largest) trials,[44,47] in agreement with the notion that thrombolysis-related bleeding rates may be lower when noninvasive imaging methods are used to diagnose PE. Noninvasive diagnostic strategies have increasingly been adopted over the past 10 years thanks to the technical advances in computed tomographic (CT) pulmonary angiography.[24] On the other hand, retrospective cohort studies and registries have suggested a 36% incidence of major bleeding events and a 4% rate of intracranial/fatal hemorrhage following thrombolysis for PE.[4,5,56,57] These rates may be inappropriately high, because registries are likely to include patients who have received thrombolysis despite the presence of formal contraindications.[5] At the same time, however, registry data may better reflect everyday clinical practice compared with controlled trials. In any case, all the results presented here highlight the importance of carefully selecting the candidates for thrombolysis in acute PE, being particularly cautious in those who appear hemodynamically stable at presentation.

CURRENT USE OF THROMBOLYSIS IN ACUTE PE WITH HIGH RISK FOR EARLY DEATH

Although the angiographic and hemodynamic benefits of thrombolysis are unequivocal, at least over the short term, the (presumed) favorable effects of thrombolysis on the clinical outcome of patients with PE have thus far not been convincingly demonstrated. As already mentioned, this partly relies on the fact that the majority of thrombolysis trials in PE were too small to address clinical end points. Even the most recent and largest of these trials failed to show a survival benefit,[44,47] possibly because they included "low-risk" patients whose mortality rate in the acute phase could not be further reduced by immediate recanalization.

Pooled data from 5 trials that included hemodynamically unstable patients have suggested a significant reduction of death or PE recurrence after thrombolysis in this group (from 19.0% to 9.4%; odds ratio [OR], 0.45; 95% confidence interval [CI], 0.22–0.92).[58] In this regard, hemodynamic instability is commonly defined as need for cardiopulmonary resuscitation, systolic blood pressure <90 mm Hg or a drop of systolic blood pressure by ≥40 mm Hg for ≥15 minutes with signs of end-organ hypoperfusion, or need for catecholamine infusion to maintain adequate organ perfusion and a systolic blood pressure ≥90 mm Hg. If PE is clinically suspected, such patients should immediately receive a weight-adjusted bolus of unfractionated heparin while awaiting the results of further diagnostic workup; as soon as PE is confirmed, thrombolysis should be administered without delay. As many as 92% of these patients may respond favorably to thrombolysis, judging by their clinical and echocardiographic improvement within the first 36 hours.[59] The greatest benefit is observed when treatment is initiated within 48 hours of symptom onset,[39] but thrombolysis can still be beneficial to patients who have had symptoms for as long as 6 to 14 days.[60] If thrombolysis is absolutely contraindicated or has failed, surgical embolectomy or catheter-based thrombus fragmentation and aspiration is a valuable alternative.[33,34] Thrombolysis may also be considered in patients with PE and free-floating thrombi in the right heart if the risk of open heart surgery is deemed extremely high.[61,62]

Validated and tested regimens of thrombolytic agents are shown in **Table 1**, which also reviews the absolute and relative contraindications to thrombolysis. Regarding the performance of various thrombolytic regimens in head-to-head comparisons, the Urokinase-Streptokinase Pulmonary Embolism Trial (USPET) documented similar

Table 1
Thrombolytic agents, regimens, and contraindications

Agent	Regimen	Contraindications to Thrombolysis[25]
Streptokinase[a]	250,000 U as a loading dose over 30 min, followed by 100,000 U per hour over 12–24 h	*Absolute* History of hemorrhagic stroke or stroke of unknown origin Ischemic stroke in previous 6 months Central nervous system neoplasms Major trauma, surgery, or head injury in previous 3 weeks
	Accelerated regimen: 1.5 million IU over 2 h[b]	
Urokinase[a,c]	4400 U/kg body weight as a loading dose over 10 min, followed by 4400 U/kg/h over 12–24 h	*Relative* Transient ischemic attack in previous 6 months Oral anticoagulation
	Accelerated regimen: 3 million U over 2 h[b]	Pregnancy or first postpartum week Noncompressible puncture sites
Alteplase[a]	100 mg over 2 h[d]	Traumatic resuscitation Refractory hypertension (systolic blood pressure >180 mm Hg)
	Accelerated regimen: 0.6 mg/kg over 15 min	Advanced liver disease Infective endocarditis Active peptic ulcer
Reteplase[a,e]	Two bolus injections of 10 U 30 min apart	
Tenecteplase[f]	30–50 mg bolus over 5–10 s adjusted for body weight:	
	<60 kg: 30 mg	
	≥60 to <70 kg: 35 mg	
	≥70 to <80 kg: 40 mg	
	≥80 to <90 kg: 45 mg	
	≥90 kg: 50 mg	

[a] Unfractionated heparin should not be infused together with streptokinase or urokinase; it can be given during alteplase or reteplase administration. Low molecular weight heparins have not been tested in combination with thrombolysis in patients with pulmonary embolism.
[b] Short (2-hour) infusion periods are generally recommended.
[c] Urokinase is available in some European countries, not in the United States.
[d] Food and Drug Administration–approved regimen.
[e] Off-label use of reteplase.
[f] Off-label use of tenecteplase; this is the regimen recommended for acute myocardial infarction. A recent randomized pilot trial[67] found it to be safe and effective in nonhigh-risk PE.

Adapted from Konstantinides S. Clinical practice. Acute pulmonary embolism. N Engl J Med 2008;359(26):2804–13; with permission.

efficacy of urokinase (UK) and streptokinase (SK) infused over a period of 12 to 24 hours.[54] In more recent randomized comparison trials,[51,52] 100 mg of recombinant tissue plasminogen activator (rtPA) infused over 2 hours led to faster angiographic and hemodynamic improvement compared with UK infused over 12 or 24 hours at the rate of 4400 U/kg/h. However, the results no longer differed at the end of the UK infusion. Similarly, the 2-hour infusion of rtPA appeared to be superior to a 12-hour SK infusion (at 100,000 U/h), but no difference was observed when the same SK dosage was also given over 2 hours.[63,64] Furthermore, 2 trials that compared the 2-hour, 100-mg rtPA regimen with a short infusion (over 15 minutes) of 0.6 mg/kg rtPA reported a slightly faster improvement with the 2-hour regimen at the cost of slightly (nonsignificantly) higher bleeding rates.[49,65] Thus, the thrombolytic regimens tested to date appear to be more or less comparable in terms of efficacy, but long infusions periods of the older thrombolytics SK or UK should generally be avoided.

Satisfactory hemodynamic results have also been obtained with double-bolus reteplase given as 2 injections (10 U) 30 minutes apart.[66] Furthermore, a multicenter randomized pilot trial demonstrated the feasibility and safety of tenecteplase, given as a weight-adjusted bolus corresponding to the regimen recommended for acute myocardial infarction, in acute nonhigh-risk PE.[67] However, neither reteplase nor tenecteplase are officially approved for treatment of PE at present.

POTENTIAL ROLE OF THROMBOLYSIS IN INTERMEDIATE-RISK (SUBMASSIVE) PE

At present, low molecular weight heparin or fondaparinux is considered adequate treatment for most normotensive patients with pulmonary embolism, whereas routine thrombolysis is generally not recommended as a first-line therapeutic option.[25,35] However, the results of the most recent randomized thrombolysis trial[47] can be interpreted as indicating that early thrombolysis may be considered in selected patients with "nonmassive," non-high-risk PE including, for example, those with comorbidities predisposing to an adverse outcome provided that these patients have no contraindications to thrombolytic treatment.

Who might then be a candidate for thrombolysis besides patients with high-risk PE? As already emphasized, RV dysfunction and failure is a crucial pathophysiological event and the main determinant of prognosis in acute PE (**Fig. 1**). Therefore, its early detection and reversal before the patient develops hemodynamic instability and shock should have high priority in the management of the disease. Based on this concept, currently available tools and emerging strategies for identifying normotensive intermediate-risk patients with RV dysfunction and/or myocardial injury are discussed below. These tools might extend the indications for thrombolysis in acute PE in the future.

Diagnosis of RV Dysfunction in Normotensive Patients

Echocardiography is an imaging modality capable of detecting the changes occurring in the morphology and function of the right ventricle as a result of acute pressure overload. Several registries and cohort studies were able to demonstrate an association between various echocardiographic parameters and a poor in-hospital outcome in terms of PE-related death and complications.[14,28,44,68,69] The post hoc analysis of a large international registry further suggested that echocardiographically detected RV dysfunction is an independent predictor of adverse outcome in normotensive patients.[70] Nevertheless, the potential prognostic and, particularly, therapeutic implications of cardiac ultrasound findings for non-high-risk PE remain the subject of debate. The persisting uncertainty is mainly due to the lack of standardization of the echocardiographic criteria and the absence of adequately powered, controlled

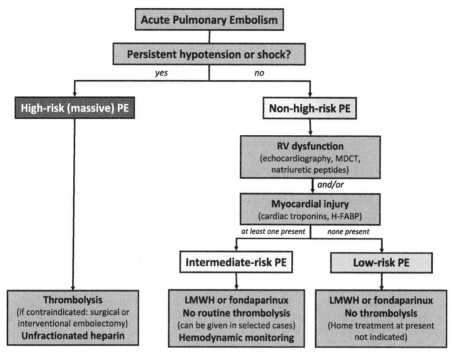

Fig. 1. Proposed risk-adjusted management algorithm for acute pulmonary embolism. H-FABP, heart-type fatty acid-binding protein; LMWH, low molecular weight heparin or fondaparinux; MDCT, multidetector-row computed tomography (pulmonary angiography); PE, pulmonary embolism; RV, right ventricle; UFH, unfractionated heparin.

studies focusing on normotensive (rather than unselected) patients with PE.[71] Accordingly, a recent meta-analysis of 5 studies including a total of 475 normotensive patients with PE reported an only moderate overall negative (60%; 95% CI, 55%–65%) and positive (58%; 95% CI, 53%–63%) value of echocardiography for predicting early death, while also emphasizing the limitations due to the clinical and methodological diversity of the pooled publications.[72] The largest randomized thrombolysis trial in PE to date, which included 256 normotensive patients with RV dysfunction (mainly) detected by echocardiography, reported a significantly reduced incidence of the primary end point (30-day mortality or need for treatment escalation) in patients who underwent early thrombolysis as opposed to those treated with heparin alone. However, there was no significant influence of the type of treatment on mortality rates during the acute phase of PE.[47] It is thus likely that additional information beyond echocardiographic findings may be needed before the decision can be made to treat aggressively (with thrombolytic agents) a normotensive patient with acute PE. Recent preliminary reports suggest that the prognostic value of echocardiography can be improved if combined with biomarkers of myocardial injury.[73–75]

Four-chamber views of the heart on MDCT, which is currently the preferred method for diagnosing PE in most institutions, may detect RV enlargement due to PE. In a large retrospective series of 431 patients, 30-day mortality was 15.6% in patients with RV enlargement (reconstructed 4-chamber views), defined as right/left ventricular dimension ratio >0.9, on MDCT, compared with 7.7% in those without this finding.[76] A meta-analysis of 2 studies (with 2 different right/left ventricular diameter thresholds, 1.5 and 1.0) including a total of 191 normotensive patients with PE reported an overall 58% (95% CI, 51%–65%) negative predictive value and a 57% (95% CI, 49%–64%) positive predictive value of RV dilatation on CT for identifying early PE deaths.[72] Of course, these rates strongly depend on the characteristics of the populations studied, and a prospective evaluation of the prognostic value of CT indicators of RV dysfunction is still missing.

Natriuretic peptides are released as a result of cardiomyocyte stretch and are very sensitive indicators of neurohormonal activation due to ventricular dysfunction. The biologically active C-terminal peptide 77-108 (BNP) and the inactive N-terminal fragment 1-76 (NT-proBNP) are detectable in human plasma, and their levels have been determined and evaluated in patients presenting with acute PE.[77–80] In general, both BNP and NT-proBNP are characterized by very high prognostic sensitivity and a negative prognostic value, which is probably even higher than that of the cardiac troponins.[81] On the other hand, they exhibit a very low specificity and positive prognostic value in the range of 12% to 25%.[81] Furthermore, the optimal cut-off levels of BNP (or NT-proBNP) for distinguishing between a prognostically "favorable" versus "unfavorable" result in patients with PE have not yet been prospectively determined.[82] A recent meta-analysis of 13 studies found that 51% of the 1132 patients included had elevated BNP or NT-proBNP levels, and these were associated with an increased risk of early death (OR, 7.6; 95% CI, 3.4–17) and a complicated in-hospital course (OR, 6.8; 95% CI, 4.4–10).[83] Nevertheless, elevation of natriuretic peptides alone does not, by itself, justify more invasive treatment regimens. Evolving concepts of risk stratification suggest that the prognostic value of natriuretic peptides may be improved if they are combined with echocardiography,[73] or integrated into risk scores that also include clinical parameters and echocardiography.[84]

Biomarkers for Detecting Myocardial Injury

Elevated cardiac troponin I or T levels, a sensitive and specific indicator of myocardial cell damage and microscopic myocardial necrosis, are found in up to 50% of patients with acute PE.[85] Twenty studies published since 1998 with a total of 1985 patients were included in a meta-analysis, which showed that cardiac troponin elevation was associated with an increased risk of death (OR, 5.24; 95% CI, 3.28–8.38) and major adverse events (OR, 7.03; 95% CI, 2.42–20.43) in the acute phase.[86] However, the positive predictive value of cardiac troponin I or T elevation has been consistently low in cohort studies, so that troponin elevation does not necessarily indicate a poor prognosis.[81] Moreover, a recent meta-analysis that focused only on normotensive patients (a total of 1366 patients included in 9 studies) was unable to confirm the prognostic value of cardiac troponins in non-high-risk PE.[87] Thus, based on the available data, the current opinion is that troponin elevation alone does not suffice to risk-stratify normotensive patients with PE, and particularly to identify intermediate-risk patients who might necessitate early aggressive (for example, thrombolytic) treatment. A large ongoing randomized trial is currently investigating whether normotensive patients with RV dysfunction, detected by echocardiography or CT, plus evidence of myocardial injury indicated by a positive troponin test, may benefit from early thrombolytic treatment.[88]

Fatty acid–binding proteins (FABPs) are small cytoplasmic proteins that are abundant in tissues with active fatty acid metabolism, including the heart.[89] Heart-type FABP (H-FABP) is particularly important for myocardial homoeostasis, because 50% to 80% of the heart's energy is provided by lipid oxidation, and H-FABP ensures intracellular transport of insoluble fatty acids. Following myocardial cell damage, this small protein diffuses much more rapidly than troponins through the interstitial space and appears in the circulation as early as 90 minutes after symptom onset, reaching its peak within 6 hours.[90] These features make H-FABP an excellent candidate marker of myocardial injury,[91] and preliminary data suggested that it may provide prognostic information superior to that of cardiac troponins in acute PE.[92,93] These data were recently confirmed by a study focusing on nonhigh-risk patients with acute PE.[94]

Growth-differentiation factor 15 (GDF-15), a distant member of the transforming growth factor β cytokine family, is an emerging biomarker for patients with cardiovascular disease. In particular, GDF-15 appears capable of integrating information both on RV dysfunction and myocardial injury in patients with acute PE. In a cohort study of 123 consecutive patients with confirmed PE, elevated levels of GDF-15 on admission were strongly and independently related with an increased risk of death or major complications during the first 30 days after diagnosis. Moreover, the prognostic information provided by GDF-15 appeared to be additive to that of cardiac troponins and natriuretic peptides, and to echocardiographic findings of RV dysfunction. GDF-15 also emerged as an independent predictor of long-term mortality.[95]

THROMBOLYSIS IN CURRENT AND EMERGING CONCEPTS OF PE MANAGEMENT

Experts and recently updated guidelines agree that thrombolysis is indicated patients with acute PE who are at high risk for early death, that is, in patients presenting with arterial hypotension and shock or refractory hypoxemia. On the other hand, heparin (unfractionated or low molecular weight) or fondaparinux is adequate treatment for most normotensive patients with PE (see **Fig. 1**). Recombinant tissue plasminogen activator (alteplase), given as a 100-mg infusion over 2 hours, is considered the treatment of choice for patients with PE, although regimens using urokinase or streptokinase were also shown to be efficacious in the past. Reteplase and tenecteplase, if eventually approved for PE, may turn out to be practical alternatives. However, beyond the relatively small population of PE patients at high risk for death (5% of all patients) as a target population for thrombolysis, there is increasing awareness of the need for risk stratification of normotensive patients and the search for an intermediate-risk group (previously defined as having "submassive" PE).[96] Recent meta-analyses of cohort studies suggest that imaging of the right ventricle or biomarkers of myocardial injury alone may be insufficient for guiding therapeutic decisions. Instead, accumulating evidence appears to support strategies that combine the information provided by an imaging procedure (RV dysfunction on echocardiography or CT) with a biomarker test (RV myocardial injury indicated by elevated troponin I or T, or possibly H-FABP, GDF-15). Accordingly, a large multinational randomized trial has set out to determine whether normotensive, intermediate-risk patients with RV dysfunction, detected by echocardiography or CT, plus evidence of myocardial injury indicated by a positive troponin test, may benefit from early thrombolytic treatment (EudraCT number, 2006-005,328-18).[88] The primary efficacy end point is a clinical composite end point of all-cause mortality or hemodynamic collapse within the first 7 days. Safety end points are total strokes (intracranial hemorrhage or ischemic stroke) within 7 days, and major bleeds (other than intracranial hemorrhage) within 7 days. Six-month follow-up is also being conducted. This study, which is already underway in 12 European countries, plans to enroll a total of 1000 patients and will be completed in 2011.

REFERENCES

1. Silverstein MD, Heit JA, Mohr DN, et al. Trends in the incidence of deep vein thrombosis and pulmonary embolism: a 25-year population-based study. Arch Intern Med 1998;158(6):585–93.
2. Anderson FA Jr, Wheeler HB, Goldberg RJ, et al. A population-based perspective of the hospital incidence and case-fatality rates of deep vein thrombosis and pulmonary embolism. The Worcester DVT Study. Arch Intern Med 1991;151(5):933–8.
3. White RH. The epidemiology of venous thromboembolism. Circulation 2003;107(23 Suppl. 1):I4–8.
4. Goldhaber SZ, Visani L, De Rosa M. Acute pulmonary embolism: clinical outcomes in the International Cooperative Pulmonary Embolism Registry (ICOPER). Lancet 1999; 353(9162):1386–9.
5. Kasper W, Konstantinides S, Geibel A, et al. Management strategies and determinants of outcome in acute major pulmonary embolism: results of a multicenter registry. J Am Coll Cardiol 1997;30(5):1165–71.
6. British Thoracic Society Optimum duration of anticoagulation for deep-vein thrombosis and pulmonary embolism. Research Committee of the British Thoracic Society. Lancet 1992;340(8824):873–6.
7. Carson JL, Kelley MA, Duff A, et al. The clinical course of pulmonary embolism. N Engl J Med 1992;326(19):1240–5.
8. Aujesky D, Jimenez D, Mor MK, et al. Weekend versus weekday admission and mortality after acute pulmonary embolism. Circulation 2009;119(7):962–8.
9. Laporte S, Mismetti P, Decousus H, et al. Clinical predictors for fatal pulmonary embolism in 15,520 patients with venous thromboembolism: findings from the Registro Informatizado de la Enfermedad TromboEmbolica venosa (RIETE) Registry. Circulation 2008;117(13):1711–6.
10. Internet Communication. Available at: http://www.surgeongeneral.gov/news/pressreleases/pr20080915.html. Accessed June 23, 2010.
11. Cohen AT, Agnelli G, Anderson FA, et al. Venous thromboembolism (VTE) in Europe. The number of VTE events and associated morbidity and mortality. Thromb Haemost 2007;98(4):756–64.
12. Cohen AT, Edmondson RA, Phillips MJ, et al. The changing pattern of venous thromboembolic disease. Haemostasis 1996;26(2):65–71.
13. Lindblad B, Sternby NH, Bergqvist D. Incidence of venous thromboembolism verified by necropsy over 30 years. BMJ 1991;302(6778):709–11.
14. Kasper W, Konstantinides S, Geibel A, et al. Prognostic significance of right ventricular afterload stress detected by echocardiography in patients with clinically suspected pulmonary embolism. Heart 1997;77(4):346–9.
15. Konstantinides S. Pulmonary embolism: impact of right ventricular dysfunction. Curr Opin Cardiol 2005;20(6):496–501.
16. Miller RL, Das S, Anandarangam T, et al. Association between right ventricular function and perfusion abnormalities in hemodynamically stable patients with acute pulmonary embolism. Chest 1998;113(3):665–70.
17. McIntyre KM, Sasahara AA. Determinants of right ventricular function and hemodynamics after pulmonary embolism. Chest 1974;65(5):534–43.
18. McIntyre KM, Sasahara AA. The hemodynamic response to pulmonary embolism in patients without prior cardiopulmonary disease. Am J Cardiol 1971;28(3):288–94.
19. Greyson C, Xu Y, Cohen J, et al. Right ventricular dysfunction persists following brief right ventricular pressure overload. Cardiovasc Res 1997;34(2):281–8.

20. Schmitto JD, Doerge H, Post H, et al. Progressive right ventricular failure is not explained by myocardial ischemia in a pig model of right ventricular pressure overload. Eur J Cardiothorac Surg 2009;35(2):229–34.

21. Chung T, Connor D, Joseph J, et al. Platelet activation in acute pulmonary embolism. J Thromb Haemost 2007;5(5):918–24.

22. Smulders YM. Pathophysiology and treatment of haemodynamic instability in acute pulmonary embolism: the pivotal role of pulmonary vasoconstriction. Cardiovasc Res 2000;48(1):23–33.

23. Konstantinides S, Geibel A, Kasper W, et al. Patent foramen ovale is an important predictor of adverse outcome in patients with major pulmonary embolism. Circulation 1998;97(19):1946–51.

24. Konstantinides S. Clinical practice. Acute pulmonary embolism. N Engl J Med 2008;359(26):2804–13.

25. Torbicki A, Perrier A, Konstantinides SV, et al. Guidelines on the diagnosis and management of acute pulmonary embolism: The Task Force for the Diagnosis and Management of Acute Pulmonary Embolism of the European Society of Cardiology (ESC). Eur Heart J 2008;29:2276–315.

26. Kucher N, Rossi E, De Rosa M, et al. Massive pulmonary embolism. Circulation 2006;113(4):577–82.

27. Stein PD, Henry JW. Prevalence of acute pulmonary embolism among patients in a general hospital and at autopsy. Chest 1995;108(4):978–81.

28. Grifoni S, Olivotto I, Cecchini P, et al. Short-term clinical outcome of patients with acute pulmonary embolism, normal blood pressure, and echocardiographic right ventricular dysfunction. Circulation 2000;101(24):2817–22.

29. Righini M, Le Gal G, Aujesky D, et al. Diagnosis of pulmonary embolism by multidetector CT alone or combined with venous ultrasonography of the leg: a randomised non-inferiority trial. Lancet 2008;371(9621):1343–52.

30. Stein PD, Fowler SE, Goodman LR, et al. Multidetector computed tomography for acute pulmonary embolism. N Engl J Med 2006;354(22):2317–27.

31. van Belle A, Buller HR, Huisman MV, et al. Effectiveness of managing suspected pulmonary embolism using an algorithm combining clinical probability, D-dimer testing, and computed tomography. JAMA 2006;295(2):172–9.

32. Torbicki A, Galie N, Covezzoli A, et al. Right heart thrombi in pulmonary embolism: results from the International Cooperative Pulmonary Embolism Registry. J Am Coll Cardiol 2003;41(12):2245–51.

33. Eid-Lidt G, Gaspar J, Sandoval J, et al. Combined clot fragmentation and aspiration in patients with acute pulmonary embolism. Chest 2008;134(1):54–60.

34. Kucher N, Goldhaber SZ. Mechanical catheter intervention in massive pulmonary embolism: proof of concept. Chest 2008;134(1):2–4.

35. Kearon C, Kahn SR, Agnelli G, et al. Antithrombotic therapy for venous thromboembolic disease: American College of Chest Physicians Evidence-Based Clinical Practice Guidelines (8th edition). Chest 2008;133(Suppl 6):454S–545.

36. Miller GA, Sutton GC, Kerr IH, et al. Comparison of streptokinase and heparin in treatment of isolated acute massive pulmonary embolism. Br Heart J 1971;33(4):616.

37. The urokinase pulmonary embolism trial. A national cooperative study. Circulation 1973;47(Suppl 2):II1–108.

38. Tibbutt DA, Davies JA, Anderson JA, et al. Comparison by controlled clinical trial of streptokinase and heparin in treatment of life-threatening pulmonary embolism. Br Med J 1974;1(904):343–7.

39. Ly B, Arnesen H, Eie H, et al. A controlled clinical trial of streptokinase and heparin in the treatment of major pulmonary embolism. Acta Med Scand 1978;203(6):465–70.

40. Marini C, Di Ricco G, Rossi G, et al. Fibrinolytic effects of urokinase and heparin in acute pulmonary embolism: a randomized clinical trial. Respiration 1988;54(3): 162–73.

41. Levine M, Hirsh J, Weitz J, et al. A randomized trial of a single bolus dosage regimen of recombinant tissue plasminogen activator in patients with acute pulmonary embolism. Chest 1990;98(6):1473–9.

42. Tissue plasminogen activator for the treatment of acute pulmonary embolism. A collaborative study by the PIOPED Investigators. Chest 1990;97(3):528–33.

43. Dalla-Volta S, Palla A, Santolicandro A, et al. PAIMS 2: alteplase combined with heparin versus heparin in the treatment of acute pulmonary embolism. Plasminogen activator Italian multicenter study 2. J Am Coll Cardiol 1992;20(3):520–6.

44. Goldhaber SZ, Haire WD, Feldstein ML, et al. Alteplase versus heparin in acute pulmonary embolism: randomised trial assessing right-ventricular function and pulmonary perfusion. Lancet 1993;341(8844):507–11.

45. Dalen JE, Banas JS Jr, Brooks HL, et al. Resolution rate of acute pulmonary embolism in man. N Engl J Med 1969;280(22):1194–9.

46. Konstantinides S, Tiede N, Geibel A, et al. Comparison of alteplase versus heparin for resolution of major pulmonary embolism. Am J Cardiol 1998;82(8):966–70.

47. Konstantinides S, Geibel A, Heusel G, et al. Heparin plus alteplase compared with heparin alone in patients with submassive pulmonary embolism. N Engl J Med 2002;347(15):1143–50.

48. Kanter DS, Mikkola KM, Patel SR, et al. Thrombolytic therapy for pulmonary embolism. Frequency of intracranial hemorrhage and associated risk factors. Chest 1997; 111(5):1241–5.

49. Sors H, Pacouret G, Azarian R, et al. Hemodynamic effects of bolus vs 2-h infusion of alteplase in acute massive pulmonary embolism. A randomized controlled multicenter trial. Chest 1994;106(3):712–7.

50. Goldhaber SZ, Kessler CM, Heit JA, et al. Recombinant tissue-type plasminogen activator versus a novel dosing regimen of urokinase in acute pulmonary embolism: a randomized controlled multicenter trial. J Am Coll Cardiol 1992;20(1):24–30.

51. Meyer G, Sors H, Charbonnier B, et al. Effects of intravenous urokinase versus alteplase on total pulmonary resistance in acute massive pulmonary embolism: a European multicenter double-blind trial. The European Cooperative Study Group for Pulmonary Embolism. J Am Coll Cardiol 1992;19(2):239–45.

52. Goldhaber SZ, Kessler CM, Heit J, et al. Randomised controlled trial of recombinant tissue plasminogen activator versus urokinase in the treatment of acute pulmonary embolism. Lancet 1988;2(8606):293–8.

53. Verstraete M, Miller GA, Bounameaux H, et al. Intravenous and intrapulmonary recombinant tissue-type plasminogen activator in the treatment of acute massive pulmonary embolism. Circulation 1988;77(2):353–60.

54. Urokinase-streptokinase embolism trial. Phase 2 results. A cooperative study. JAMA 1974;229(12):1606–13.

55. Konstantinides S, Marder VJ. Thrombolysis in venous thromboembolism. In: Colman RW, Marder VJ, Clowes AW, et al, editors. Hemostasis and thrombosis. Philadelphia: Lippincott Williams and Wilkins; 2006. p. 1317–29.

56. Hamel E, Pacouret G, Vincentelli D, et al. Thrombolysis or heparin therapy in massive pulmonary embolism with right ventricular dilation: results from a 128-patient monocenter registry. Chest 2001;120(1):120–5.

57. Meyer G, Gisselbrecht M, Diehl JL, et al. Incidence and predictors of major hemorrhagic complications from thrombolytic therapy in patients with massive pulmonary embolism. Am J Med 1998;105(6):472–7.

58. Wan S, Quinlan DJ, Agnelli G, et al. Thrombolysis compared with heparin for the initial treatment of pulmonary embolism: a meta-analysis of the randomized controlled trials. Circulation 2004;110(6):744–9.

59. Meneveau N, Seronde MF, Blonde MC, et al. Management of unsuccessful thrombolysis in acute massive pulmonary embolism. Chest 2006;129(4):1043–50.

60. Daniels LB, Parker JA, Patel SR, et al. Relation of duration of symptoms with response to thrombolytic therapy in pulmonary embolism. Am J Cardiol 1997;80(2):184–8.

61. Rose PS, Punjabi NM, Pearse DB. Treatment of right heart thromboemboli. Chest 2002;121(3):806–14.

62. Chartier L, Bera J, Delomez M, et al. Free-floating thrombi in the right heart: diagnosis, management, and prognostic indexes in 38 consecutive patients. Circulation 1999; 99(21):2779–83.

63. Meneveau N, Schiele F, Metz D, et al. Comparative efficacy of a two-hour regimen of streptokinase versus alteplase in acute massive pulmonary embolism: immediate clinical and hemodynamic outcome and one-year follow-up. J Am Coll Cardiol 1998;31(5):1057–63.

64. Meneveau N, Schiele F, Vuillemenot A, et al. Streptokinase vs alteplase in massive pulmonary embolism. A randomized trial assessing right heart haemodynamics and pulmonary vascular obstruction. Eur Heart J 1997;18(7):1141–8.

65. Goldhaber SZ, Agnelli G, Levine MN. Reduced dose bolus alteplase vs conventional alteplase infusion for pulmonary embolism thrombolysis. An international multicenter randomized trial. The Bolus Alteplase Pulmonary Embolism Group. Chest 1994; 106(3):718–24.

66. Tebbe U, Graf A, Kamke W, et al. Hemodynamic effects of double bolus reteplase versus alteplase infusion in massive pulmonary embolism. Am Heart J 1999;138(1 Pt 1): 39–44.

67. Becattini C, Agnelli G, Salvi A, et al. Bolus tenecteplase for right ventricle dysfunction in hemodynamically stable patients with pulmonary embolism. Thromb Res 2010; 125(3):e82–6.

68. Kucher N, Goldhaber SZ. Management of massive pulmonary embolism. Circulation 2005;112(2):e28–32.

69. Ribeiro A, Lindmarker P, Juhlin-Dannfelt A, et al. Echocardiography Doppler in pulmonary embolism: right ventricular dysfunction as a predictor of mortality rate. Am Heart J 1997;134(3):479–87.

70. Kucher N, Rossi E, De Rosa M, et al. Prognostic role of echocardiography among patients with acute pulmonary embolism and a systolic arterial pressure of 90 mm Hg or higher. Arch Intern Med 2005;165(15):1777–81.

71. ten Wolde M, Sohne M, Quak E, et al. Prognostic value of echocardiographically assessed right ventricular dysfunction in patients with pulmonary embolism. Arch Intern Med 2004;164(15):1685–9.

72. Sanchez O, Trinquart L, Colombet I, et al. Prognostic value of right ventricular dysfunction in patients with haemodynamically stable pulmonary embolism: a systematic review. Eur Heart J 2008;29(12):1569–77.

73. Binder L, Pieske B, Olschewski M, et al. N-terminal pro-brain natriuretic peptide or troponin testing followed by echocardiography for risk stratification of acute pulmonary embolism. Circulation 2005;112(11):1573–9.

74. Scridon T, Scridon C, Skali H, et al. Prognostic significance of troponin elevation and right ventricular enlargement in acute pulmonary embolism. Am J Cardiol 2005;96(2): 303–5.

75. Kucher N, Wallmann D, Carone A, et al. Incremental prognostic value of troponin I and echocardiography in patients with acute pulmonary embolism. Eur Heart J 2003; 24(18):1651–6.
76. Schoepf UJ, Kucher N, Kipfmueller F, et al. Right ventricular enlargement on chest computed tomography: a predictor of early death in acute pulmonary embolism. Circulation 2004;110(20):3276–80.
77. Kucher N, Printzen G, Doernhoefer T, et al. Low pro-brain natriuretic peptide levels predict benign clinical outcome in acute pulmonary embolism. Circulation 2003; 107(12):1576–8.
78. Kucher N, Printzen G, Goldhaber SZ. Prognostic role of brain natriuretic peptide in acute pulmonary embolism. Circulation 2003;107(20):2545–7.
79. Pruszczyk P, Kostrubiec M, Bochowicz A, et al. N-terminal pro-brain natriuretic peptide in patients with acute pulmonary embolism. Eur Respir J 2003;22(4):649–53.
80. ten Wolde M, Tulevski II, Mulder JW, et al. Brain natriuretic peptide as a predictor of adverse outcome in patients with pulmonary embolism. Circulation 2003;107(16): 2082–4.
81. Kucher N, Goldhaber SZ. Cardiac biomarkers for risk stratification of patients with acute pulmonary embolism. Circulation 2003;108(18):2191–4.
82. Giannitsis E, Katus HA. Risk stratification in pulmonary embolism based on biomarkers and echocardiography. Circulation 2005;112(11):1520–1.
83. Klok FA, Mos IC, Huisman MV. Brain-type natriuretic peptide levels in the prediction of adverse outcome in patients with pulmonary embolism: a systematic review and meta-analysis. Am J Respir Crit Care Med 2008;178(4):425–30.
84. Sanchez O, Trinquart L, Caille V, et al. Prognostic factors for pulmonary embolism: the PREP study, a prospective multicenter cohort study. Am J Respir Crit Care Med 2010;181(2):168–73.
85. Korff S, Katus HA, Giannitsis E. Differential diagnosis of elevated troponins. Heart 2006;92(7):987–93.
86. Becattini C, Vedovati MC, Agnelli G. Prognostic value of troponins in acute pulmonary embolism: a meta-analysis. Circulation 2007;116(4):427–33.
87. Jimenez D, Uresandi F, Otero R, et al. Troponin-based risk stratification of patients with acute nonmassive pulmonary embolism: systematic review and metaanalysis. Chest 2009;136(4):974–82.
88. Lankeit M, Konstantinides S. Tenecteplase can be given to patients with intermediate-risk pulmonary embolism – but should it? Thromb Res 2010;126(6):e407–8.
89. Storch J, Thumser AE. The fatty acid transport function of fatty acid-binding proteins. Biochim Biophys Acta 2000;1486(1):28–44.
90. Alhadi HA, Fox KA. Do we need additional markers of myocyte necrosis: the potential value of heart fatty-acid-binding protein. QJM 2004;97(4):187–98.
91. Pelsers MM, Hermens WT, Glatz JF. Fatty acid-binding proteins as plasma markers of tissue injury. Clin Chim Acta 2005;352(1-2):15–35.
92. Puls M, Dellas C, Lankeit M, et al. Heart-type fatty acid-binding protein permits early risk stratification of pulmonary embolism. Eur Heart J 2007;28(2):224–9.
93. Kaczynska A, Pelsers MM, Bochowicz A, et al. Plasma heart-type fatty acid binding protein is superior to troponin and myoglobin for rapid risk stratification in acute pulmonary embolism. Clin Chim Acta 2006;371(1-2):117–23.
94. Dellas C, Puls M, Lankeit M, et al. Elevated heart-type fatty acid-binding protein levels on admission predict an adverse outcome in normotensive patients with acute pulmonary embolism. J Am Coll Cardiol 2010;55(19):2150–7.

95. Lankeit M, Kempf T, Dellas C, et al. Growth differentiation factor-15 for prognostic assessment of patients with acute pulmonary embolism. Am J Respir Crit Care Med 2008;177(9):1018–25.

96. Lankeit M, Konstantinides S. Thrombolysis for hemodynamically stable patients with pulmonary embolism: still searching for the intermediate-risk group. Thromb Res 2009;124(6):647–8.

Index

Note: Page numbers of article titles are in **boldface** type.

A

Age
  as factor in PE, 910–911
Air travel
  VTE related to, 915
Angiography
  pulmonary
    in diagnostic approach to PE in critical care setting, 857
Antibodies
  HIT
    laboratory detection of, 807–808
Anticoagulants
  endogenous
    loss of function of
      inherited hypercoagulable states due to, 935–938
  in PE management, 825–828
    complications of, 828
    LMWH, 827
    new oral anticoagulants, 827
    UFH, 826
    warfarin, 827
  in VTE prevention in critically ill patients with renal insufficiency, 774
Antiphospholipid antibody syndrome
  acquired hypercoagulable states related to, 939–940
Antithrombin deficiency, 935
  acquired
    causes of, 935
Arterial blood gases
  in diagnostic approach to PE in critical care setting, 851
Arthritis
  rheumatoid
    VTE related to, 921
Aspiration embolectomy
  for acute PE, 831

B

Balloon angioplasty
  for acute PE, 832
Bariatrics
  VTE in, 789

Crit Care Clin 27 (2011) 969–980
doi:10.1016/S0749-0704(11)00081-9
0749-0704/11/$ – see front matter © 2011 Elsevier Inc. All rights reserved.

criticalcare.theclinics.com

United States Postal Service

Statement of Ownership, Management, and Circulation
(All Periodicals Publications Except Requestor Publications)

1. Publication Title	2. Publication Number	3. Filing Date
Critical Care Clinics	0 0 0 - 7 0 8	9/16/11

4. Issue Frequency	5. Number of Issues Published Annually	6. Annual Subscription Price
Jan, Apr, Jul, Oct	4	$179.00

7. Complete Mailing Address of Known Office of Publication (Not printer) (Street, city, county, state, and ZIP+4®)

Elsevier Inc.
360 Park Avenue South
New York, NY 10010-1710

Contact Person
Amy S. Beacham
Telephone (Include area code)
215-239-3687

8. Complete Mailing Address of Headquarters or General Business Office of Publisher (Not printer)

Elsevier Inc., 360 Park Avenue South, New York, NY 10010-1710

9. Full Names and Complete Mailing Addresses of Publisher, Editor, and Managing Editor (Do not leave blank)

Publisher (Name and complete mailing address)

Kim Murphy , Elsevier, Inc., 1600 John F. Kennedy Blvd. Suite 1800, Philadelphia, PA 19103-2899

Editor (Name and complete mailing address)

Patrick Manley, Elsevier, Inc., 1600 John F. Kennedy Blvd. Suite 1800, Philadelphia, PA 19103-2899

Managing Editor (Name and complete mailing address)

Barton Dudlick, Elsevier, Inc., 1600 John F. Kennedy Blvd. Suite 1800, Philadelphia, PA 19103-2899

10. Owner (Do not leave blank. If the publication is owned by a corporation, give the name and address of the corporation immediately followed by the names and addresses of all stockholders owning or holding 1 percent or more of the total amount of stock. If not owned by a corporation, give the names and addresses of the individual owners. If owned by a partnership or other unincorporated firm, give its name and address as well as those of each individual owner. If the publication is published by a nonprofit organization, give its name and address.)

Full Name	Complete Mailing Address
Wholly owned subsidiary of	4520 East-West Highway
Reed/Elsevier, US holdings	Bethesda, MD 20814

11. Known Bondholders, Mortgagees, and Other Security Holders Owning or Holding 1 Percent or More of Total Amount of Bonds, Mortgages, or Other Securities. If none, check box ☐ None

Full Name	Complete Mailing Address
N/A	

12. Tax Status (For completion by nonprofit organizations authorized to mail at nonprofit rates) (Check one)
The purpose, function, and nonprofit status of this organization and the exempt status for federal income tax purposes:
☐ Has Not Changed During Preceding 12 Months
☐ Has Changed During Preceding 12 Months (Publisher must submit explanation of change with this statement)

PS Form 3526, September 2007 (Page 1 of 3 (Instructions Page 3)) PSN 7530-01-000-9931 **PRIVACY NOTICE:** See our Privacy policy in www.usps.com

---

13. Publication Title	14. Issue Date for Circulation Data Below
Critical Care Clinics	July 2011

15. Extent and Nature of Circulation			Average No. Copies Each Issue During Preceding 12 Months	No. Copies of Single Issue Published Nearest to Filing Date
a. Total Number of Copies (Net press run)			1713	1839
b. Paid Circulation (By Mail and Outside the Mail)	(1)	Mailed Outside-County Paid Subscriptions Stated on PS Form 3541. (Include paid distribution above nominal rate, advertiser's proof copies, and exchange copies)	779	714
	(2)	Mailed In-County Paid Subscriptions Stated on PS Form 3541 (Include paid distribution above nominal rate, advertiser's proof copies, and exchange copies)		
	(3)	Paid Distribution Outside the Mails Including Sales Through Dealers and Carriers, Street Vendors, Counter Sales, and Other Paid Distribution Outside USPS®	275	291
	(4)	Paid Distribution by Other Classes Mailed Through the USPS (e.g. First-Class Mail®)		
c. Total Paid Distribution (Sum of 15b (1), (2), (3), and (4))		▶	1054	1005
d. Free or Nominal Rate Distribution (By Mail and Outside the Mail)	(1)	Free or Nominal Rate Outside-County Copies Included on PS Form 3541	82	77
	(2)	Free or Nominal Rate In-County Copies Included on PS Form 3541		
	(3)	Free or Nominal Rate Copies Mailed at Other Classes Through the USPS (e.g. First-Class Mail)		
	(4)	Free or Nominal Rate Distribution Outside the Mail (Carriers or other means)		
e. Total Free or Nominal Rate Distribution (Sum of 15d (1), (2), (3) and (4))		▶	82	77
f. Total Distribution (Sum of 15c and 15e)		▶	1136	1082
g. Copies not Distributed (See instructions to publishers #4 (page #3))		▶	577	757
h. Total (Sum of 15f and g)		▶	1713	1839
i. Percent Paid (15c divided by 15f times 100)			92.78%	92.88%

16. Publication of Statement of Ownership
☐ If the publication is a general publication, publication of this statement is required. Will be printed in the **October 2011** issue of this publication. ☐ Publication not required

17. Signature and Title of Editor, Publisher, Business Manager, or Owner

Amy S. Beacham — Senior Inventory Distribution Coordinator

Date: September 16, 2011

I certify that all information furnished on this form is true and complete. I understand that anyone who furnishes false or misleading information on this form or who omits material or information requested on the form may be subject to criminal sanctions (including fines and imprisonment) and/or civil sanctions (including civil penalties).

PS Form **3526**, September 2007 (Page 2 of 3)

Printed and bound by CPI Group (UK) Ltd, Croydon, CR0 4YY

03/10/2024

01040461-0002